IN CHANGING TIMES

IN CHANGING TIMES

GAY MEN AND LESBIANS ENCOUNTER HIV/AIDS

EDITED BY

MARTIN P. LEVINE

PETER M. NARDI

JOHN H. GAGNON

THE UNIVERSITY OF CHICAGO PRESS   CHICAGO AND LONDON

Martin P. Levine was a pioneer gay studies researcher who died of AIDS in 1993. Peter M. Nardi teaches sociology at Pitzer College. John H. Gagnon is a sociologist at the State University of New York, Stony Brook.

The University of Chicago Press, Chicago 60637
The University of Chicago Press, Ltd., London
© 1997 by The University of Chicago
All rights reserved. Published 1997
Printed in the United States of America
06 05 04 03 02 01 00 99 98 97   1 2 3 4 5

ISBN: 0-226-27856-5 (cloth)
ISBN: 0-226-27857-3 (paper)

Library of Congress Cataloging-in-Publication Data

In changing times : gay men and lesbians encounter HIV/AIDS /
    editors, Martin P. Levine, Peter M. Nardi, and John H. Gagnon.
        p.   cm.
    Includes bibliographical references and index.
    ISBN 0-226-27856-5 (alk. paper).—ISBN 0-226-27857-3 (pbk.
alk. paper)
    1. AIDS (Disease)—Social aspects—United States.   2. Gay men—
United States.   3. Lesbians—United States.   I. Levine, Martin P.
II. Nardi, Peter M.   III. Gagnon, John H.
RA644.A25I49   1997
362.1′969792′008664—dc21   97-3414
                                                   CIP

Chapter 5 © 1997 by Gayle S. Rubin.
Chapter 7 © 1995 by Temple University.

⊗ The paper used in this publication meets the minimum requirements of the American National Standard for Information Sciences—Permanence of Paper for Printed Library Materials, ANSI Z39.48-1984.

CONTENTS

PREFACE

John H. Gagnon

The idea for the conference that led to this book emerged in 1991, when two of the editors (Levine and Gagnon) were members of a small working group undertaking an exploratory case study of the impact of the human immunodeficiency virus (HIV)/acquired immune deficiency syndrome (AIDS) epidemic in New York City. This working group had been assembled as part of an effort by the Panel on the Social Impact of the HIV/AIDS Epidemic (a subcommittee of the Committee on AIDS Research in the Social and Behavioral Science—of which I was a member—that had been created by the Commission on Behavioral and Social Sciences and Education of the National Research Council) to understand the differing impacts of the epidemic in various geographical and social communities in the United States. It was clear to the members of that panel that the epidemic was developing in multiple ways socially and epidemiologically in these communities. A case study of the situation in New York City was one of three studies that were discussed. Unfortunately, due to limits on funding and time, only the New York study was completed, and that report was published in a truncated version in the volume *The Social Impact of AIDS* (Jonson and Stryker, 1993). The completed case study, which treated a larger set of issues than the gay community, was primarily the result of the work of Shirley Lindenbaum of the Department of Anthropology at the Graduate Center of City University of New York and me.

Even on the basis of this limited case study, it was clear that there was not just one unified epidemic that could be properly represented by a single rising curve of reported AIDS cases and the message of equal and universal risk to all members of the society. What was immediately evident was that there were a number of microepidemics epidemiologically centered primarily around (1) men who had sex with men, (2) injection drug users (IDUs), their sexual partners, and their children, and (3) those infected through contaminated blood products. From a sociological perspective these three epidemiological categories offered only a gross version of reality, since they concealed important differences in the social characteristics of the individuals and communities that made up these three focal groups. In New York City alone, the category "men who have sex with men" (MSM) included members of the publicly identified "gay community," which was composed of a majority of White men with smaller numbers of African American and Latino gay-identified men, in addition to collectivities of African American and Latino men whose connection with a gay identity ranged from "none" to "in the process of formation."

Without a recognition of these within group differences, neither the course of the epidemic (i.e., where was it going and how fast) nor how to construct appropriate prevention programs could be understood. A serious response to these differences between the epidemics involving gay men and injection drug users or the differences in the epidemics among gay men in New York, San Francisco, and Houston (for example) seemed to be absolutely critical. However, in our view, even these recognitions appeared insufficient and a deeper set of understandings was required.

From the beginning of the epidemic, the biomedical emphasis in AIDS research, even that research conducted by behavioral and social scientists, seemed sensitive to only limited aspects of the gay community or gay life. How many partners men had, whether they had anal sex, and what their serostatus might be loomed large in the rapidly growing literature. The major cohort studies that were conducted in a variety of cities with differing gay communities were analyzed as if they existed in some abstract and uniform territory. Interventions were discussed, designed, and compared as if they were intended for some uniform gay man who differed only by race or ethnicity or age. The relation or lack of relation of the man who had sex with other men to his local gay community and the relation of that community to the larger nongay community in which it was embedded went unaddressed. Yet it was these gay communities, with their specific histories of relations with the institutions of the surrounding urban place, that were the primary vehicles for behavior change and prevention.

How the HIV/AIDS epidemic was reshaping the practices and culture of gay and lesbian communities and the identities of gay men and lesbians did not appear on the social science agenda. Except for a few maverick anthropologists and sociologists, it was left to journalists and novelists to record the texture and quality of these changes. It may be possible as part of some larger metanalysis to take all of these fragmentary medicalized journal articles on "homosexuals and bisexuals" or "men who have sex with men" to understand the actual lives and subjectivities of the primarily White gay men who willingly participated in so many studies. But this would be a task of extraordinary subtlety and imagination.

As a consequence of these recognitions, Martin Levine and I worked together and consulted widely with other researchers to put together a list of social science participants for a small conference on various aspects of the impact of the epidemic on the gay male and lesbian communities. We chose a format that would have the participants prepare papers prior to the conference so we could devote the conference itself to discussion. Marty had been working with the community advisory board of the Burroughs Welcome Company for a number of years, attempting to influence the way in which that company related not only to the gay community, but also to communities of color. Using that specific entree to Burroughs Welcome, he was able to secure a small grant that would be used to support the conference itself.

The conference was held in December 1992 in Rancho Santa Fe, near San Diego, California. It was administered and managed by Laurie Obbink, who used her experience organizing conferences with the Wenner Gren Foundation to create a smoothly running and comfortable environment for the conferees. Except for the intellectual ferment and collegial warmth, the conference was uneventful.

A tragedy of the conference was that Martin Levine was unable to participate. Over the course of 1992 when the conference was being organized, his health grew more perilous from the complications of HIV disease. Up until the very last moment before the conference, he had hoped to be well enough to take the long trip to California from New York City. Just before the journey to the airport, he decided that he could not make the trip.

HIV/AIDS was with us in a variety of other ways. One participant could not come because his lover was entering the final crisis stage of the disease. Charles Silverstein, whom we invited to the conference to talk about the process of grieving, refused our invitation with the following letter:

> August 11, 1992
> Dear John,
>   I have tried, and I simply cannot do it. Perhaps not so simply. There have been too many deaths, too many memorials, and too many more deaths to come for me to write the paper you've asked for.
>   William has AIDS. Though in good health, we both know that

it's a matter of time. We're trying to bring an old friend, currently in Houston, to live with us, because he has AIDS, and there is no one to take care of him there.

I spoke at John Martin's memorial service. As I spoke I could see the faces of so many patients, friends, colleagues, as if they all sat quietly waiting for my words—for what I would say about them and their deaths. I even saw the face of a young man, now dead, who was a student of mine when I taught fifth grade.

For awhile I thought I might write a personal statement about AIDS, about the experience of watching so many people die. I thought it might be therapeutic to do so. But as I charted an outline in my mind, I thought it much too self-absorbed, too depressing, and would clash with the tone of sociological inquiry. So I am not able to write the paper and it feels like a great weight has been taken off my shoulders. I'm disappointed that I won't be meeting with you and the others. Perhaps we can have lunch one day soon.

Charles

All of the participants at the conference were in various ways AIDS activists and academics, everyone had had significant losses from the epidemic. The invited participants and their affiliations at the time were: Barry Adam, University of Windsor; Lourdes Arguelles, Pitzer College; Rafael Miguel Diaz, Center for AIDS Prevention Studies, University of California, San Francisco; John H. Gagnon, State University of New York at Stony Brook; Gilbert Herdt, University of Chicago; Gregory Herek, University of California, Davis; Amber Hollibaugh, Gay Men's Health Crisis, New York City; Nan Hunter, Brooklyn Law School; Stuart Michaels, University of Chicago and NORC; Peter Nardi, Pitzer College; Jay Paul, Center for AIDS Prevention Studies; John Peterson, Center for AIDS Prevention Studies, University of California, San Francisco; Anne Rivero, Kaiser Permanente Hospital, Montclair, California; Gayle Rubin, independent scholar, San Francisco; Beth Schneider, University of California, Santa Barbara; Nancy Stoller, University of California, Santa Cruz; Carole Vance, Columbia University School of Public Health; Vera Whisman, Ithaca College; and Paul Whitaker, Center for AIDS Prevention Studies, University of California, San Francisco. Unfortunately, Stuart Michaels and John Peterson were unable to attend at the last moment. Not all of the participants have been able to revise the papers that they presented at the conference and so are not represented in the chapters of the book, though they made important contributions to the discussions at the conference.

Given the perilous state of Martin Levine's health in December 1992 and the difficulties he was having with his illness, he proposed that we ask Peter Nardi to join with us in the final editing of the book. This turned out to be an important decision in making sure the book was completed. During the winter, Marty's condition grew more grave, and in late March 1993, he decided to cease all medication except for palliative treatment to make him comfortable. Martin Levine died on April 3, 1993.

Peter Nardi took major responsibility for the completion of the essays that make up this book and has been a key person in bringing this work to fruition. He has commented in detail on the essays and has pressed the contributors to get their work completed.

The editors owe a debt of gratitude to the Burroughs Welcome Company for funding this conference and especially to Fred Gregg, group manager for professional and community relations and HIV, who sponsored this activity. Mr. Gregg and Martin Levine were friends as well as collaborators in promoting better relations between the pharmaceutical company and the afflicted communities. Fred Gregg has referred to Marty as "a dear friend and mentor." As noted before, Laurie Obbink made an important contribution in her successful management of the conference itself.

The participants in the volume have received a small stipend from the grant from Burroughs Welcome for their contribution and have agreed that all royalties from the volume will be paid to the Martin P. Levine Memorial Dissertation Award, which is supervised by the Sex and Gender Section of the American Sociological Association. These fellowships are open to students from all disciplines in the social sciences, including persons doing social science research in the professions.

A word about Martin Levine, his professional career and this book. Marty devoted much of the last years of his life to AIDS activism and AIDS education. He tirelessly taught about AIDS in a variety of contexts and helped others do the same. He conducted research on gay men with HIV/AIDS and consulted widely. Fighting the epidemic became an organizing principle of the last years of his life. Like many other gay men and lesbians who have made the epidemic their cause, Marty did not have the opportunity to fulfill his early intellectual promise. His dissertation on "clone culture" and the gay ghetto in New York City (see Levine's chapter in Herdt's *Gay Culture in America*, 1992) was a detailed study of a major transition in the history of gay life in the United States. The masculinization of gay men's desire was an important step in changing both the character of the gay community

and gay identity. Like all important changes, these may well have facilitated the unknowing spread of the virus in the late 1970s and the early
1980s and played an equally important role in facilitating the changes
in behavior that reduced its toll. Marty was one of the first to recognize
this irony.

Marty was always proud of being gay and always open about his
HIV status after he knew it. He was out as a gay man and out as a
person living with AIDS. It is not enough to say he will be missed. No
one who loved him will recover from his absence.

INTRODUCTION

JOHN H. GAGNON AND
PETER M. NARDI

An understanding of the dramatic changes within what is now called the gay and lesbian communities (and other persons who have same-gender sex, but who are not self-identified as gay or lesbian) since the onset of the public phase of the HIV/AIDS epidemic around 1981 is profoundly difficult to attain. Even more difficult to characterize is how the epidemic and the response to the epidemic by gays and lesbians have changed the relationship between these complex minority communities and the larger collectivity of those whose sexuality is defined as "heterosexual." The purpose of the essays in this book is to understand how the epidemic has played a role in creating and changing sites of focused interaction (communities and social movements as well as specific institutions and organizations), systems of intersubjective meaning (culture), and the content and salience of novel identities (agency).

An analysis of the impact of what are defined as exogenous events (extrasocial or social) on ongoing bounded social systems usually involves (1) an assessment of the state of the social system at a time prior to the moment of impact, (2) a characterization of the dimensions of the exogenous event (such as earthquake, drought, or dam collapse), and (3) an assessment of how critical features of individual lives and collectivities that made up the affected social system were modified or changed in the short and long term. The large literature on "natural" disasters has followed this pattern of research (preevent conditions, event, postevent sequelae) (Erikson, 1976), as has research on the evaluation of programs that are meant to induce community or individual change (for a review of intervention program research methods specific to HIV/AIDS, see Coyle, Boruch, & Turner, 1991). Although most disaster research is ex post facto in its assessment of both the preevent conditions and of the event, research on planned interventions may take measures prior to the introduction of the intervention itself.[1]

The HIV/AIDS epidemic is both like and unlike other disasters that are commonly interpreted as entirely "natural" in their origins and that therefore offer a morally neutral status for those affected. Thus a hurricane, an earthquake, a forest fire, or a flood are understood *as if* they come from an unpredictable and sometimes malign "nature" and those affected are treated as being immediately deserving of disaster relief in a variety of forms.[2] Even though the HIV/AIDS epidemic is equally a "natural" disaster in the sense that a change in the nonhuman world has unexpectedly affected people going about their usual business, the majority of those afflicted by the virus has been treated as morally culpable. This, of course, is a consequence of the prior marginalized status of the collectivities affected and the primary modes of transmission of the virus, certain sexual practices and injection drug use. Particular moral condemnation is aimed at those who relapse to "unsafe practices," given that they have knowledge of the risks of transmission.[3] Similar condemnation is not aimed at those persons who either move to regions of high risk for "natural disasters" or to those who rebuild their devastated homes and businesses in areas where they know there will be earthquakes, mud slides, floods or forest fires.

This moral distinction between those affected by HIV and those affected by other natural disasters is the crucial difference that has shaped the entire course of the epidemic. Although all presidents and governors rush to the scene of other "natural" disasters, promising on national television immediate relief to those affected, none have made such an appearance with gay men or injection drug users.[4] This failure of political will, however, should not prevent the use of the disaster model as a way of understanding the consequences of the epidemic in more neutral terms than are commonly employed.

The disaster analogy has its merits in identifying what people with AIDS (PWAs) and others affected by the epidemic have in common with those subpopulations of citizens who have been equally selectively affected by "natural" disasters during the HIV/AIDS era. Consider those who survived the floods in the Mississippi River valley, Hurricanes Hugo and Andrew, the brush fires of the Pacific Coast, the earthquakes of Santa Cruz, San Francisco, Oakland, and Northridge, as *citizens* they differed not one whit from those who have been infected with the virus.

True differences between these other "natural" disasters and the HIV/AIDS epidemic are that the former are geographically concentrated and of short duration. There is a disaster event that is a "spike in time" that lasts at most a few minutes in the case of an earthquake or several weeks in the case of a flood. The geographical concentration allows for dramatic television coverage of the impact on the material environment and for human interest stories about the local population. The HIV/AIDS disaster is an example of what can be recognized as a new class of disasters that develop slowly (often exhibiting a phase structure) and in more geographically dispersed ways (one could think of cigarette smoking, exposure to environmental and occupational hazards, etc.). In such dispersed and slow-developing disasters, there are substantial social and cultural transformations in the character of the disaster itself, including the development of moral and cultural calls as the disaster becomes more normalized and its costs diffused into various bureaucracies. This is what has happened to the HIV/AIDS epidemic in the fifteen years of its public phase: it has changed from an acute disease, ill understood and without a specialized and responsive medical and social infrastructure, to a "chronic" disease with a range of stable social practices at the individual and personal network levels and from local communities to the highest levels of the federal government.

From Homosexuals to Gay and Lesbian: The Confluence of Agency and Opportunity

The collectivities of men and women who composed the emergent self-identified gay and lesbian collectivities in the 1960s and 1970s were subjects and objects in the process of formation. New relationships and social structures would begin to characterize "open communities" that signaled changes not only to those who were not gay- or lesbian-identified yet having same-gender sex with women or men, but also to those who acted out the conventional scripts of woman-man sexual relations. The complexity and density of possible relations with non-gays and nonlesbians were changing in the spheres of religion, economics, professional organizations, and politics. At the same time the subject of gay and lesbian life became the terrain of gay and lesbian scholars, artists, writers, and intellectuals, rather than those who were not gay- and lesbian-identified (except for the religious right).

This wave of change prior to the epidemic has accumulated its master narratives. The gay man's story is the transition from queen, fairy, and closet to clone, hot men, and the dance floor (Chauncey, 1994; Levine, 1992). If one examines only the evidence of Christopher Street in New York, Lakeview in Chicago, Santa Monica Boulevard in Los Angeles/West Hollywood, and the Castro in San Francisco at the height of the 1970s, the public face of middle-class, White, gay male culture had dramatically changed into a more open, casually sexual, and masculine world. Hot sex between men was the dominant media image. At the same time many men, even living in immediate proximity to "the public gay scene," lived in long-term sexual/affectional couples, with cliques of like-minded friends, and shared quiet lives of mutual affection and support (Bell & Weinberg, 1978). They were that invisible face of gay men's lives that is the search for constancy, stability, and love that was not highlighted in the 1970s representations. Some men found the fast lane too fast; others found it too far away; others in small towns and cities found living partially in a closet was safest; and many of different races and social classes were often excluded. The world of gay men was marching to many drummers, some political, some consumerist, some erotic, not all of which added up to a solidary social movement or culture of gay men.

The master narrative of the relations between lesbians and gay men in this period has centered on conflicts between gay men and lesbians on the importance of casual and erotic sex as a community focus and what appeared to be the avid participation of gay men in consumer culture (Wolf, 1979). Viewed through these two critiques, the ties between the lesbian and gay male communities appeared to have loosened and, in the public spotlight and hurly-burly of separate community-building and attendant identity formation, a cultural split between some gay men and some lesbians did emerge. This master narrative does not take into account solid political ties between those lesbians and gay men who shared the gay liberation movement, the ties that existed between lesbians and gay men around the potentials of sexual experimentation, and the long history of slightly amused and slightly hostile relationships that had existed between two minorities forced to share some of the same spaces and subjectivities.

The situation of these collectivities was (and is) much the same as other collectivities in United States society. They are, as the political scientist Norton Long (1968) once said, "an ecology of games." By this he meant that a community, territorial or symbolic, involves a vast array of social ties of greater or lesser durability and that individuals could play a few too many roles in this social collectivity. Some of these roles are reinforcing in ideology and social participation, others are contradictory—contradictions that actors sometimes recognize and at other times do not. The implications of this model of community for identity formation are that the flow of influence is bidirectional, that individuals have ambitions for certain identities and seek to shape the community to accommodate them, even though the community of others may accept or resist such attempts at forming new identities. The process involves individual agency, structural opportunity and constraint, and cultural acceptance and resistance.

Thus the quasi-public homosexual communities and the illness-and-crime-dominated ideologies of the 1950s offered to the *majority* of homosexual men and women a subterranean way of life, defensively constructed against the police, employers, parents, the mass media, even close nonhomosexual friends and relatives. Some men and women were being blackmailed, assaulted, fired from jobs, expelled from the military, attacked by thugs, rejected by parents, imprisoned in jails and mental hospitals, and targeted by homophobic biomedicine well into the early 1970s. Even if these punishments were not experienced by everyone, nearly everyone knew someone who had had such experiences (Gagnon & Simon, 1973). These repressive conditions of daily life became for many the normal conditions of identity formation (Duberman, 1991 on the acceptance of the need for therapy).

The transformation of the homosexual community of the 1950s and 1960s into the 1970s and 1980s communities of gay men and lesbians changed the basis for identity formation of both current participants as well as future generations. In part these changes emerged from the writing and actions of a variety of gay activists, intellectuals, and academics who were critical of the medical and law-enforcement approaches to what is now known as sexual difference (the individual ambitions for change and new identities) and in part from the opportunities presented by a general climate of resistance to social marginalization by other groups in the society, primarily ethnic minorities and women, as well as the antiwar movements of the Vietnam era (the existence of structural and cultural options).

Examined from one perspective, say from that of occupation or religion, the individuals who formed the homosexual community often looked much like the people around them; examined from another, their sexual/affectional preferences represented foci of interest and a sense of difference (even while performing conventional roles) out of which both communities and identities could be built. Some of the seeds of early community formation linked to civil rights and citizenship grew around what were meliorist and accommodational groups such as One, the Mattachine Society, and the Daughters of Bilitis. During the later 1960s, gay and lesbian organizations became more oriented toward direct action (particularly in larger cities) and within the professions, in which caucuses and networks were formed (Bayer, 1981).

Entering the 1970s both the communities of gay men and lesbians, taken together and separately, had found open spaces in the society, in which new gay and lesbian communities and identities could be structured. In the larger metropolises such as New York, San Francisco, Los Angeles, Miami, and Houston, quite diverse "gay communities" were being put together. The existence of an open community with ancillary social support attracted more men who were reconstituted as being gay rather than homosexual. There was a powerful sexual underpinning, particularly among gay men, that supported this transition, and sexual styles became both a source of social networks and components of identity. Both the everyday and the exotic began to flourish especially in the larger urban, middle-class centers—gay travel agencies, bookstores, physicians, newsstands—as well as speciality bars and venues serving diverse sexual tastes and sometimes specific ethnic groups, races, and social classes.

By the early 1980s the entire collectivity of persons who were having sex with the same gender in the United States were now more directly implicated by the existence of a newly structured public gay and lesbian world. A gay and lesbian world had emerged that was more visible to all, a world in which more people could identify as gay or lesbian as part of their public personas. The direction of attention was more toward the metropolises and more and more men made the odyssey to the gay centers during this period for both sexual activity and identity work. The direction of developments among some lesbian women had a more ideological cast with the growth of a vocal separatism, from all men, or from all men and women who associated with men. The role of "gay" or "lesbian" became the central reference point in everyday life, passing from isolated and hidden desire or a constricted role to a touchstone of identity.

In the late 1970s, as HIV was becoming seeded among sexually active gay men in some large cities (as well as among injection drug users, their sexual partners, in some cases their children, and among persons exposed to contaminated blood products), gay men and lesbians, unaware of the virus, were working out the new directions of a more visible and politically active community. Civil rights, antidiscrimination efforts, and community organizing were the foci of the lives of politically active gay men and lesbians.

Even at the end of the 1970s, however, the lives of the majority of gay men and lesbians were not directly related to gay politics or activism. Like most members of the society, they were primarily interested in their friends, lovers, children, parents, jobs, vacations, and leisure time. Edmund White's (1981) informative volume on the conditions of some gay men's sexuality across the United States in the late 1970s suggested enormous variations in "gay communities" even among the more gay areas of New York, Los Angeles, and San Francisco. Of course, gay life in other regions in the late 1970s was different from that of the 1950s, since it was influenced by the changes in the major cities. Even so, a bar in Salt Lake City or in southern Georgia to this day may provide a sudden sense of recognition to those old enough to have been adults in the 1940s and 1950s (Whittier, 1995).

The Virus and its Secret Spread

Estimates of when the virus was first seeded and its rate of spread in gay communities in the United States suggest the degree to which the epidemic took hold among populations that were unaware of its existence. In addition, these estimates suggest how quickly gay men and the gay community responded to the epidemic in terms of behavior change. All estimates of when infections with HIV occurred have only limited precision since they are based on the dates when AIDS cases were reported, which is only variably related to the date of HIV infection. The long latency period between infection and the clinical manifestations of AIDS has been a crucial problem in determining the size and direction of the epidemic, since reported AIDS cases reflect only infections that took place, on average, eight to ten years earlier.

The statistical method most often used to make estimates of when HIV infections took place is back-projection. This method takes the diagnosed AIDS cases reported in a given year and projects into the past when these infections should have occurred. This requires an estimate of the distribution of when the infections in a given year should have reached a stage in the HIV disease process that would be identified as AIDS. The accuracy of such estimates is reduced by underreporting of persons with AIDS (Centers for Disease Control [CDC] estimates that from 15 to 20 percent of all persons infected with HIV are not included in the AIDS registry). These underestimates were probably particularly large among injection drug users and in the early stages of the epidemic for all persons (Stoneburner et al., 1988). A second major factor is variation in the estimates of the average time between infection and diagnosis resulting from (1) actual changes in the duration of latency time from HIV infection to AIDS depending on the year of infection, or (2) differences of the survival time among different subpopulations due to variations in availability of health care or preinfection health status (e.g., hemophiliacs in contrast to poor, drug-using women).

Despite these difficulties it is possible to make reasoned estimates of when HIV infections occurred so as to estimate how much of the infection epidemic occurred under conditions of varying levels of ignorance. Don Des Jarlais provided the *New York Times* with his best personal estimate of when HIV infections occurred (Kolata, 1995).[5]

What this graph in Fig. 1 suggests is that of the approximately 1 million persons who were infected by HIV by the end of 1989 (The CDC [1990] estimate; the Des Jarlais figure is somewhat higher, perhaps 1.14 million by this same date), some forty percent were infected prior to the end of 1981, which was the year that the first cases of Kaposi's sarcoma (KS) and Pneumocystis carinii pneumonia (PCP) were reported publicly by the CDC (1981a, 1981b) in the *Morbidity and Mortality Weekly Report*. During the long mainstream media silence about the epidemic from 1982 to 1987, an additional 50 percent of those infected by the end of 1989 had been infected (Kinsella, 1990). Even if we accept the extremely unreliable estimates of infections after 1988 (CDC estimates of new infections growing at a *constant* rate of 40,000 to 80,000 per year for every year from 1988 to 1995 should not inspire much confidence in the surveillance system), it is clear that by the time Ronald Reagan addressed the American Foundation for AIDS Research (AmFAR) in Washington, D.C., on the occasion of the International AIDS Conference in June 1987, the vast majority of per-

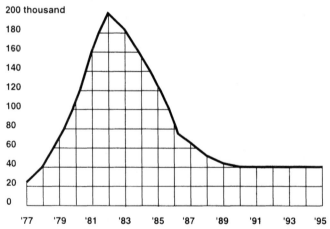

Fig. 1. One estimate of the incidence of HIV infections by year. The estimated rate of new HIV infections has been constant since 1988. Adapted from Don Des Jarlais of Beth Israel Hospital, New York; *New York Times*, February 28, 1995.

sons who were infected in the epidemic had already been infected. Other studies, although not locating the peak of infections as early as had Des Jarlais, also estimate that the peak of infections occurred before the end of 1984 (Rosenberg, 1995).

This rapid decline in the numbers of new infections prior to most major public health initiatives of the federal and state governments suggests that in addition to the exhaustion of the susceptibles in any specific location (e.g., networks of injection drug users in limited areas of central cities, men having frequent anal sex with many other men in various venues), behavior change at the individual and collective level was well underway in the early 1980s, particularly among gay men. The recognition of the prevalence of nonlethal sexually transmitted infections and the first evidence of AIDS may already have triggered behavior change at the individual level (Shilts, 1987).[6] Additionally, gay and lesbian community-based institutions devoted to AIDS prevention were formally in place by 1982. Given the time from the first awareness that a disaster is impending to construction of operating institutions, this means that a preliminary informal awareness was already in existence in 1981. There is considerable ethnographic and local community evidence to suggest this is true (i.e., there is considerable evidence of a very rapid decline in the incidence of rectal gonorrhea during this period).

The point here is that the pre-epidemic state of the gay and lesbian communities provided the basis for the rapid start-up of collective responses to the epidemic. The prior level of political organization, economic prosperity, and community building during the 1970s could be called upon during the 1980s. These pre-AIDS developments were the basis for prevention and care activities as well as the ability to press city, state and federal agencies, the health care industry (from insurance companies to private providers), private businesses, and foundations to institute new practices and policies with respect to HIV disease and PWAs. The specific histories (mostly unwritten yet) of these efforts are quite different for various cities and states depending on the characteristics of the gay and lesbian communities and their relation to the nongay communities in which they were embedded (McKenzie, 1991).

The Demographic Impact of the Epidemic

The exact number of gay men who have been (or will be) infected with HIV and who will have become ill and die may never be known. But it is this number that most tellingly expresses the role of the epidemic in transforming the communities of gay men of the AIDS generation and the successive generations of gay men. The sheer volume of sickness and death affects not only those who have been infected and those persons closest to them, but also the successive circles of relationships inside and outside of the gay and lesbian communities. Further, the size of the epidemic determines the degree of institutional change and resource reallocation that might be required to deal with this disaster. The phrase "might be required" was chosen to indicate the struggle that has emerged about how much institutional change and resource reallocation the HIV/AIDS epidemic *deserves*. Indeed, in the early stages of the epidemic, debates about how many AIDS cases there were, how many would occur, the cost to treat PWAs, the protection of the citizenship rights of those who were infected, whether HIV testing should be mandatory and so forth were also debates about institutional change and resource allocation. These answers—depending on the outcome of political struggles—could have ranged from a little to a great deal and, as might have been expected, could have varied in actual practice in different areas over this response range from none to little to some.

In a more focused manner, an examination of how many gay men have become ill and have died gives a first approximation of the impact on the communities themselves. Similar to great demographic catastrophes caused by recent wars that cut great notches in specific age grades in the population (Marwick, 1965; Winter, 1986), the AIDS epidemic has primarily affected thirty- to thirty-nine-year-old gay men, followed by those who are twenty-five to twenty-nine and forty to forty-four years old (CDC, 1995a). Although the exact number is not known, it is possible to estimate how many gay men have been infected, how many have been diagnosed with AIDS, how many have died, and how this relates to contemporary estimates of the numbers of gay-identified men in the society. These assessments are necessarily crude, but based on publicly available data and assumptions.

In addition to cases of gay men dying undiagnosed early in the epidemic, the actual number of *gay-identified men* is lost in the CDC categories "homosexual and bisexual" and "homosexual and bisexual men who use injection drugs." The more recent CDC label "men who have sex with men" (MSM) at least has the virtue of not making implicit conjectures about the sexual orientation of those infected. In addition, there is the complication presented by the intersection of ethnicity and gay identity. Close to one-half of all Latin- and African-origin men who have been diagnosed with AIDS are described as "men who have sex with men." But how many of these men self-identify as "gay men" in the same sense of gay community participation that characterizes White middle-class men is a matter of contention. An indication of the separation of these communities in social and sexual terms is that the epidemic among Latin- and African-origin men who have sex with men started later than did the epidemic of European-origin gay men. The separation of the epidemics is a measure of the social separation of the communities.

The first 500,000 (actually 501,310) AIDS cases were reported in the United States by October 31, 1995 (CDC, 1995b). This number represents close to one-half or more than one-half of *all* of those estimated by the CDC to be infected with HIV by the end of 1989 (CDC, 1990) or 1993 (Rosenberg, 1995). This indicates that there are between 400,000 and 600,000 persons living with HIV, but not diagnosed with AIDS at the present time. Rosenberg (1995) estimated that the total number of persons ever infected with HIV was between 870,000 to 1,200,000 by the end of 1993.

Of these half-million reported AIDS cases, some 51 percent (256,000) were men who had sex with men (MSM) and 7 percent (35,000) had joint exposure from sex with men and injection drug use. If we accept that persons who are infected with HIV are underreported in the AIDS registry by some 18 percent (as did Rosenberg, 1995), this would mean that the number of cases in the MSM category would be around 300,000 and in the MSM/IDU group about 41,000.

Although not all of these men are members of gay communities (regardless of their ethnic origins), it is not unreasonable to argue that the majority are gay-identified and participate in gay community life. Thus there are more than 210,000 men of European origin, 75,000 men of African origin, and 45,000 men of Latin origin who had sex with men who have been diagnosed with AIDS (in this case we have combined MSM with MSM/IDU). These figures, which total 330,000, have not been corrected for underreporting, but if we use the 18 percent figure to account for underreporting, the total would be 390,000 men who had sex with men of all ethnicities who have been diagnosed with AIDS. If we assume that about 60 percent of those infected have already died (CDC, 1995a) then close to 240,000 MSMs (included those who were IDUs) have died since the epidemic began.

The deaths of this many people and the expected deaths of many more would represent a national tragedy; but at the level of the local gay communities, it looms much larger. If we accept the figures from recent national surveys of the number of men who have sex with men (figures that minimally range from 3 percent to 5 percent of the national population) as closely depicting the numbers of gay-identified men in the society, the AIDS death figures represent a major catastrophe for the gay communities. There are 90,000,000 men 18 and over in the United States and if 4 percent of these men are gay-identified there would be 3,600,000 gay men in the United States over 18 (this figure could range between 2,700,000 and 4,500,000). This means that 1 gay man in 9 (390,000 diagnosed/3,600,000 total gay men = 11%) has been diagnosed with AIDS and that 1 gay man in 15 (240,000 deceased/3,600,000 = 7%) has died.

The concentration of the epidemic is, however, greater than these figures express, yet much smaller than antigay groups and religious right organizations lead one to believe when they equate AIDS with homosexuality. The epidemic among gay men is concentrated in the gay communities of two dozen cities and primarily among men 25 to 44 years old. Although these ages include 46 percent of all gay men 18 and over, about three-quarters of men diagnosed with AIDS are in this age range. This means that the impact of these age groups is much greater still, decimating a large portion of a cohort of gay men. If one assumes that 4 percent of the population of men in the United States is gay-identified, then of the 1,600,000 gay-identified men between 25 and 44, about 1 in 10 have died by 1995, a number that will rise to 1 in 3, absent any change in the "natural course" of the disease.

The secondary and tertiary waves of the first epidemic are still upon us. The first wave was that of infection (the HIV epidemic), the second is the falling ill phase (the AIDS epidemic), and the third is the epidemic of mortality. It is important to mention some costs that will never be measured or recovered in addition to the loss of life: the redirection of lives of those who have been living with HIV, as well as of their entire personal social networks and the institutions that have been reorganized to meet the needs of the epidemic. It should also be noted that some have profited from the epidemic, both in economic terms and in social prestige. There has been a large transfer of wealth from the gay community (or its insurers) to the health care industry (in all its guises), as well as the creation of opportunity for a variety of professional unknowns in various fields to become well-rewarded AIDS warriors.

The Normalcy of AIDS and Changes in Gay and Lesbian Agendas

As we move into the fourth quinquennium of the AIDS era in the United States, it is clear that AIDS has become a "post-popular cause" in the larger society (Jonsen & Stryker, 1993). The coverage of AIDS in the press and on television has declined steadily and the notice given to popular figures who have been infected with HIV has assumed far less significance. Within "AIDS Inc.," service agencies are searching for new ways to raise funds and chart directions for action. Even AmFAR has lost its cachet along with its primary spokesperson, Elizabeth Taylor (Jacobs, 1996). CDC now publishes its AIDS surveillance journal every quarter instead of every month and Peter Jennings's televised *AIDS Quarterly* is now the *Health Quarterly*. Major newspapers such as the *New York Times* no longer have dedicated AIDS reporters, but relegate local stories to the minority desk or to the science desk.

Even within the gay and lesbian movements, HIV/AIDS is no longer the central issue. At the lesbian and gay march on Washington, D.C., in 1993, only a few speakers addressed the AIDS epidemic and mention of it was entirely missing in a number of speeches. And the 1994 New York march remembering the twenty-fifth anniversary of the Stonewall rebellion was criticized for ignoring AIDS issues, resulting in a counter-march of over ten thousand people. New issues—gays in the military, domestic partner benefits, gay and lesbian marriage, parenting, and state and local antigay initiatives by the radical right—have become more and more significant to gay men and lesbians.

In this new agenda, HIV/AIDS has slid from first place in the panoply of gay issues; this is true even though many gay men are living with HIV infection and many have been diagnosed as having AIDS. The difficulty of balancing the needs of the three-hundred thousand to four-hundred thousand gay men living with HIV and the millions of gay men who are HIV negative creates a special cleavage in the community. This can be seen especially among the young men who have come into the gay communities and the gay movements since the height of the epidemic (perhaps since 1987)—older men infected with HIV/AIDS seem part of the past—even though at least some of these young men are probably the most likely to become infected in the next few years.

This transition between the era of AIDS and the era of post-AIDS is happening as this volume is being published. It will be a difficult transition because it involves continuing the caretaking of large numbers of gay men who are infected and ill from the virus, as well as responding to those who are grieving for the men who are dying each day. The gay communities' institutions—many of which were formed in the midst of the infection wave of the epidemic—need to continue to accentuate prevention, protect the rights of the ill, put pressure on government, prevent discrimination, and provide services as they are being refashioned to meet the needs of a changing epidemic. At the same time, the lesbian and gay communities need to address non-HIV/AIDS issues.

The Essays

Over the past two decades, an infrastructure of organizations, communication systems, neighborhoods, and economic and political power has contributed significantly to the responses many gays and lesbians made to the encounter with HIV/AIDS. In the face of indifference and opposition from political, media, religious, and medical institutions, gay men and lesbians were forced to deal with the realities of the hegemonic organizational structures of the society in ways that many racial and class minorities had already done for decades. The church, schools, media, health care systems, economic agencies, and the legal structure, in turn, were forced to reconsider fundamental assumptions about homosexuality, sexuality, and heterosexism. This dialectic became one of the central dynamics characterizing the relationship among gay men, lesbians, and the social system.

And in the process, a restructuring of gay people's lives, identities, and cultural practices has been occurring. The chapters in this reader are discussions and analyses of this encounter with HIV/AIDS and of the restructuring that continues in these changing times. The original focus of the conference, for which these papers were prepared, was to assess the ways HIV/AIDS changed the lives and practices of gay men and lesbians, their communities and social worlds, and their collective and individual identities—and how all these, in turn, changed HIV/AIDS and the ways it was discussed. Thus we have arranged the papers into three general areas: *Practices, Communities,* and *Identities.* Although the papers deal with all of these issues in various degrees, the chapters have been grouped according to the articles' primary theme.

Part 1, *Practices,* focuses on the impact of HIV/AIDS on several basic social institutions and organizational arrangements. Barry Adam's paper, for example, analyzes the dynamics of collective mobilization around AIDS, the ways various AIDS organizations have affected state, medical, corporate, and social service bureaucracies, and how these institutions have helped shape AIDS activism. In the process, according to Adam, AIDS has become "normalized" and assimilated, contained, and institutionalized by the welfare, health, and education systems.

But state health care and social service systems are not the only institutions affected by the encounter with HIV/AIDS. Law and politics have been affected as well. Nan Hunter develops an analysis of the history of the complicated relationship between expression and equality in lesbian and gay rights law. Hunter discusses how AIDS brought issues of self-representation of gay identity, openness, and state regulation of desire and sexuality into the public arena. She traces the development of identity concepts in law and the shift in claims from privacy to equality. According to Hunter, AIDS disrupted the social contract of complicity in silence, thereby elevating and demonizing homosexuality as a national political issue.

How people practiced, discussed, and created structures of interpersonal relationships is the central concern of Peter Nardi's paper on AIDS's impact on romantic, sexual, familial, and friendship relationships. Nardi discusses assumptions of monogamy, coupling, and sexual partner reduction that dominated the AIDS discourse of the mid- and late-1980s. He then focuses on the history of the concept of gay marriage as reported in archival documents and gay publications, and on the impact of AIDS on restructuring concepts of family and friendship networks.

As Lourdes Arguelles and Anne Rivero report, spiritual and religious systems, mental health practices, and healing techniques are also seriously affected by HIV/AIDS. They discuss the spiritual emergencies faced by some Latino gay men and the psycho-spiritual strategies they and their clinicians and traditional healers have developed to cope with the virus. How the encounter with AIDS has raised spiritual and psychological issues, especially among the Latino population, is a central theme of their paper.

Just as HIV/AIDS affected cultural practices and institutions, it has also restructured communities and interactions among various subcultures. Part 2, *Communities,* includes articles that focus on the changes in different gay and lesbian communities and their relationship to the larger social system. Gayle Rubin's chapter, for example, looks at the impact of HIV/AIDS on a gay male leather community in San Francisco during the 1980s. She discusses how the effects of AIDS have been mediated through complex layers of signification, public policy decisions, and preexisting economic conditions. Despite assumptions that AIDS eradicated the San Francisco leather community, Rubin explains how some dimensions of its social structure were reinforced and others were profoundly changed, especially by geographic competition in the South of Market neighborhood.

Although much attention has been given to the HIV/AIDS epidemic in large urban centers by both the dominant and gay media, Beth

Schneider considers the impact on small communities and the extent to which lesbian and gay communities take "ownership" of AIDS in small cities and rural areas. Some responses to the epidemic closely resemble those made in the larger cities during the first years of HIV/AIDS, but it becomes clear that in such cities as Bismarck, North Dakota; Gainesville, Florida; Lexington, Kentucky; and Santa Barbara, California, gay men and lesbians have been at the center of AIDS-related organizations, even when state agencies are dominant.

AIDS has mostly spared lesbians from the epidemic, yet many lesbian communities have been profoundly affected by HIV/AIDS. Nancy Stoller analyzes the involvement of lesbians in the crisis and the ways the culture of lesbian communities has changed from the 1970s through the 1980s. The values, social location, and occupations of lesbians are related to the possibilities of involvement in AIDS work. Stoller considers these economic conditions, the feminist movement, coalition perspectives, and generational differences in lesbian communities.

Finally, Gregory Herek's chapter sets the broader cultural context by describing the impact of the HIV epidemic on heterosexuals' attitudes toward gay men and lesbians. Cultural constructions of AIDS are shaped by public attitudes toward homosexuality, as evidenced by the connections between AIDS-related stigma and antigay prejudice. Herek presents important longitudinal trends in attitudes toward homosexuality and then analyzes data from a two-stage panel study of public reactions to AIDS. He concludes by discussing the relationship between AIDS-related attitudes and attitudes toward gay men and lesbians.

Since so much of the early gay and lesbian social movements depended on a form of identity politics, it would be impossible to overlook the impact of HIV/AIDS on gay and lesbian identities. Part 3, *Identities*, assesses how the encounter with AIDS affects and is affected by issues of identity in three different groups. Rafael Diaz focuses his chapter on Latino gay men, the integration of their Latino and gay identities, and the apparent inconsistency between AIDS knowledge and risk behavior. He argues that many Latino gay men have conceptualized their identities in terms of gender rather than sexual orientation. Issues of masculinity, dominance, machismo, *simpatia,* and *familismo* need to be analyzed to understand better the culture of non-acculturated Latino men who engage in same-sex sexual behavior. In so doing, AIDS prevention strategies and the psycho-cultural factors that can act as barriers can be clarified more accurately.

Identity is also strongly connected to age and to coming out strategies and practices. As Gilbert Herdt demonstrates, gay adults and gay
youth were united in the same cultural spaces to share a common purpose, namely halting HIV/AIDS. He assesses the impact of AIDS on
gay identity development in terms of the increasingly normative process of individual identity formation for a newer generation and the
process of culture-building among older gay adults socializing gay
youth. AIDS-related activities promoted an intergenerational discourse
and structural changes that have altered the coming out and identity-
formation processes in a new generation of American youth.

Finally, John Peterson's chapter focuses on African American same-
sex behaviors and HIV/AIDS and the relative absence of research on
the topic. He reviews the major findings from a few (mostly psychological) studies and suggests the methodological issues that need to be
considered when doing research on African American gay and bisexual
men. Peterson offers some important ideas about definitions of sexual
identity among African American men and how these might relate to
risky sexual behavior.

Well into the second decade of a worldwide pandemic, our societies
and their social structures have been profoundly altered in ways that
will continue to have significant implications for generations. Not just
a biological and viral agent, HIV has demonstrated itself to be an opportunistic social invader, making headway into the core elements of
our complex cultures. In addition to the psychological toll HIV/AIDS
has taken in individuals' lives and personal experiences, in addition to
the countless deaths and grief shared by friends and families, our ways
of living, thinking, and creating meaning, cultures, communities, and
identities have been severely altered. In short, our encounters with
HIV/AIDS have restructured the very basic organizational and personal systems of our societies.

The stories of HIV/AIDS have yet to be finished; they remain incomplete documents of sad and terrifying times. Yet they also report the
heroism and incredible responses of resistance that have taken shape
in these changing times. These complex encounters are described
within the chapters, written by those who have experienced, survived,
and analyzed the impact—and by those whose absence makes it quite
clear what the impact has really been about.

Notes

1. In some circumstances, data relevant to the assessment of an outcome will have
been gathered for other purposes before the event, or detailed records of the event will

have been recorded at the time. This will be fortunate for the researchers if not the afflicted.

2. HIV has often been demonized or anthropomorphized, but this has largely been directed at the difficulties that it has presented to the biomedical scientist.

3. The problem of relapse to unsafe sex or of young gay men practicing unsafe sex has received a great deal of attention in the last few years. Over and above the fear of new infections, there is the anxiety that those who become infected during the 1990s will be accused of knowingly "taking risks" and therefore undeserving of care.

4. Even with the best of will, relations between the powerful and gay activists often go wrong. Thus in a meeting between gay community leaders and President Bill Clinton at the White House, the White House guards wore rubber gloves to "prevent" HIV infection.

5. This figure is based on a reading of the statistical evidence, including various projections; John Gagnon's long-term participation in various scientific committees; and Des-Jarlais's intimate knowledge of HIV infection among injection drug users and their sexual partners (personal communication, Don Des Jarlais, 1995).

6. Shilts (1987) makes a very strong case that he (and only a few others) were responsive to the epidemic of sexually transmitted infections among sexually active gay men in the mid- to late-1970s. If the early declines in anal gonorrhea (and HIV) are any evidence, other men had noticed this epidemic as well and behavior change may have predated the knowledge of HIV (Shilts, 1987).

References

Bayer, Ronald. (1981). *Homosexuality and American Psychiatry.* New York: Basic Books.

Bell, Alan & Martin Weinberg. (1978). *Homosexualities: A Study of Diversity Among Men and Women.* New York: Simon and Schuster.

Centers for Disease Control. (1981a). "Pneumocystis pneumonia—Los Angeles." *Morbidity and Mortality Weekly Report, 30,* 250–252.

———. (1981b). "Kaposi's Sarcoma and Pneumocystis pneumonia among homosexual men—New York City and California." *Morbidity and Mortality Weekly Report, 30,* 305–308.

———. (1990). "HIV seroprevalence estimates and AIDS case projections in the United States. Report based on a workshop." *Morbidity and Mortality Weekly Report, 39*(110), 1–31.

———. (1995a). *HIV/AIDS Surveillance Report,* 7(2), 39.

———. (1995b). "First 500,000 AIDS Cases—United States, 1995." *Morbidity and Mortality Weekly Report, 44,* 46.

Chauncey, George, (1994). *Gay New York.* New York: Basic Books.

Coyle, Susan, Robert Boruch, & Charles F. Turner, eds. 1991. *Evaluating AIDS Prevention Programs,* Washington, DC: The National Academy Press.

Duberman, Martin. (1991). *Cures: A Gay Man's Odyssey.* New York: Dutton.

Erikson, Kai T. (1976). *Everything in Its Path.* New York: Simon and Schuster.

Gagnon, John H. & William Simon. (1973). *Sexual Conduct.* Chicago: Aldine.

Jacobs, Andrew. (1996). "Can AmFAR survive AIDS?" *New York,* April 8.

Jonsen, Albert & Jeffrey Stryker, eds. (1993). *The Social Impact of AIDS in the United States.* Washington, DC: The National Academy Press.

Kinsella, James. (1990). *Covering the Plague: AIDS and the American Media.* New Brunswick, NJ: Rutgers University Press.

Kolata, Gina. (1995). "New picture of who will get AIDS is dominated by addicts." *New York Times,* February 8.

Levine, Martin P. (1992). The life and death of gay clones. In Gilbert Herdt (Ed.), *Gay Culture in America* (pp. 68–86).

Long, Norton. (1968). "The community as an ecology of games." *American Journal of Sociology, 63*(3), 251–261.

Marwick, Arthur. (1965). *The Deluge: British Society and the First World War.* London: Macmillan.

McKenzie, Nancy F., ed. (1991). *The AIDS Reader: Social, Political, Ethical Issues.* New York: Meridian.

Rosenberg, Philip S. (1995). "The scope of the AIDS epidemic in the United States." *Science, 270*(24), 1372–1375.

Shilts, Randy. (1987). *And the Band Played On.* New York: St. Martin's Press.

Stoneburner, R. L., et al. (1988). "A larger spectrum of severe HIV-1-related disease in intravenous drug users in New York City." *Science, 242,* 916–919.

White, Edmund. (1980). *States of Desire.* New York: Dutton.

Whittier, David. (1995). *Gay Life in a Southern Town.* Ph.D. dissertation, Department of Sociology, State University of New York at Stony Brook.

Winter, J. M. (1986). *The Great War and the British People.* Cambridge, MA: Harvard University Press.

Wolf, Deborah. (1979). *The Lesbian Community.* Berkeley: University of California Press.

PART ONE

PRACTICES

ONE

Mobilizing Around AIDS: Sites
of Struggle in the Formation of
AIDS Subjects

Barry D. Adam

This chapter probes the dynamics
of collective mobilization around AIDS to examine the ways in which
AIDS organizations have affected "business as usual" among state,
medical, corporate, and social service bureaucracies. An equal concern
is to consider the ways in which these institutions have, in turn, shaped
AIDS activism. Any social movement presupposes a constituency and
its adversaries; much of the story of AIDS organization emerges from
the ongoing clash of the so-called "risk groups" with the pre-existing
social institutions. Though one might begin simply by populating the
contemporary stage with these preconstituted actors to produce an
account of AIDS activism, the intent here is to unravel some of the
tangled "multiplicity of practices at play on intersecting and disjunc-
tive sites" (Patton, 1990: 125) that generate AIDS "subjects."

Just who might become mobilized into a constituency for AIDS activism is not self-evident. Collective mobilization of any sort rests upon
preexisting social networks and self-identification of commonality
among a group that can be mobilized. This sense must be reinforced
through shared narratives that construct common identities and meanings. These accounts must be effectively communicated to call upon
and indeed generate the subjectivity that makes mobilization possible.
Yet "AIDS" has been organized through several competing and partially incompatible discourses that, in some cases, impel the processes
of subjective identification and movement formation and, in others,
dissipate potential constituencies into alternative and depoliticized
channels.

This paper benefited from the comments of workshop participants Lourdes Arguelles, Rafael Díaz, John Gagnon, Amber Hollibaugh, Nan Hunter, Peter Nardi, Jay
Paul, Anne Rivero, Gayle Rubin, Beth Schneider, Nancy Stoller, Carole Vance, Vera
Whisman, and Paul Whitaker, at a seminar held in Rancho Sante Fe, California, in December 1992.

Discontinuous AIDS discourses have emerged from diverse social networks and communities affected by the syndrome. Black and White, male and female, heterosexual and homosexual people draw on a sometimes-incompatible range of personal and collective histories and languages in making sense of AIDS.[1] Social institutions, in turn, take up these discursive disjunctures in the organization of experiences around AIDS, frequently transform and recontextualize them, and then purvey them back to new seropositives—who employ the reworked narratives in making sense of their own experiences with HIV disease. In this way, the subjectivity of AIDS, emerging in heterogeneous, inchoate, and fragmented ways, becomes reorganized into systematic narratives that provide its subjects a location and orientation in the world. For the purposes of this chapter, only some of these discursive/institutional complexes can be indicated, and even then somewhat cursorily.

AIDS Life-worlds

Steven Epstein (1991:38) has enumerated several of the social factors that underlie contemporary AIDS mobilization. AIDS struck an already organized gay community that included a middle class with significant cultural capital. The disease itself presents the clearly alarming characteristics of threatening life and heavily affecting a relatively young population through a lengthy incubation period. These are the sorts of factors that answer many of the questions posed by resource mobilization theory (McAdam, 1982:21) as to how a social movement gets under way. The premise of this form of AIDS mobilization rests, as Cindy Patton (1990:9) has pointed out, on "the 'coming out' experience of gay liberation . . . mobilized as a model for people with AIDS, who, it is believed can create an identity and group unity by claiming the common experience of living with AIDS." AIDS activism is generated out of the "PWA" ("persons with AIDS") identity, itself built on an especially North American model of gay politics that parallels ethnic organization (Adam, 1992c, 1995). Here people self-label, identify, build networks and solidarity, and fight back—a model that sets seropositivity apart, organizes an AIDS subject, and creates a social force capable of confronting established social and political institutions. Though this discourse and organizational model are founded solidly in gay and lesbian communities, there is no easy one-to-one connection from gay identity to PWA identity. There is no lack of seropositive gay men who avoid the PWA identity and yet, at the same time, this model attracts some support from seropositive people traditionally marginal to or outside of gay worlds.

This mobilization model also draws people together from a wide ambit encompassing those who, although seronegative, are "living with AIDS" in their own ways, including many gay men who are "at risk" according to epidemiological criteria; friends, lovers, household and family members of people with HIV disease; lesbians; and some front line medical and social service workers. At the same time, many HIV-positive people, including homosexually interested men, disavow gay identification (as the increasingly common phrase "men who have sex with men" implies) and feel little connection to the gay/PWA identity complex.

In contrast, for many women, Blacks, Latinos, and aboriginal people (always highly overlapping categories), PWA identity lacks an easy fit with experience. HIV disease may present itself as "another trouble" among people already struggling to survive unemployment, poverty, addiction, and poor medical services while attempting to provide for children and other dependents (see Patton, 1990:9). Melinda Cuthbert's (1992) work on San Francisco street youth reveals a similar pattern: AIDS may present itself as simply another risk among a number of imminent dangers ranging from violence to homelessness. The threat of AIDS as a possible outcome ten years away from the point of contraction of HIV infection, may seem relatively "theoretical" to people concerned with meeting immediate problems of food, shelter, and personal security. Organizing one's identity around AIDS as a first priority makes less sense in this context. For Black men with homosexual experience in our study (Adam & Sears, 1996), this orientation to AIDS was common, though gay discourse influenced some. As a result, African American, Latino, and aboriginal communities often deal with AIDS as one problem added to the crowded agenda of overburdened health and social service agencies. Specific AIDS projects similarly must respond with a multi-issue agenda because addressing AIDS means addressing other medical and social problems.

HIV-positive hemophiliacs have other strong disincentives against embracing PWA identity. Located at the opposite end of the public moral hierarchy from gay men and drug users, and having successfully won compensation for damages from a number of governments, they have more to lose than gain through association with the other marginalized and subordinated people who make up the overall PWA population. Hemophilia is a category that has "worked" better than "PWA" in securing state resources and most hemophiliacs with HIV have avoided the PWA model.

Complicating all of this is the very powerful and pervasive discourse of therapy (see Patton 1990:10). Especially for people who have experienced drug rehabilitation, twelve-step programs, or professional counseling, therapeutic language offers a complete conceptual universe in which to place AIDS. Therapeutic discourse is particularly salient in the lives of injection drug users, who are usually otherwise unorganized, but is also influential among many gay men who have encountered one of the many professional programs. As well, many people discover their serostatus as part of a therapeutic process, whether in substance abuse counseling or another clinical setting. HIV enters this narrative track as part of the conversion experience from an addictive existence that denies itself as addiction, to a newfound overcoming of addiction through (a dialectical) identification with it. In this system, HIV often plays a redemptive role as the impetus to people "getting their act together." Therapy psychologizes and depoliticizes AIDS, thereby producing quite another AIDS subjectivity that is much less susceptible to mobilization. Like AIDS activism, therapy offers an experience of empowerment, but it is an individual liberation that presents little challenge to outside institutions.

Nor do these discourses exhaust the myriad "conceptual inputs" that can be drawn upon in making sense of AIDS. For people in touch with Caribbean, Latin American, or aboriginal healing traditions, the narratives of *santería, candomblé, juju/voudun,* or aboriginal traditions may enter into personal meanings of disease causation and death (see chapter 4). Folk theology, familial idiolects, sexual-romantic scripts (Adam & Sears, 1994; 1996; chapter 4), and others have their places.

Given these heterogeneous and discontinuous forms of AIDS subjectivity, it cannot be entirely surprising that such AIDS activism as ACT-UP (AIDS Coalition to Unleash Power) protest has been typified as a "white, middle-class gay and lesbian" undertaking (Gamson, 1989: 356). ACT-UP's lack of representativeness of the full epidemiological profile of those affected by AIDS has often given rise to both external and internal criticism. Indeed, it is less an inclusive organization than a new social movement preoccupied by inclusiveness. Yet whatever its explicit intentions, underlying discursive/institutional complexes will likely continue to limit the scope of its support base.

The Welfare State and AIDS Service Organizations

AIDS service organizations stand at the interface between the life worlds of people with HIV disease and various state and social welfare systems. Arising in the early 1980s as the community-based response to the new health menace, AIDS service organizations have undergone a variable process of institutionalization within the context of social welfare delivery in advanced capitalist societies. Like the many popular movements that have preceded it, community-based AIDS mobilization has represented a popular claim to "new social rights limiting the heretofore unrestrained power of capital" (Fraser, 1987:47) by demanding state and corporate accountability in the face of widespread death. The first AIDS organizations educated a new class of critical medical consumers who would not presume that the medical establishment acts automatically in its interests. They demanded entitlement to medical and social services, which have always been taken for granted by the middle class, and in their time of greatest need, they have pressed for a return on the taxes they had invested in the welfare state.

At the same time, engagement with the state has made AIDS organizations vulnerable to a well-established process of "rendering [PWAs] dependent on bureaucracies and therapeutocracies, and preempting their capacities to interpret their own needs, experiences and life-problems." (Fraser, 1987:48). As Jürgen Habermas (1987) and many other observers of the welfare state have noted, the strategy of modern state systems is to convert political problems into administrative ones, to reduce civil society to media management, to limit politics to elections, and to convert citizens into social welfare clients. The overall effect is to deny preexisting community and indigenous cultural forms by treating citizens/clients/consumers as a series of unconnected, "strategically-acting, self-interested monads" (Fraser, 1987: 50; see Fraser, 1989). For women, who make up the majority of social welfare clients, this extension of state management further presses patriarchal money- and power-mediated relations into the domestic sphere. For gay men and Black people (once again, overlapping categories), whose household relationships tend to stray far from the iconic "family" promoted especially by Republican and Christian right ideologies, this constitutes a failure to take account of or support the primary relationships on the front line of the epidemic (see, e.g., Levine, 1991). As Gary Kinsman (1992:219,225) remarks in his critical review of the 1990 National Policy on AIDS developed by the Conservative government of Canada, the policy amounts to "a hegemonic administrative framework for incorporating community-based groups into a state regulatory strategy" with "still more emphasis on palliative care—compassion while dying in dignity and AIDS as a necessarily fatal disease—than on developing the capacity of people to live longer and resist HIV/AIDS."

AIDS services organizations today continue to manifest their hybrid origins, preserving a gay-positive enclave in the midst of a homophobic social context, while restructuring themselves along the explicitly nonpolitical lines required by government grants and charitable registration. Their mediating position between the state and the communities in which people with AIDS live has involved them in innovating gay-positive safer sex and needle exchange projects while preserving the human rights of its recipients (Adam, 1992b). But although some organizations—especially those lacking state funding—press state structures entirely from the outside, others have become partially or primarily state-funded, thereby "allow[ing] governments to avoid confronting some AIDS issues themselves" (Rayside & Lindquist, 1992:41). Cindy Patton (1990:22) notes that the introduction of the HIV antibody test in 1985 hastened this institutionalization process by differentiating "at-risk" populations into "service users" (primarily HIV-positive gay men) and "volunteers" (HIV-negative gay men and women) while opening the door for a new class of "experts" (inevitably mostly heterosexual White men with institutional power and no organic connection to the issue).

The trajectory of contemporary AIDS service organizations has been both toward the proliferation of culturally sensitive, specialized, autonomous projects directed toward women, aboriginal, Black, Asian, Latino, and sex worker populations, and toward increased professionalization of service. Although clients have benefited from the experience and training that professionals have brought to AIDS service, the result has been movement toward increased reproduction of therapeutic strategies and retrenchment of a depoliticized style of the "management" of AIDS. In ten years, a great many AIDS organizations have evolved from manifestos to mission statements and from community mobilization to "volunteerism."

Mobilization and Militance

It is here that Doug McAdam's (1982:37) advocacy of a "political process" model of social movements comes into its own, where movements are seen as "rational attempts by excluded groups to mobilize sufficient political leverage to advance collective interests through non-institutionalized means." Stated somewhat ideal-typically, a fundamental aim of the AIDS movement is to democratize the struggle against AIDS, to promote "health from below" (Sears, 1991; Adam, 1992b) by mobilizing affected communities to take measures against the transmission of HIV, and to provide care for those suffering from it. Accomplishing this aim entails action to gain a share of state resources for medical research and for PWA support in opposition to the state's record of traditional neglect and exclusion of the high risk groups. These notions inhere in the movement slogan, "silence = death" (Russo, 1989:67). Josh Gamson (1989:354) sums up ACT-UP objectives this way:

> [It] pushes for greater access to treatments and drugs for AIDS-related diseases; culturally sensitive, widely available, and explicit safe-sex education; and well-funded research that is "publicly accountable to the communities most affected."

And certainly, a primary objective of militant AIDS action has been to break away from the pacification of AIDS evident in institutionalized AIDS service organizations. Larry Kramer (1989:102–103) laid this criticism at the doorstep of New York's Gay Men's Health Crisis in the formative days of ACT-UP:

> The bigger you get, the more cowardly you become; the more money you receive, the more self-satisfied you are. No longer do you fight for the living; you have become a funeral home. . . . [GMHC] was not founded to help those who are ill. It was founded to protect the living, to help the living go on living, to help those who are still healthy to stay healthy, to help gay men stay alive. . . . to bargain with, to fight with, to negotiate with—to use this strength to confront our enemies, to *make* them help us.

PWA groups, organized by and for people with HIV and AIDS, have become alarmed about the apparent slide toward "grief, palliative care and prevention" (LeBourdais, 1991:151) in medical, social welfare, and AIDS service organizations, emphasizing instead, to anyone who will listen, its preference for emphasis on "quality of life and . . . AIDS as a chronic disease." They have resisted being reduced to welfare clients, by asserting their participation in defining their needs in treatment and services.

New social movement theory typically postulates that popular mobilization in the current era has been characterized by a shift toward:

- attempts to decolonize the lifeworld of intrusions by the economic and political spheres (Habermas, 1987:392),
- the mobilization of largely middle class constituencies, and
- the rise of a new "cultural politics" oriented less to "bread-and-butter" issues than to questions of identity, rights, and autonomy.

This portrait of the new social movements suffers from several defects when applied to the full range of contemporary movements, including AIDS activism. The decolonization thesis renders a "too-defensive" image of new social movement activity that, in fact, shows many pro-active and innovative initiatives (Adam, 1993). The middle-class claim derives from a strong analytic focus on a particular face of the environmental movement; it remains to be demonstrated for other new social movements and certainly fails to recognize the very real poverty of a great many people living with AIDS, both gay and non-White, when applied to AIDS activism. The "cultural politics" thesis underestimates the fundamental engagement of the new social movements and AIDS organizations with the state.

Nonetheless, there are also grains of truth in each of these postulates, which can help illuminate the nature of AIDS activism. In the contemporary world, where public debate in civil society has become a matter of "breaking into" a corporate media monopoly, ACT-UP has succeeded at times in both attracting and forcing the media to put AIDS on the public agenda. Gamson (1989) has emphasized AIDS activists' expressive and theatrical side, but the new cultural politics is a necessary political strategy in a "mass-mediated" society. The organizer of the 1990 San Francisco AIDS conference found himself confronted with "media-savvy activists, armed with the new instruments of war—Macintosh computers, fax machines, and cellular phones—[who] produced one press release after another explaining every act of civil disobedience" (Wachter, 1991:295). Demonstrators succeeded, if only momentarily, in democratizing the monopoly media when they broke into CBS and PBS news broadcasts at the height of the Gulf War to demand, "Fight AIDS, not Arabs." Later in September 1991, with the media eye focused upon President George Bush aboard his sailboat at Kennebunkport, Maine, activists proved to be remarkably successful in putting themselves again on the public stage by occupying the president's resort village to contrast the president's leisure to their sense of urgency (Boyce, 1991:1).

Identity politics remain unavoidable in the problematic relationship of "gay" with "AIDS."

> AIDS activists find themselves simultaneously attempting to dispel the notion that AIDS is a gay disease (which it is not) while, through their activity and leadership, treating AIDS as a gay problem (which, among other things, it is). (Gamson, 1989:356).

Stephen Manning's 1990 speech to the Canadian AIDS Society about who "owns" AIDS stems from an anxiety that the colonization of AIDS work by nongay experts and professionals will ultimately result in the total engulfing of AIDS by the welfare state, thereby destroying the core of democratization and community control still alive in AIDS service organizations. Similar debates have preoccupied major AIDS organizations in the United States (see Rofes, 1990). At the same time, this reassertion of gay "ownership" denies the multiplicity of AIDS experiences, as well as the household and family members and "concerned citizens" "living with AIDS" in their own way, who turn up at the doors of AIDS service organizations to help shoulder the AIDS struggle.

Medicine, Science and the Professions

The confrontation of AIDS organizations with medical science also shows a twin movement: (a) a popular initiative to democratize the research process, and (b) the scientific colonization of gay sexuality and the lives of drug users. AIDS activists have challenged research scientists on a wide range of traditional practices borne more perhaps of complacency and historical accretion than scientific reason. They have contested the preference of the pharmaceutical industry to test only very expensive, high-tech drugs with high-profit potential while ignoring alternative treatments. They have confronted the separation of treatment accessibility from drug trial eligibility that frequently imposed a long list of arbitrary exclusions upon women, people who had taken certain treatments before, and people with certain T4-cell count thresholds. They questioned state funding directed toward drugs already favored by the pharmaceutical industry. They disputed the ethics of placebo control testing. They asserted a new range of "catastrophic rights" (Dixon, 1990), to allow consumers to try out treatments without regulatory approval and they organized buyers' clubs to import and distribute approved treatments, followed by community research initiatives to monitor their use and effects. The organizers of the 1990 San Francisco AIDS conference eventually acceded to having activists review and retrieve rejected abstracts (Wachter, 1991:49) and to sit on each of the scientific oversight committees.

People with HIV disease proved capable of breaking out of the role predetermined for them by the research enterprise as the simple objects of the scientific gaze. They "question not just the *uses* of science, not just the *control* over science, but sometimes even the very *contents* of science and the *processes* by which it is produced" (Epstein, 1991:37).

Still, as Epstein (1991:55) continues, "The more we distribute the knowledge formerly monopolized by the mainstream experts, the more, perhaps, we solidify the cultural hegemony of science *over us*." One of the internal tensions of AIDS movement groups has been between political activist tendencies, on the one hand, and treatment information groups on the other. Indeed, one of the early objectives of Toronto's AIDS Action Now! was the creation of a treatment registry to collect and distribute medical information more efficiently to community physicians and people with AIDS. When the Canadian AIDS Treatment Information Exchange became institutionalized with government funding, it separated from AIDS Action Now! As AIDS activists have won representation in scientific and state policy committees, they have been drawn into the process of interpelating AIDS subjects into medical and juridical discourses, for example, in developing punitive criminal sanctions against the "sexually irresponsible."[2] Safer sex education has also trod a fine line in attempting to shear away heterosexist moralism in favor of a sex-positive message that saves lives, all the while developing a central canon intended to domesticate a sexuality that has so long escaped the supervisory hegemony of family, church, and state (see Adam, 1992b). AIDS service organizations now shelter a wave of professional and quasi-professional psychological, spiritual, and nutritional therapists who are able to cultivate a ready-made clientele *assigned* by the power of the ELISA test. The clergy, always on the lookout for new consumers in a secular age, recasts folk cosmology into a round of commemorative rituals, healing circles, and spiritual "discoveries" for people with HIV and their caregivers.

The effects of the professions on AIDS have been two-edged. Without them, AIDS activists could not have made their inroads into state funding, the research establishment, or social services. With them, they invite incorporation into the state-and-scientific panopticon that extends over the "at-risk" populations (Adam, 1992a; 1992b). The outcome may be some unexpected realignments of tactical coalitions. Robert Wachter (1991:79) notes that new relationships—even alliances—may be supplanting old antagonisms: for example, medical researchers may now "leak" information to activists, essentially using them as a radical arm in a common campaign to advance research into treatments.

The State and Corporate Regulation

In the larger scheme of things, AIDS service organizations, social service professionals, and medical researchers are easy targets of criticism and relatively powerless actors caught in historical contradictions and ironies often not of their own making. It is the state and the corporations, primarily the pharmaceutical and health insurance companies, that prove to be most powerful and thus most intractable of all. These struggles expose the limitations of social movement politics and the need for much larger alliances and radical changes if the structural underpinnings of AIDS dilemmas are to be addressed.

The greatest successes of AIDS activism in confronting state apparatuses have been in securing legal protection for people with HIV by working *within* well-established legal frameworks developed around the rights of the disabled. Litigation and government commissions have generally won the inclusion of people with AIDS within the coverage of rights to treatment and rights conferring protection against discrimination due to disability. Gaining access to those rights has proved more problematic as people facing life-threatening illness, uncertain availability of medical services, and potential rapid downward social mobility, must decide whether to add legal expenses to their lives to combat discrimination (Adam & Sears, 1996). Challenging existing legal frameworks has proved far more difficult.

One of the most persistent issues of AIDS activism has been the effort to break through the procedural tangle that impedes the development and approval of new treatments to meet the AIDS emergency. The first demonstration by ACT-UP in 1987 focused on demanding that the Food and Drug Administration accelerate its drug testing and approval process (Kramer, 1989:138). In 1988, demonstrators laid siege to the FDA and the Department of Health and Human Services in Washington (Russo, 1989:65). Many demonstrations throughout the United States, Canada, and Australia campaigned for the release of specific drugs, first aerosolized pentamidine, then ddl and ddC. Yet successes in this area have less to do with pressure-group politics than with the structural organization of the capitalist state. As Harold Edgar and David Rothman (1991:97) wryly observe:

> large parts of the AIDS advocates' critique of the FDA could have
> been scripted by the Pharmaceutical Manufacturers Association

.... Sick gay men, abandoned by a president who refused publicly to acknowledge their disease on all but one occasion, provided the shock troops to move forward his administration's de-
regulatory drug control program.

AIDS activist rhetoric provided a humanistic veneer for the Reagan
administration to present its corporate agenda of facilitating profit-
making with minimal state or consumer oversight. Demands directed
toward government succeeded to the degree that they conformed to the
structural prerequisites of the capitalist state by (inadvertently) coin-
ciding with the corporate agenda for state expenditure.

On other fundamental issues the state-corporate complex remains
obdurate, though AIDS activists have done all in their power to advance them into the public arena. Limited successes have been
achieved, as when Burroughs Wellcome dropped the price of zidovud-
ine (AZT) by twenty percent following demonstrations embarrassing
to corporate management (Wachter, 1991:65). The tactic was tried
again in 1992 to embarrass Astra into cutting its price for Foscarnet.
But in the delivery of health services, the obstacles are formidable.
AIDS activists have picketed the convention of the National Council
Against Health Fraud to protest insurers' refusal to reimburse experimental and alternative treatments (Nealon, 1990:1). They have challenged the Medical Information Bureau, which enables insurers to
deny medical coverage on the basis of information compiled by the
bureau on applicants' sexual orientation (Briggs, 1990:2). They have
attacked insurance companies for dropping or capping treatment costs
for HIV disease, for covering AIDS only when acquired through transfusion, and for redlining gay neighborhoods (Gould, 1990:1; Zeh,
1991:1; Yukins, 1991:1). Ultimately these challenges strike at the heart
of a profit-making system whose insurers have greatest incentive to
cover those least in need, having created a panoply of ruses and regulations to abandon people with AIDS (Adam & Sears, 1996: ch.7). Only
full participation in a much bigger coalition to secure national health
insurance will offer any chance of solving these problems. By comparison, AIDS politics in Canada, which does have a universal medical care
system, are relatively more conciliatory and focused on improving the
quality of service.

Still, federal policy in both Canada and the United States under conservative administrations through the 1980s and early 1990s has been
characterized by truculence, neglect, and stigmatization. Since the introduction of the HIV antibody test in 1985, the state has contributed
to the construction and reproduction of people with AIDS as the

"other" (Adam, 1992b). Kinsman (1992:218) sums up Canadian federal policy as "palliative care and defending the 'general public' from 'infection' from PLWAs and affected communities." The United States shows its most repressive face toward the most powerless members of society: noncitizens and prisoners. As the nation with the largest number of HIV-positive people in the world, the United States has few grounds to regard itself as threatened by the importation of HIV. Yet despite a boycott by the International AIDS Society because of the country's discriminatory immigration policy, the U.S. Congress prefers to be seen acting against AIDS through the harassment, detention, and expulsion of HIV-positive visitors and immigrants. AIDS workers from the Netherlands, Canadian visitors to the Names Project Quilt in Washington, and refugees from the military dictatorship in Haiti have all been subject to imprisonment and expulsion.

In the prison system, where state organs have greatest direct control over citizens, Gregory Smith, a gay Black PWA, was sentenced to twenty-five years in Philadelphia for "attempted murder" for biting a jail guard in 1989; Curtis Weeks was sentenced to life for spitting at a jail guard in Texas in 1989; Shaquita Johnson was charged with murder for spitting at a jail guard in Texas in 1989; Adam Brock was sentenced to fifteen years for biting an Alabama prison guard (subsequently overturned on appeal); Madline Rodrigues was convicted of second-degree assault for spitting on a police officer in Minnesota in 1990; Donald Haines was convicted of attempted murder for biting a police officer in Indiana in 1989; and Gregory Scroggings was sentenced to ten years for biting a police officer in Georgia (McKnight, 1990:1).

The state reflex has been to promote the family of nostalgia while refusing to recognize, legally secure, and support the primary relationships on the frontlines of the AIDS crisis: gay male couples, families with gay members, and Black, Latino, aboriginal, and working-class households eking out an existence on transitory employment and transfer payments.

Conclusion

The uniqueness and indeed genius of contemporary AIDS mobilization has been its success in organizing a collective identification of a shared fate around AIDS and its achievement of an international set of urban nuclei willing to jump the traces imposed by contemporary state systems. AIDS organizations have made noteworthy gains in leaping beyond the roles of patient/client/voter/consumer assigned by modern state systems for people suffering from disabling illnesses. In this, AIDS movement organizations have distinguished themselves in creating strategies that contrast with those of other disease groups fully contained by the nonpolitical, charitable organization model.

At the same time, these gains have been won through a fragile organizational structure with unsure footing. The diversity of experiences occasioned by the impact of HIV on everyday lives far exceeds the possibilities of any one interpretive framework. The result is that AIDS movement groups (like most other social movements) attract only a small fraction of their potential constituency and remain open to the charge of partiality. Furthermore, the dissenting and reformative initiatives pressed by AIDS organizations face formidable forces of bureaucratization and pacification endemic to advanced capitalist societies.

Perhaps most remarkable of all in the interminable advance of HIV disease has been its successful routinization. This holocaust-scale death force, surging through gay, Black, and Latino communities in the first world, and the Caribbean, southern Asia, and sub-Saharan Africa in the third world, has become increasingly "normalized" and, once integrated into the usual state mechanisms, deprioritized in turn. Once assimilated as just another task for health, education, and welfare systems, it becomes vulnerable to the larger problem of the fiscal crisis of the state as international corporate elites respond to the geopolitics of the modern world system by demanding more efficient capital accumulation by stripping state services to ordinary citizens. The neoconservative turn of governments in the 1990s toward the dismantling of social services in the name of deficit reduction makes even routinization vulnerable to new policies of neglect or abandonment. State disengagement from research funding, treatment subsidies, and education for prevention can now be justified as part of a general policy of downsizing and privatization. The recent history of AIDS is subject to the same force as a thousand other popular initiatives: containment and pacification of its support base at the same time as the resolution of the fundamental problem seems no closer.

Notes

1. Many of the observations in this section are further developed in *Experiencing HIV* (1996). This study comprised 100 HIV-positive people and their caregivers in southeastern Michigan and southwestern Ontario and was funded by the Canadian Foundation for AIDS Research.

2. See Leeming (1992). The paper is an example, rather than an analysis, of this process.

References

Adam, Barry D. (1992a). "Sociology and People Living With AIDS." In Joan Huber & Beth Schneider, (Eds.) *The Social Context of AIDS* (pp. 3–18). Newbury Park, CA: Sage.

———. (1992b). "The State, Public Policy, and AIDS Discourse." In James Miller (Ed.), *Fluid Exchanges* (pp. 305–320). Toronto: University of Toronto Press.

———. (1992c). "Sex and Caring Among Men." In Ken Plummer (Ed.), *Modern Homosexualities*, (pp. 175–183). London: Routledge.

———. (1993). "Post-Marxism and the New Social Movements." *Canadian Review of Sociology and Anthropology, 30*(3), 316–336.

———. (1995). *The Rise of a Gay and Lesbian Movement.* Revised edition. New York: Twayne.

Adam, Barry, & Alan Sears. (1994). "Negotiating Sexual Relationships after Testing HIV-Positive." *Medical Anthropology, 16,* 63–77.

———. (1996). *Experiencing HIV.* New York: Columbia University Press.

Boyce, Ed. (1991). "Protest in Kennebunkport." *Gay Community News, 19*(8), 1.

Briggs, Laura. (1990). "ACT UP Closes Down Medical Information Office." *Gay Community News, 18*(16), 2.

Cuthbert, Melinda. (1992). "A Population in Peril." Presented to the Society for the Study of Social Problems, Pittsburgh.

Dixon, John. (1990). *Catastrophic Rights.* Vancouver: New Star.

Edgar, Harold, and David Rothman. (1991). "New Rules for New Drugs." In Dorothy Nelkin, David Willis & Scott Parris (Eds.), *A Disease of Society* (pp. 84–115). New York: Cambridge University Press.

Epstein, Steven. (1991). "Democratic Science?" *Socialist Review, 91* (2), 35–64.

Fraser, Nancy (1987). "What's Critical about Critical Theory?" In Seyla Benhabib & Drucilla Cornell (Eds.), *Feminism as Critique.* Minneapolis: University of Minnesota Press.

———. (1989). *Unruly Practices.* Minneapolis: University of Minnesota Press.

Gamson, Joshua. (1989). "Silence, Death, and the Invisible Enemy." *Social Problems, 36*(4), 351–367.

Gould, Debbie. (1990). "Chicago Actions Slam U.S. Health Care." *Gay Community News, 17*(41), 1.

Habermas, Jürgen. (1987). *The Theory of Communicative Action.* Vol. 2 Boston: Beacon.

Kinsman, Gary. (1992). "Managing AIDS Organizing." In William Carroll (Ed.), *Organizing Dissent,* (pp. 215–231). Toronto: Garamond.

Kramer, Larry. (1989). *Reports from the Holocaust.* New York: St. Martin's.

LeBourdais, Eleanor. (1991). "AIDS Patients' Concerns at Centre Stage during Vancouver Conference." *Canadian Medical Association Journal, 145*(2), 151–152.

Leeming, William. (1992). "On Assuming the Responsibility of Living With AIDS/HIV." Presented to the Canadian Sociology and Anthropology Association, Charlottetown, Prince Edward Island.

Levine, Carol. (1991) "AIDS and Changing Concepts of Family." In Dorothy Nelkin, David Willis, & Scott Parris (Eds.), *A Disease of Society* (pp. 45–70) New York: Cambridge University Press.

McAdam, Doug. (1982). *Political Process and the Development of Black Insurgency, 1930–1970.* Chicago: University of Chicago Press.

McKnight, Jennie. (1990). "Is Saliva a Murder Weapon?" *Gay Community News, 17*(40), 1.

Nealon, Chris. (1990). "Demos in Kansas City and S. F. Blast Medical Bigwigs." *Gay Community News, 18* (14), 1.

Patton, Cindy. (1990). *Inventing AIDS.* New York: Routledge.

Rayside, David, & Evert Linquest. (1992). "AIDS Activism and the State in Canada." *Studies in Political Economy, 39,* 37–76.

Rofes, Eric. (1990). "Gay Lib vs. AIDS." *Out/Look, 8,* 8–17.

Russo, Vito. (1989). "State of Emergency." *Radical America, 21* (6), 64–68.

Sears, Alan. (1991). "AIDS and the Health of Nations." *Critical Sociology, 18*(2), 31–50.

Wachter, Robert. (1991). *The Fragile Coalition.* New York: St. Martin's Press.

Yukins, Elizabeth. (1991). "Insurance Firm Bows to ACT UP." *Gay Community News, 18* (46), 1.

Zeh, John. (1991). "ACT UP Blasts Insurance Bias." *Gay Community News, 18*(42), 1.

**Censorship and Identity in
The Age of AIDS**

NAN D. HUNTER

For lesbians and gay men, the price of inclusion in the body politic has been silence. In the absence of self-identifying speech, most persons are assumed to be heterosexual. Indeed, one might paraphrase the ACT-UP slogan as silent = straight. Because of this, because we become gay in some real social sense only when we speak as gay, there is an important and complicated relationship between expression and equality in lesbian and gay rights law.

The emergence of lesbian and gay identity politics has further complicated the expression-equality dynamic. Increasingly, gay and lesbian equality claims center on notions of identity, an idea that encompasses expression. To be openly gay, when the closet is an option, is to function as an advocate as well as a symbol. Self-representation of one's sexual identity necessarily includes a message that one has not merely come out, but that one intends to *be* out, to act and live out that identity.

These aspects of gay politics remained largely subterranean, however, until AIDS. With its urgency, mystery and fear, the topic of AIDS forced itself into public debate. In the process, AIDS transformed American discourse about sexuality. Homosexuality emerged as an identity that could be claimed as a part of public discourse and in public space. Debates over the content of safe-sex educational programs exemplified the battle over attempted state regulation of desire, and of the expressions not only of desire but also of identity, an identity constituted at least partially by desire.

The old social contract about sexual deviance—that we will permit your secrecy if you collude in our silence—was already starting to erode at the end of the 1970s and the beginning of the 1980s. AIDS shattered it, simultaneously elevating and demonizing homosexuality as an issue in national politics.

This chapter was published in substantially similar form in *Virginia Law Review* 79, no. 7, 1993. Reprinted with permission of Fred B. Rothman & Co.

Prehistory

Until 1958, the law treated representational speech about homosexuality as obscenity. Under the tendency-to-corrupt-morals test for obscenity that preceded the current standard,[1] courts treated promotion or advocacy of homosexuality as obscene. For example, in finding Radclyffe Hall's *The Well of Loneliness* obscene in 1929, a New York judge wrote that "[t]he book can have no moral value, since it seeks to justify the right of a pervert to prey upon normal members of a community, and to uphold such a relationship as noble and lofty."[2]

In a ruling nearly thirty years later, the Ninth Circuit Court of Appeals found the Mattachine Society's monthly political and literary magazine *One* to be obscene and thus not mailable.[3] The court based its finding on one short story described as "nothing more than cheap pornography calculated to promote lesbianism" and one poem about gay male sexual activities that "pertains to sexual matters of such a vulgar and indecent nature that it tends to arouse a feeling of disgust and repulsion."[4] The equivalency of affirmation of homosexuality with obscenity ended when, without opinion, the Supreme Court reversed the appeals court in early 1958, citing its then-new obscenity standard that had dropped moral corruption as its touchstone.[5]

Beginning in the early 1970s, cases in which the plaintiffs sought recognition for lesbian and gay organizations—often student groups—marked the first step in the law toward the effort to seek an open existence in American society.[6] Simultaneously, individuals began to come out in a self-consciously political way, and then to sue if employers or others retaliated against them with dismissals and other reprisals.[7] Activists in a handful of the more progressive cities won amendments to local civil rights laws that added sexual orientation as a ground on which employers and landlords could not discriminate.[8]

The Briggs Initiative: "No Promo Homo" Begins

By consensus, the Stonewall rebellion in June 1969 marks the beginning of the lesbian and gay political movement.[9] One result of the growing political consciousness of gay rights was the enactment of the first civil rights ordinances in a handful of cities. These breakthroughs in turn led to a series of repeal campaigns in 1977, in which voters eliminated civil rights protections in Dade County, Florida; St. Paul, Minnesota; Wichita, Kansas; and Eugene, Oregon, in rapid succession.[10] Speech of various sorts obviously facilitated these events, but did not appear openly as a constituent part of what was at stake. It was nearly ten years after Stonewall, in 1978, in the first political debate about homosexuality that extended beyond urban centers or limited enclaves such as universities, that expression rather than conduct formed the core of the issue.

The Briggs initiative appeared on the November 1978 California ballot as a referendum question that would have permitted the firing of any school employee who engaged in "advocating, soliciting, imposing, encouraging or promoting private or public sexual acts" as defined in the state criminal code "between persons of the same sex in a manner likely to come to the attention of other employees or students."[11] It was widely understood to be a vote on whether the state should fire gay teachers and thus purge that group from the schools and from contact with children.[12] This understanding of the meaning of Briggs was consistent with the older, purge-the-homosexuals theme that had dominated debates since the McCarthy era.

In fact, however, the Briggs initiative was much more complicated. On one hand, to come out is to implicitly, often explicitly, affirm the value of homosexuality. For that reason, a Briggs-style law could be used to target all lesbian and gay school employees who had expressed their sexual orientation, except in the most furtive contexts. But the Briggs initiative was configured to play a double role. It was framed in terms of banning a viewpoint, the "advocating" or "promoting" of homosexuality, rather than the exclusion of a group of persons. The proposed statute targeted anyone, gay or straight, who voiced the forbidden ideas.

Early opinion polls indicated that the initiative was likely to pass.[13] In efforts that became a model for the later response to AIDS, the California lesbian and gay community mobilized on a scale that it had never before attempted. Thousands of volunteers, many politically active for the first time, joined the anti-Briggs crusade, and massive fundraising supported a sophisticated advertising and public relations campaign.[14] The full range of gay politics surfaced: more sexually radical groups based in San Francisco conducted speak-out-type campaigns aimed at directly confronting homophobia and linking it to other forms of oppression;[15] David Goodstein, then publisher of *The Advocate*, warned that all was lost unless openly gay people stayed in the background and let straight teachers lead the campaign;[16] and the National Log Cabin Federation, the first gay Republican organization, was born.[17] These efforts combined with the ineptness and underfunding of the pro-Briggs campaign and statements opposing the initiative from a series of conservative political leaders, most famously Ronald Reagan.[18] The initiative was defeated by 58 to 42 percent.[19]

The Briggs initiative campaign marks the moment when American politics began to treat homosexuality as something more than deviance, conduct or lifestyle; it marks the emergence of homosexuality as an openly political claim and as a viewpoint. That, in turn, laid the foundation for the emergence of a new analysis of speech about homosexuality. Instead of treating such speech as the advocacy of conduct, courts shifted to a consideration of gay speech as the advocacy of ideas. The once-bright boundary between sexual speech and political speech began to fade.

A year after the Briggs vote, the California Supreme Court ruled that statements of homosexual identity constituted political speech protected by the state's labor code.[20] In a conclusion still unique in judicial decisions, the court ruled that a complaint that the defendant discriminated against "manifest" homosexuals and homosexuals who make " 'an issue of their homosexuality' " stated a cause of action that defendants violated the labor code by trying to pressure employees to " 'refrain from adopting [a] particular course or line of political . . . activity.' "[21]

> Measured by these standards, the struggle of the homosexual community for equal rights, particularly in the field of employment, must be recognized as a political activity. . . [O]ne important aspect of the struggle for equal rights is to induce homosexual individuals to 'come out of the closet,' acknowledge their sexual preferences, and to associate with others in working for equal rights.[22]

This was the first ruling treating self-affirming "identity speech" as political because of—rather than despite of—its expression regarding sexuality.[23]

By contrast, the federal courts, in adjudicating the constitutionality of language identical to the Briggs initiative, relied on reasoning that avoided the question of whether promoting homosexuality could qualify as political expression. Legislators in Oklahoma enacted the same language rejected by voters in California, after Anita Bryant, a former Miss Oklahoma who led the effort to repeal the Dade County civil rights provision, urged them to protect schoolchildren from persons who "profess homosexuality."[24] The Tenth Circuit found the Oklahoma statute overbroad because it had the potential to reach such conventional political speech as a teacher's out-of-classroom arguments in favor of adopting a civil rights law or repealing a sodomy law.[25] The dissent attempted to create a rule against incitement to sexual conduct, arguing that although advocacy of "violence, sabotage and terrorism" was protected under the First Amendment, advocacy of "a crime *malum in se*," "a practice as universally condemned as the crime of sodomy" did not qualify for First Amendment protection.[26] Bryant's own phrase had captured the paradox, however: one "professes" a belief, not an act.

Testing as Speech, Speech under Test

With the advent of the HIV epidemic, courts, Congress and state legislatures began a fight over which new social understanding about homosexuality would supersede silence. At issue were the questions of which information would comprise public knowledge and how the government would define and enforce the boundaries of public discourse. Framed in this way, many aspects of AIDS law that we think of as falling within the doctrinal category of privacy are grounded instead in expression.

This contest over public knowledge and discourse was fought first, and most significantly, in the policy debate over education versus testing. It quickly became a commonplace in AIDS policy discussions to note that, in the absence of a cure, prevention was the only weapon against the spread of HIV.[27] The contest became how to define "prevention": would that term be interpreted to mean testing or education?[28] The question became, in effect, which form of knowledge would be available in the public realm.

Education efforts, including safe-sex education, required a public discourse that was nonjudgmental of the individual and agnostic toward sexual practices. It sought to promote greater knowledge about sexualities and incited public discussion about specific sexual acts. By contrast, advocates of mandatory testing emphasized a private procedure that led to identification of those who were HIV-infected and often to reporting of that information to public health authorities.

Two competing "right-to-know" campaigns began. Conservatives argued that the public most urgently needed to know who was infected and thus who posed a danger. The gay community used public health arguments to justify opening public fora such as schools and broadcast media to an unprecedented discussion of male homosexuality.

Each side in the debate produced dual arguments. AIDS activists argued for widespread knowledge and openness at the collective level and anonymity at the individual level, especially in the context of the individual reporting information to the state. Conservatives countered with arguments for revealing information about individuals to a state authority, together with silence about sexuality in the public, collective discourse.

At the level of individual knowledge, HIV testing in the early years of the epidemic, before treatments became available, functioned as exposure of (usually) homosexuality with little or no benefit to the persons being tested. As a result, some gay rights groups attempted unsuccessfully to dissuade the Food and Drug Administration from licensing the antibody test in 1985.[29] Licensure of the antibody test saved the nation's blood supply and, in the process, probably averted what would have been a far worse social panic had contaminated blood remained a real threat. But the test also began to be used in exactly the way that rights advocates feared—as a marker for identification and exclusion.[30]

The testing debate within the federal government climaxed in 1987. In February of that year, the CDC held a massive conference in Atlanta on mandatory testing proposals for a variety of populations. Hundreds of persons attended: CNN broadcast the major sessions and billed its daylong coverage as the "national AIDS meeting." Proponents of forced testing lost the battle of the conference; the panelists' recommendations emphasized voluntariness and confidentiality and urged the adoption of antidiscrimination protections.[31]

The CDC toned down these recommendations before transmitting them upward in the federal chain of command, but retained the basic focus on consent and confidentiality.[32] The issue reached the Domestic Policy Council that spring. Surgeon General C. Everett Koop won acceptance of a let-the-states-decide position on a number of testing proposals, but could not stop the Reagan administration from undertaking mandatory testing of federal prisoners and immigrants, groups characterized by their vulnerability to government control rather than by any logical relationship to a heightened risk of transmission.[33]

For both sides in the debate over testing, knowledge of individuals' status became an important commodity in and of itself. For social conservatives, screening and identification of the HIV infected became a kind of justified stigmata, a rite of expulsion, and a method of defining the boundary of community and politics to reject the alien. For AIDS activists, resistance to testing served as both a protective barrier against those expulsions and a bargaining chip. Public health officials desperately needed the cooperation of the gay community for any prevention programs to succeed, and activists tacitly or explicitly sought to trade cooperation in exchange for support of new laws banning discrimination based on HIV status or on sexual orientation.

Although the struggles over individual testing continue and remain important, the framework of the debate has changed. In the same year—1987—that the testing controversy peaked, the focus of debates about AIDS shifted from a contest primarily about knowledge of individual status to one increasingly about the content of public discourse.

In 1985, the CDC had begun funding educational programs aimed at behavior change, including support for some innovative programs undertaken by Gay Men's Health Crisis, which promoted safe-sex practices. GMHC and other AIDS service organizations had always developed their most provocative materials, which sought to eroticize condom use and other safe-sex practices, with private funds. But officials at CDC became alarmed by the potential for conservative backlash against the agency for support of anything controversial.[34] In January 1986, the CDC first promulgated restrictions on the content of federally funded programs, requiring that all such materials use language that "would be judged by a reasonable person to be unoffensive [sic] to most educated adults."[35]

In 1987, this issue reached Congress. In October, Senator Jesse Helms introduced an amendment to the appropriations bill for the Department of Health and Human Services that forbade use of any CDC funds "to provide AIDS education, information, or prevention materials and activities that promote or encourage, directly or indirectly, homosexual sexual activities." The bill was unstoppable. Opponents succeeded only in deleting the term "indirectly," thus arguably limiting its scope to the most graphic materials.[36]

The Helms amendment cleverly drew on the most successful argument of the antiabortion movement: that public funds should not be used to "subsidize" activity associated with what conservatives painted as sexual permissiveness. Here the target group was gay men rather than indigent women. And unlike abortions, the funded activity of education was thoroughly public in its nature, raising the questions of how and on what terms the nation would discuss AIDS. In fact, gay-targeted educational campaigns were very unlikely to be seen outside gay venues, but the right launched an attack that spread from the safe-sex comics and erotic videos distributed in gay bars to sex education and condom availability in the schools.

The debate on the Helms amendment centered on Helms's objections to AIDS education efforts within the gay male community, spe-

cifically those of Gay Men's Health Crisis. Helms made clear, repeatedly, that his objections were based on his views of what was moral,
and that the purpose of his amendment was to insure that the content
of AIDS education be made to conform to what he believed to be moral
precepts of behavior (i.e., an opposition to homosexuality or to tolerance for it).

Helms paraphrased the GMHC proposal, noting that AIDS education sessions (all of which were specifically targeted for gay male participants) included discussions of " 'a positive sense of gay pride.' " [37]
He continued:

> Then ... we get to sessions 5 and 6 ... This is entitled "Guide-
> lines for Healthy Sex." ... The behavioral objectives of these two
> sessions included the ability to "list satisfying erotic alternatives
> to high-risk sexual practices; identify erogenous areas of the
> body," and here I get embarrassed—"other than the genitals that
> produce an erotic response."
> Oh boy ...
> There is no mention of any moral code ... Good Lord, Mr.
> President, I may throw up. [38]

Helms reiterated throughout the debate his intent that the amendment was designed to forbid publicly funded AIDS education materials
from advocacy:

> Yes, it will require us to make a moral judgment. I think it is about
> time we started making some moral judgments and stop playing
> around with all those esoteric things and saying "Yes but." I be-
> lieve, Mr. President, it is time to draw the line. [39]
> I think this is a moral question, and I will be accused of trying
> to impose my morality on somebody else. If someone wants to say
> that, that's fine. [40]
> Mr. President, some Senators want to compromise with a moral
> stand because it is so often said that we talk too much about mo-
> rality. I say to the Senator we can never talk too much about mo-
> rality. We are not going to solve this problem or a lot of others in
> this country unless we get that through our heads ...
> What the amendment does is to propose that we ensure that
> any money spent for such purposes is not spent in such a way that
> it even comes close to condoning or encouraging or promoting
> intravenous drug use or sexual activity outside of sexually monog-
> amous marriage including homosexual activities ... [41]

Immediately before the final vote, Helms summed up the provision:

> Earlier, Mr. President, on this floor, I read from grant presentation
> documents prepared by the Gay Men's Health Crisis of New York
> City. That is a corporation. It is unmistakably clear that those ac-

tivities are being federally funded and are promoting and encouraging homosexuality . . . Therefore, Mr. President, it should be
clear that in adopting this amendment, if in fact it is adopted, this
Senate is prohibiting further funding for programs such as those
sponsored, operated by the Gay Men's Health Crisis Corp. that
promote or encourage homosexual sexual relations.[42]

The following year, Congress rejected the Helms language in favor
of a provision that neutralized its antigay focus while retaining some
limitations on speech. The new language, known as the Kennedy-
Cranston amendment, limited funding only if AIDS educational materials were "designed" to encourage sexual activity, whether heterosexual or homosexual.[43] Under this intent requirement, materials that
were designed to reduce HIV transmission, and that were erotic only
as a by-product of that purpose, were supposed to be exempt from the
limitation because they were not "solely and specifically" intended to
encourage sexual activity.[44] Helms vehemently fought the new language, declaring that it would render his own approach "nugatory."[45]
In fact, however, despite the Kennedy-Cranston amendment, the CDC
retained its own "offensiveness" restrictions until they were ruled invalid by a federal court in 1992.[46]

In the context of AIDS education, sexual explicitness became difficult to separate from expressions of gay male identity. AIDS educators
who produced and distributed safe-sex materials understood that the
explicitness served the function not only of making safe sex seem attractive and inviting, but also of reaffirming the sense of worth of the
gay men at whom the materials were aimed. Representations of sexual
culture marked otherwise nonspecific imagery as gay. As the education
director of the San Francisco AIDS Foundation noted, the posters "really are about who we are. To say these materials are inappropriate is
to say *we* are inappropriate."[47]

In sum, although few of the judicial texts addressing AIDS-related
issues focus on expression, the politics of speech profoundly shaped
AIDS policy. AIDS policies, in turn, transformed public discourse on
homosexuality, more so than any other event, including Stonewall,
Briggs or the battles over municipal and state civil rights laws.

By the end of the 1980s, the angle of right-wing attack was clearly
directed at a concept of advocacy as embodied in the idea of gay identity, and not simply at gay persons as such. Dozens of AIDS service
organizations, many openly affiliated with gay community groups, received millions of dollars of government funding for education and
other prevention efforts. Neither the Reagan administration nor Helms
ever attempted to exclude all gay persons or groups as grantees; even

if there had been the desire for such exclusion, it was practically infeasible and politically implausible. The attack on gay identity centered on advocacy, rather than on either acts or status per se. "No promo homo" was its theme song.

After Stonewall, Beyond AIDS

The "no promo homo" language that originated in the Briggs initiative and was used to restrict AIDS education became the model for many antigay legislative initiatives, in the United States and beyond. Arizona enacted criteria for AIDS education materials in public schools that prohibit any local district from including "instruction which promotes a homosexual lifestyle, portrays homosexuality as a positive alternative lifestyle, [or] suggests that some methods of sex are safe methods of homosexual sex."[48] Alabama adopted similar legislation.[49] In Britain, Clause 28 of the Local Government Act of 1988 stated that local governments could not "promote homosexuality or publish material for the promotion of homosexuality" or "promote the teaching . . . of the acceptability of homosexuality as a pretended family relationship."[50] Nor could government funding go to private entities engaged in those acts.[51] Members of Congress also seemingly became fond of the "no promo homo" principle, reinvoking it when various issues pertaining to homosexuality have surfaced.

In spring 1988, a family planning clinic in New Hampshire finished work on a federally funded sex education program for adolescents, especially males, whom researchers found believed that impregnating their girlfriends and becoming fathers proved to peers that they were not homosexual.[52] The manual written for teachers stated that "[g]ay and lesbian adolescents are perfectly normal and their sexual attraction to members of the same sex is healthy."[53] Senator Gordon Humphrey of New Hampshire introduced legislation that would have prohibited federal funding support for sex education materials "that promote or encourage homosexuality, or use words stating that homosexuality is 'normal,' 'natural,' or 'healthy.'"[54] The legislation passed the Senate, but died in the House-Senate conference committee. That same year, Congress attempted to force the District of Columbia to alter its municipal civil rights law, one of the first to include sexual orientation as a protected category, to exempt religious colleges from its scope. Reacting to a ruling of D.C.'s highest court that Georgetown University had violated the law by refusing to extend benefits to a lesbian and gay student group,[55] Congress conditioned federal appropriations to the district on the City Council's allowing religious schools to

deny benefits or recognition to "any person or persons that are organized for, or engaged in, promoting, encouraging, or condoning any
homosexual act, lifestyle, orientation or belief."[56] Congress never defined "homosexual belief," but the inclusion of that term signifies a
recognition of and a desire to suppress something more than either
conduct ("act") or status ("orientation").

In 1989, in response to public outcry over reports that National Endowment for the Arts (NEA) funds had supported an exhibit of homoerotic Robert Mapplethorpe photographs and other controversial art,
Congress enacted legislation prohibiting the NEA from funding "obscene materials including but not limited to depictions of sadomasochism, homoeroticism, the sexual exploitation of children, or individuals engaged in sex acts."[57] As anthropologist Carole S. Vance has
pointed out, this linguistic construction collapsed homoeroticism
and obscenity, making the former appear to be a synonym for the
latter.[58] Although homoerotic materials are simply one example of
what might meet the legal test for obscenity, the NEA restriction came
full circle from 1950s obscenity case law by seeming to the casual
reader to equate the two, although legally it did not do so. Like the
pre-*Roth* obscenity cases, its implicit message was that homoeroticism
was obscene—indeed, in contemporary terms, that gay identity was
obscene.

Ironically, it was a case in which the Supreme Court ruled against
the gay plaintiffs that led it to accept finally and fully expressions of
gay identity as legitimate political speech. In ruling that the organizers
of Boston's St. Patrick's Day Parade could legitimately exclude a lesbian
and gay Irish group,[59] the court described the content of the gay march-
ers' message as:

> to celebrate its members' identity as openly gay, lesbian and bisex-
> ual descendants of the Irish immigrants, to show that there are
> such individuals in the community and to support the like men
> and women who sought to march in the New York parade. . . .
> [A] contingent marching behind the organization's banner would
> at least bear witness to the fact that some Irish are gay, lesbian or
> bisexual, and the presence of the organized marchers would sug-
> gest their view that people of their sexual orientations have as
> much claim to unqualified social acceptance as heterosexuals and
> indeed as members of parade units organized around other identi-
> fying characteristics.[60]

Thus the U.S. Supreme Court recognized in 1995 what the California
Supreme Court had declared in 1979: that expressions of gay identity
are core political speech.

Conclusion

AIDS talk—with its morally urgent demand to save lives—forced open the door for a politics of (homo)sexuality to enter the national conversation. Since the late 1980s, AIDS itself had lapsed as a focus of media attention, but its effect continues. Although the flashpoints of today's sexual politics—gays in the military, gay marriage, pro- and anti-gay civil rights campaigns—have no direct connection to the epidemic, the passion of a community mobilized by AIDS has forced those issues into the political mainstream.

Notes

1. See *Roth v. United States*, 354 U.S. 476 (1957), abandoning the morality test. The current standard was adopted in *Miller v. California*, 413 U.S. 15 (1973).

2. *People v. Friede*, 233 N.Y.S. 565, 567 (Magis. Ct. 1929).

3. *One v. Olesen*, 241 F.2d 772 (9th Cir. 1957), *rev'd* 355 U.S. 371 (1958). For a description of the magazine and its role in the homophile movement, see John D'Emilio, "Gay Politics and Community in San Francisco since World War II," in Martin Duberman, Martha Vicinus, & George Chauncey Jr. (Eds.), *Hidden from History: Reclaiming the Gay and Lesbian Past*, p. 469 (New York, 1989).

4. *One v. Olesen* (supra n. 3), 241 F.2d at 777.

5. The Supreme Court's ruling consisted of one sentence reversing the lower court and a citation to *Roth v. United States* (supra n. 1). The court's opinion thus did not address the specific question of whether promotion of homosexuality, at least if eroticized, could be a component of obscenity. In *Manual Enterprises Inc. v. Day*, 370 U.S. U.S. 478 (1962), however, the court ruled that nudity in gay male-oriented body-building magazines was "no more objectionable" than comparable female nudity "that society tolerates." Ibid. at 490. The *Day* decision laid the groundwork for the growth of a national gay press. Arthur S. Leonard, *Sexuality and the Law: An Encyclopedia of Major Legal Cases* (New York, 1993) at 209 (hereinafter, Leonard).

6. See, for example, *Gay and Lesbian Students Ass'n v. Gohn*, 850 F.2d 361 (8th Cir. 1988); *Gay Students Services v. Texas A & M University*, 737 F.2d 1317 (5th Cir. 1984); *Gay Lib v. University of Missouri*, 558 F.2d 848 (8th Cir. 1977), *cert. denied sub nom; Ratchford v. Gay Lib*, 434 U.S. 1080 (1978), *reh. denied* 435 U.S. 981 (1978); *Gay Alliance of Students v. Matthews*, 544 F.2d 161 (4th Cir. 1976); *Gay Students Organization of the Univ. of New Hampshire v. Bonner*, 509 F.2d 652 (1st Cir. 1974); *Student Coalition for Gay Rights v. Austin Peay University*, 477 F.Supp. 1267 (M.D. Tenn. 1979); *Wood v. Davison*, 351 F.Supp. 543 (N.D. Ga. 1972).

7. *Van Ooteghem v. Gray*, 628 F.2d 488 (5th Cir. 1980), *aff'd en banc* 654 F.2d 304 (1981), *cert. denied*, 455 U.S. 909 (1982); *Singer v. U.S. Civil Service Comm'n*, 530 F.2d 247 (9th Cir. 1976), *vacated and remanded*, 429 U.S. 1034 (1977); *Acanfora v. Board of Education of Montgomery Cty.*, 491 F.2d 498 (4th Cir. 1974); and *McConnell v. Anderson*, 451 F.2d 193 (8th Cir. 1971), *cert. denied*, 405 U.S. 1046 (1972).

8. Nan D. Hunter, Sherryl E. Michaelson & Thomas B. Stoddard, *The Rights of Gay People* (Carbondale, 1992), pp. 21–22.

9. The event occurred at the Stonewall bar in Greenwich Village, when the bar's patrons spontaneously resisted what the police no doubt considered a routine raid. The resistance was all the more dramatic because most of the patrons were drag queens in full dress, although one observer credits a lesbian among the crowd with being the first

to call on her comrades to fight back. The ensuing struggle became a pitched battle between gays and police that continued for hours in the streets of the Village. Lucian Truscott, "Gay Power Comes to Sheridan Square," *The Village Voice,* July 3, 1969.

10. Randy Shilts, *The Mayor of Castro Street: The Life and Times of Harvey Milk* (New York, 1982), p. 222.

11. "School Employees. Homosexuality—Initiative Statute: Official Title and Summary Prepared by the Attorney General."

12. See, for example, Shilts (supra n. 10), 212–251, and "California Referendums; Witch-hunting," *The Economist,* October 28, 1978, p. 50.

13. Shilts (supra n. 10), p. 242; David B. Goodstein, "The California Teachers Initiative Battle: An Appraisal," *The Advocate,* June 14, 1978, p. 6; "Poll Shows a Major Shift on Prop 6," *Gay Community News,* October 21, 1978, p. 1.

14. See, for example, Scott Anderson, "After Victories, Leaders Ponder the Next Step," *The Advocate,* December 27, 1978, pp. 8–9.

15. D'Emilio, p. 469.

16. Goodstein, (supra n. 13).

17. Kay Longcope, "Weld Moves to Add Gays to the GOP," *Boston Globe,* February 17, 1991, p. 40.

18. Shilts (supra n. 10), pp. 245–249; Sasha Gregory-Lewis, "California Faces Proposition 6 and Will it Be Written, *Mene, Mene, Tekel Upharsin?*", *The Advocate,* November 15, 1978, pp. 7–12; "Victory in California, Seattle; Miami Defeat" *The Advocate,* December 13, 1978, p. 9.

19. "Victory in California" (supra n. 18).

20. *Gay Law Students Assn. v. Pacific Telephone and Telegraph Co.,* 24 Cal.3d 458 (Cal. 1979).

21. Ibid., 488.

22. Ibid.

23. The *Pacific Telephone* case was settled with a $5 million payment to the plaintiff class and the adoption by defendant of an anti-discrimination policy. Leonard (supra n. 5), at 417. In a later case, the California Court of Appeal, First District, ruled that the Labor Code provision did protect against discrimination based on sexual orientation. *Soroka v. Dayton Hudson Corp.,* 235 Cal. App. 3d 654, 1 Cal. Rptr 2d 77 (1st Dist. 1991), appeal dismissed as moot, 24 Cal. Rptr 2d 587 (1993). In 1992, the Labor Code was amended to add an explicit protection. Cal. Lab. Code Sec. 1102.1 (1993).

24. Brief of Appellees in *Board of Education of Oklahoma City v. National Gay Task Force* (No. 83-2030) at 2–3 n. 3.

25. *National Gay Task Force v. Board of Education of Oklahoma City,* 729 F.2d 1270 (10th Cir. 1984), *aff'd per curiam* 470 U.S. 903 (1985). The Supreme Court ruled by an evenly divided vote; Justice Powell took no part in the case because of illness. Leonard (supra n. 5), at 616.

26. 729 F.2d at 1277.

27. See, for example, Report of the National Commission on Acquired Immune Deficiency Syndrome, *America Living with AIDS,* p. 19 (Washington, D.C., 1991).

28. Dennis Altman, "Legitimation through Disaster: AIDS and the Gay Movement," in Elizabeth Fee & Daniel M. Fox (Eds.), *AIDS: The Burdens of History,* p. 305 (Berkeley, 1988). See also, for example, Jeffrey Levi, Testimony on PHS AIDS Budget for Fiscal Year 1989, House Appropriations Committee, Subcommittee on Labor-HHS-Education, April 26, 1988 at 3.

29. Ronald Bayer, *Private Acts, Social Consequences: AIDS and the Politics of Public Health,* pp. 89–93 (New York, 1989); Dennis Altman, *AIDS and the New Puritanism,* pp. 74–78 (London, 1986).

30. Almost immediately after licensure, the U.S. military began mass HIV screening of all recruits and active-duty personnel. Recruits who tested positive were rejected for

the service, often informed of their HIV status with no counseling or information about the disease. Military use of the test was followed by adoption of mandatory testing programs by the Foreign Service and the Job Corps. Bayer (supra n. 29), pp. 158–162. See *Local 1812, American Federation of Government Employees v. U.S. Department of State,* 662 F. Supp. 50 (D.D.C. 1987) (Foreign Service policy).

31. Conference on the Role of AIDS Virus Antibody Testing in the Prevention and Control of AIDS, Atlanta, GA, Closing Plenary Session: Reports from the Workshops, Transcript of the Proceedings, February 24–25, 1987.

32. United States Dept. of Health and Human Services, Recommended Additional Guidelines for HIV Antibody Counseling and Testing, April 30, 1987.

33. Bayer (supra n. 29), p. 164. The final recommendations were published at 36 *Morbidity and Mortality Weekly Report* 509 (Aug. 14, 1987).

34. Marlene Cimons, "AIDS Education Grants Frozen," *Los Angeles Times,* December 4, 1985.

35. 51 Fed Reg 3431, January 27, 1986.

36. The Labor-Health and Human Services Appropriations Act for Fiscal Year 1988, P.L. No. 100-202. Section 514(a) provided that: "[N]one of the funds made available under this Act to the Centers for Disease Control shall be used to provide AIDS education, information, or prevention materials and activities that promote or encourage, directly, homosexual activities."

37. 133 Cong. Rec. S 14203 (October 14, 1987).

38. Ibid.

39. Ibid. at S14204 (October 14, 1987).

40. Ibid. at S14205.

41. Ibid. at S14208.

42. Ibid. at S14219.

43. The Kennedy-Cranston amendment stated: "Notwithstanding any other provision of this Act, AIDS education programs funded by the Centers of Disease Control and other education curricula funded under this Act dealing with sexual activity (1) shall not be designed to promote or encourage, directly, intravenous drug abuse or sexual activity, homosexual or heterosexual . . ."

44. See statement of Sen. Cranston, 134 Cong. Rec. S10025 (July 27, 1988); statement of Sen. Kennedy, 134 Cong. Rec. S17005 (October 20, 1988).

45. 134 Cong. Rec. S10027 (July 27, 1988).

46. *Gay Men's Health Crisis v. Sullivan,* 792 F.Supp. 278 (S.D.N.Y. 1992).

47. Chuck Frutchey, presentation to American Association of Law Schools, program on "Sex and Censorship in the Age of AIDS," January 7, 1993, San Francisco.

48. Ariz. Rev. Stat. Title 15, Ch. 7, Sec. 15-716 (1991).

49. Alabama requires that sex education programs include "an emphasis, in a factual manner and from a public health perspective, that homosexuality is not a lifestyle acceptable to the general public and homosexual conduct is a criminal offense under the laws of the state." Code of Ala., Sec. 16-40A-2(a)(8) (1992).

50. Simon Garfield, "The Age of Consent," *The Independent,* November 10, 1991.

51. The basic form of Clause 28 traveled back across the Atlantic in the form of an Oregon ballot initiative, rejected by voters in November 1992, that would have required that "state, regional, local governments and their properties and monies shall not be used to promote, encourage, or facilitate homosexuality." Timothy Egan, "Oregon Measure Asks State to Repress Homosexuality," *New York Times,* August 16, 1992.

52. Rorie Sherman, "Sex Education Manual Spurs Censorship," *National Law Journal,* July 18, 1988; Clare Kittredge, "Sex-education Dispute Settled by State, Clinic," *Boston Globe,* September 7, 1988.

53. Rod Paul, "Sex Education Manual Prompts Moral Outrage," *New York Times,* April 24, 1988.

54. 134 Cong. Rec. S 10,048, July 27, 1988.

55. *Gay Rights Coalition of Georgetown University Law Center v. Georgetown University*, 536 A.2d 1 (D.C.App. 1987).

56. Pub L. No. 100-462, Sec. 145(b), 102 Stat. 2269 (1988). The attempt temporarily failed when City Council members won a ruling that the provision violated their free-speech rights. *Clarke v. United States*, 886 F.2d 404 (D.C.Cir. 1989), *reh'g denied*, 898 F.2d 161, *vacated on other grounds*, 915 F.2d 699 (1990). Congress had the last word, however; it simply amended the D.C. human rights act directly, drawing on its residual power over local district government. District of Columbia Appropriations Act of 1990, Pub. L. No. 101-168, Sec. 141, 103 Stat. 1267, 1284 (1989).

57. Pub.L. No. 101-121, Sec. 304 (1989).

58. Carole S. Vance, "Misunderstanding Obscenity," *Art in America*, May 1990, pp. 49–55. As Vance (p. 50) notes, "[T]he list of sexual acts simply gives examples of depictions that *might* fall under the legal definition of obscenity, *after* the three prongs of the Miller test are met. But these sexual depictions or acts are not by themselves obscene. (Or, to take another example, more easily understood because it is not about sex, consider the phrase, 'obscene materials including but not limited to black-and-white photographs, color slides and Cibachromes.')"

59. *Hurley v. Irish-American Gay, Lesbian and Bisexual Group of Boston*, 115 S.Ct. 2338 (1995).

60. Ibid., 2347, 2348.

THREE

**Friends, Lovers, and Families:
The Impact of AIDS on Gay and
Lesbian Relationships**

PETER M. NARDI

In many Western societies, one of
the most contested cultural debates centers on lesbian and gay relationships, such as legalized same-sex unions, child custody and adoption
cases, domestic partner benefits, and social and legal redefinitions of
the concept of family and friendships. Although many of these issues
have been a part of lesbian and gay life for decades, others are a result
of the encounter with HIV/AIDS in the early 1980s. This chapter traces
the historical and contemporary ways in which many lesbians and gay
men have organized their romantic, sexual, familial, and friendship relationships and how these may have been affected by the changing
times brought about by HIV.

As the everyday lives of gays and lesbians become more visible, attention to the range of our interpersonal relationships similarly grows.
And with the appearance of HIV/AIDS, sexual, romantic, and friendship relationships have emerged as central concerns both within and
outside lesbian and gay communities. Both anecdotal evidence and
popular discourse allege that significant changes related to romantic
relationships, family life, and sex have occurred during the AIDS decades.

For example, in the early years of the growing AIDS pandemic, an
opinion piece in *The Advocate* by gay activist/writer Doug Sadownick
(1985: 8) claimed that AIDS "hasn't only changed the way gay men
make love . . . it's also made a serious dent in the way we sometimes
fall into it—and stay in it. . . . [T]he health crisis refereed as the built-
in 'marriage counselor' of the '80s." He argued that the post-Stonewall
generation looks to relationships and monogamy as one way of dealing

Special thanks to Jim Kepner and his collection at the International Gay and Lesbian
Archives in West Hollywood for providing research materials, to Ralph Bolton and Josh
Gamson for their comments on the paper, and to the Rancho Santa Fe conference parti-
cipants who helped clarify some important points in the paper.

with gay identity in an era of health concerns and survival. "How can one be sexually liberated when the answer, even from gay men, is to marry?" he asked (1985: 9).

What's interesting in Sadownick's article is not only the perceived relationship between the appearance of AIDS and the supposed turn toward monogamy and commitment, but also his use of the word "marry." That it is clearly understood to mean a committed relationship between two men, and not a legal marriage license for same-gender couples, or a reference to some heterosexual "marriage of convenience," represents a significant shift over the years of the changing concepts of marriage, relationships, and family for gays and lesbians.

But his article also represents the way in which some gay men and lesbians began to talk about their lives and communities, often as a result of the discourse used in the mainstream and gay media to construct the impact of AIDS on gay "lifestyles." Seidman (1992: 161, 165) argues that

> The liberal media has used AIDS to rehabilitate a pre-gay libera-
> tion ideal of the 'respectable homosexual': discreet, coupled, mo-
> nogamous and cohabiting, bound by love, shared responsibilities,
> and property. . . . Stories abound in the gay media . . . [that] de-
> scribe a pre-AIDS period of immaturity and indulgence, with
> AIDS marks [sic] the great turning point where, after a protracted
> period of soul-searching, one is reborn, and the profligate, self-
> destructive ways of the past given up for the new morality of
> health, romance, and monogamy.

It is a difficult task to demonstrate a direct cause-effect connection between the encounter with HIV and how gay men and lesbians changed the way they talked about and enacted their relationships. Still, it is possible to illustrate some of the differences in the language, the images, and the behavior associated with gay men's and lesbians' sexual, romantic, familial, and friendship lives before and during the HIV/AIDS years.

Friends and Families

Many of the ways in which gay men and lesbians encounter AIDS/HIV emerge when discussing the changing organization of, and discourses about, family and friends. Weston (1991: 196) states the argument succinctly:

> The emergence of gay families represents a major historical shift,
> particularly when viewed against the prevalent assumption that

claiming a lesbian or gay identity must mean leaving blood relatives behind and foregoing any possibility of establishing a family
of one's own, unless a person is willing to make the compromise
of hiding out in a marriage of convenience. . . . [T]his entire shift
has happened within a relatively brief period of time.

The concept of "chosen families," in contrast to biogenetically based
families of blood, challenges the cultural assumptions that procreation
alone determines kinship (see Maxey, 1986). Because of changes in the
social context for disclosing gay identity to others, in attempts to build
an urban gay community, and in a lesbian baby boom, images and
discourse have been transformed from "lesbians/gays = no family" to
"lesbians/gays = chosen families" (Weston, 1991). Although some
gays and lesbians—particularly those from ethnic, racial, and class
backgrounds that emphasize strong concepts of family—continue to
restrict family terminology to biological kin, the language of kinship
among friends and lovers has developed quite visibly in the past
decade.

This change, especially prominent during the AIDS decades, has its
roots in the early years of an emerging gay community. There was a
developing understanding that gays and lesbians were an oppressed
minority, imprisoned by the hegemonic heterosexual culture. For
many, the debate to organize a "highly ethical homosexual culture"
centered on issues of assimilation: whether to seek respectability
within the framework of the dominant ideologies or to create alternative socio-political structures that challenge the social order (D'Emilio,
1983). This tension—which is apparent in the issue of gay marriage—
has also persisted to the present day in discussions about sexuality
and relationships.

The language used to describe the growing sense of community and
identity among many lesbians and gay men illustrates these arguments.
Before Stonewall, the word "family" was often limited to family of
origin, as in Cory (1951). But it was not uncommon then (and even
today) for people to signal that others were also gay or lesbian by suggesting that they were "a member of the family," and sometimes with
even more explicit kinship terminology. Chauncey (1994: 291) describes how many gay men in the 1920s adopted fictive kinship relationships and called each other "sisters" (those never "married" to
each other) or "aunties" (elderly men). Both of these categories of
people remain protected by "incest" taboos from sexual involvement.

Warren (1973: 109–110) found similar kinship concepts forty years
later among the gay men she got to know in "Sun City" from 1968 to

1973: "several words used to describe community relationships are social kinship words like mother, auntie, and sister. . . . Gay people are
bound by bloodlike ties of fate and community as are aunts and neph-
ews or mothers and sisters, and their sociable interaction has the same
formal and obligatory character as visits from relatives."

Rodgers' (1972: 181) definition of "sister" in his gay dictionary
shows the "incest" taboo of these fictive kinships: "[H]e will share anything but his bed with friends. A sister is sexually neutral with his comrades; he is a chum, not a lover. Sisters are in the same business, but
only as competition." Other entries in the book include such terms as
"auntie," "sugar daddy," "brother," "mother," "mom," and "daughter," some used by lesbians and others by gay men.

For the most part, kinship terms were one way of signifying who
were nonsexual, "just friends" in opposition to those who were "more
than friends" in a sexual sense (see Nardi & Sherrod, 1994). This is
evident in Crowley's (1968: 134) play *The Boys in the Band*: "No
man's still got a roommate when he's over thirty years old. If they're
not lovers, they're sisters." Sonenschein (1968) made a similar argument that gay men separated those who met their sexual needs from
those who met their social ones. And Weston (1991: 120) observes
that "This reservation of kinship terminology for nonsexual relations
represents a very different usage from its subsequent deployment to
construct gay families that could include both lovers and friends."

Interestingly, in the years after Stonewall, as gay identity became
more politicized and as sexuality and friendship became more openly
discussed, many of these kinship terms became "camp" references to
preliberation years or were transformed into political and community
terms, such as in the gay ("we are family"), women's ("sisterhood"),
and civil rights movements ("brother to brother"). References to
"daddy" and "son" appear in sexual classified ads in gay men's publications, but not always in the same way in which "sugar daddy" was
once defined. Rather than "an auntie with money," or an older man
who supports a younger lover (Rodgers, 1972: 191), the contemporary
terms "daddy" and "son" reflect physical types, intergenerational attraction, and sometimes sexual relationships of dominance and sub-
mission.

Although kinship terminology was often used to describe others in
one's nonsexual friendship circle in the past, it could be argued that
many were not quite yet defining themselves as a family, either metaphorically or as an alternative form. Part of the move in that direction
began by reconstructing friends and lovers as two ends of a continuum

rather than as oppositional categories (see Nardi, 1992a). Weston (1991: 122) argues that "the shift from contrast to continuum laid the ground for the rise of a family-centered discourse that bridged the erotic and the nonerotic, bringing lovers together with friends under a single construct."

The importance of friends in the organization of gay identity was evident, of course, long before Stonewall, as Chauncey (1994) demonstrates, but it took on more political meanings in the 1970s and more family terminology during the AIDS years. Although she did not use the word "family" to describe the gay men she studied, Hooker (1965: 101) notes that they regularly gathered in "cliques, groups, and networks of friends" to celebrate anniversaries, birthdays, and other special occasions together. Similarly, with the rise of counterculture communities during the late 1960s and early 1970s, Barnhart (1975: 92) describes a lesbian residential community in Oregon as "a partial alternative form of family unit. . . . a psychological kin group" made up of "sisters," many of whom were lovers and ex-lovers.

Conceptualizing their relationships as alternative family forms, and not just metaphorically as brothers and sisters, has been a significant part of the "house" subculture of drag balls and vogueing for some time, best depicted in the documentary "Paris Is Burning." The predominantly Latino and African American working-class men organize a kinship structure in which a "'mother' and 'father' supervise the training and activities of their 'children'" (Goldsby, 1989: 35). For many of them, often alienated and rejected from their families of origin, these houses are not metaphors or fictive kinship structures, derivative of "real" kinship, but transformations of kinship relations organized around the principle of choice.

The saliency of families of choice was also recognized in the larger culture, especially in the therapeutic professions (see Shernoff, 1984; Stein, 1988), and the national movement in the alcohol and drug rehabilitation fields toward family therapy. Many agencies and recovery programs restructured during the late 1970s and early 1980s to incorporate family members of the client on the belief that the entire social unit contributed to the problems and that the abusing was not simply an individual pathology (Nardi, 1982). Many, if not most, of these family programs allowed for a broader definition of family, encouraging friends, lovers, and even housemates to participate in the recovery program. As Hall (1978: 380) stated almost twenty years ago in an article on lesbian families, "As the traditional nuclear family declines as the norm in this country—in numbers if not in influence—members of alternative families are appearing with greater frequency in the agency offices and clinical practices of social workers."

In the years just before AIDS was recognized, the importance of friends as family was an acknowledged part of gay and lesbian life. Vetere (1982: 61) observed that "friendship is a prime developmental and maintenance factor in the respondents' lesbian love relationships." Altman (1982: 190) also wrote:

> what many gay lives miss in terms of permanent relationships is more than compensated for by friendship networks, which often become de facto families. . . . Former lovers often are drawn into such networks, so that many gays are surrounded by a rich network of friends (often originally sexual partners) and past and present lovers, which can be far more supportive than are most nuclear families.

Thus the shift from kinship terms to indicate nonsexual friends in the pre-Stonewall years, to the ideology of family metaphors and fictive kinship to describe an identity-based sociopolitical community of lovers and friends in the 1970s, sets the stage for the AIDS years. "Friends as family" took on a variety of political, sexual, and relationship meanings (Nardi, 1992b) and, as Hayden (1995: 49) said about lesbian kinship, it "refigures the alignment of gender and power roles which have traditionally marked the American family."

The power of the chosen family is evident when AIDS becomes an issue. Often the family gets defined as those who are available to offer care, money, and emotional support during the illness, regardless of biology. For many, the family of origin was not the major source of assistance. But some gays and lesbians of color, in particular those from Latino cultures, often remain in close contact with their families, thereby creating some possible tensions around identity and illness (see Murray, 1995). Conflicts can arise over care and, if death occurs, "disputes over whether families we choose constitute 'real' or legitimate kin can affect wills, distribution of possessions . . . listings of survivors in obituaries, and dispositions of the body" (Weston, 1991: 186). Hence the rise in importance of domestic partner legislation in the 1980s.

What once was a debate within the gay and lesbian communities over what defines a family soon became larger political, religious, economic, and media issues. Newspapers were challenged to redefine family members and next of kin to include "longtime companions" in obituaries (Nardi, 1990) and courts were asked to rule on whether lesbian and gay couples were families, as the New York State Court of Appeals (in *Braschi v. Stahl Associates*) did in 1989, when it held that unmarried cohabitants constitute families under the state's rent-control law (Harvard Law Review Editors, 1990).

Part of the shift from a collective to an interpersonal kinship language is illustrated by the legal and social challenges related to the birthing and raising of children, especially among lesbians (Burke, 1993). Riley (1988: 87) argues that "Parenting relationships are perhaps the most significant changes in kinship among lesbians." Definitions of what constitutes parents and kinship, in the absence of heterosexual intercourse and both genders, have been challenged by the lesbian baby boom (Lewin, 1993) and by court cases seeking to clarify the legal rights of a same-gender coparent (Harvard Law Review Editors, 1990). Legalization of second-parent adoptions in New York and California and a New Mexico ruling granting a nonbiological parent visitation rights have led Nonas (1992: 52) to conclude that "lesbians and gay men with children are one more segment of the population redefining what constitutes a functional family."

But Crawford (1987) makes an insightful point when she argues that the lesbian family most conveniently recognized in our culture is the single-parent model, not the two-parent version, thereby avoiding the lesbian dimensions of the relationships. Still, these ideas of gay parenting are a long way from Cory's (1951: 189) characterization of gay men getting heterosexually married to fulfill a desire to have children because, as an orthodox Freudian told him, they have "a strong mother instinct, actually desiring to give birth. . . . they want to become a mother, not a father."

Advertisements in gay and lesbian publications also illustrate the shift from a collective kinship terminology to individual relationships. The back cover of the 1993 *Community Yellow Pages* (Los Angeles's lesbian and gay directory) featured an ad for a medical group claiming, "Families today are different. So are their Doctors". The tag line read "Family Practice for Today's Families" and accompanied four photographs, one of a lesbian couple with a cat, one with a male and baby, another of two women of very different ages (possibly a mother with a teenage daughter), and one of a gay male couple with dog. All imitated traditional heterosexual images (including gendered stereotypes about pets); none was a family of friends.

Soon after the 1992 Republican National Convention's attack on the lack of "traditional family values," more ads appeared appropriating the concept, but always in terms of individual relationships, rather than the collective concept that described the gay community of the

1970s. The cover of the October 8, 1992 issue of *Frontiers,* a Los Angeles gay newsmagazine, proclaimed "Family" and was illustrated with a framed photo of a Black man hugging a White man, holding their dog, with an old family photo of mom, dad, and baby in the background.

Other ads in the magazine included one encouraging people to vote for Bill Clinton for president, headlined "Defend *Our* Family Values" and illustrated with a photo of two women and their young boy; another was for gay and lesbian greeting cards stating, "Family Values to put your stamp on" and showing a card with two men walking arm in arm with their two dogs. And several chapters of the Gay and Lesbian Alliance Against Defamation put up billboards depicting a lesbian couple, one pregnant, with the phrase "Another Traditional Family."

What is missing, however, are the depictions of gay families made up of friends as well as lovers. It is also not clear how gay families are constituted by gays and lesbians of different races, ages, and social classes. Although Clunis and Green (1988: 106) claim that "for lesbians and lesbian couples, this network of friends, children, and relatives constitutes a chosen family," the discussions and images have decidedly favored the concept of gay and lesbian families primarily as a couple with child and/or pets and secondarily as a more collective one.

Whatever the configuration, the current definitions of gay and lesbian families emphasize the notion of choice over genetic ties, as Weston (1991: 202) argues: "By substituting images of creation and selection for the logic of reproduction and succession, discourse on gay families can—and does—remind people of their power to alter the circumstances into which they were born." And this has been the major change since the era when "family" typically signified a discussion of family of origin.

Romantic and Sexual Relationships

Anecdotes about the increasing emphasis among gay men on "settling down" with a lover, dating more before sex, and staying in relationships longer proliferated throughout the 1980s as responses to the AIDS pandemic. Weston (1991: 159) has argued that "The appearance of AIDS, too, had ushered in a renewed emphasis on relationships among gay men," and Marks (1988: 70) quotes a San Francisco psychologist who claims that "Everyone is looking to couple up. . . . People are coming out to settle down instead of coming out into an atmosphere to be wild."

For lesbians, anecdotal evidence appears in the popular press about the growing commercialization of sex and the increasing desire to have or raise children in reconstructed families. For example, Miller (1989: 178) claims (without much empirical evidence) that "as lesbians moved towards a more openly sexual stance, many men, facing AIDS, were retreating towards the very sexual patterns lesbians were questioning or abandoning." He observes that while gay men were confronting issues of mortality, lesbians were dealing with issues of having babies; while men were moving away from sexual experimentation, women were moving away from sexual repression; and while men moved toward questions about living a life away from the "fun and frivolity" of the '70s, lesbians were becoming less dogmatic and earnest about their lives.

The implication of these writings is that many gay men are settling down more into committed, longer-term, and monogamous relationships during the AIDS decades to a greater extent than in the 1970s or earlier, although many lesbians are becoming more sexually active. These points are not easy to verify, given the lack of longitudinal survey data. Furthermore, any variations related to class, race, and region cannot be assessed, since almost all of the studies and documents cited below emphasize White, middle-class, urban gays and lesbians. From a review of some accounts about gay romantic and sexual relationships before HIV, however, we can evaluate how discussions about same-sex coupling, "gay marriage," and sexual monogamy were presented.

Gay Marriage: Some Historical Comments

To understand romantic and sexual relationships in the AIDS era, it is important first to remind ourselves about the ways in which some gay men and lesbians organized their lives before HIV. Books and articles about gay marriage often referred to gays and lesbians getting heterosexually married. If there was a need to signify a gay relationship instead, the word "marriage" was typically put in quotation marks, as Hooker (1959: 30) did when referring to long-lasting homosexual couples as "'marriage' partners." Donald Webster Cory's *The Homosexual in America* (1951) also illustrates this distinction between heterosexual marriages of convenience and homosexual "marriages." A chapter entitled "Till Death Do Us Part" is not about committed gay relationships; it is a discussion of how some men find it necessary to marry women to cope with the hostilities of being alone and gay.

Although many gay men and lesbians found some form of community in a few large urban centers and many were in same-sex couples (Chauncey [1994] describes uses of the word "husband" and "marriage with fairies" among some working-class men in 1920s New York), for others, the "homosexual lifestyle" was a lonely, isolated experience filled with short-term sexual adventures, often out of sight of a legal spouse. Gay people needed to hear stories from each other about how they could have a committed relationship with someone of the same gender and were not just limited to a series of lonely sexual episodes. Hence a typical question of the early gay literature would phrase it as Cory (1951: 133) did: "Is it possible or desirable for two people of the same sex to be in love with each other, just as a man is in love with a woman; to show the same affection and interest, to offer the same loyalty, to form a union as permanent?" Negative answers to this question often stated that it was not impossible, but that psychological and biological barriers were more likely to prevent love and commitment. The "nature" of gay men was seen to be promiscuous, due in part to the belief in the inability of achieving real sexual pleasure with another man.

But some men were seeking permanent unions and mimicking heterosexual marriages. Stearn (1961: 215) said: "Many homosexuals living together speak of themselves as married, occasionally referring to their partners as 'my husband' or 'my wife.' And while the majority of homosexual relationships are fleeting affairs, some relationships are as enduring as heterosexual unions and the principals seem as devoted." As an outsider observing the homosexual world, however, Stearn (1961: 217) described a gay marriage ceremony as a way of providing "a twisted link with the normal world whose approval they secretly covet." For him and other writers of that era, committed gay couples were seen to be seeking traditional middle-class respectability by imitating heterosexual life. In a December 1963 *New York Times* article, headlined "Growth of Overt Homosexuality Provokes Wide Concern" Doty wrote, "Many homosexuals dream of forming a permanent attachment that would give them the sense of social and emotional stability others derive from heterosexual marriage, but few achieve it."

In much of the early gay literature, "marriage" was almost a code letting gay men and lesbians know that they, indeed, were not alone, and could find someone else such as themselves with whom to settle down and gain social respectability, difficult as it might be. It did not signify an alternative form of heterosexual marriage with its own religious ceremonies, legal recognition, and spousal benefits. Marlowe (1965: 149) believed that "homosexual 'marriage' is a very real and greatly desired experience. In general, it is impractical and nearly impossible, but not improbable."

Hauser (1962: 51) wrote that "Only the homosexuals who have a lasting affair and are faithful to one another will be considered 'married'. . . . [T]hese couples do not normally mix with other homosexuals." Because of the belief in fidelity as an essential characteristic of marriage, Hauser felt that the chances were slim for homosexuals to form relationships, since it is rare to remain faithful. But, as Plummer (1963: 55) wrote, "most homosexuals regard the 'married' state or 'affair' as the ideal for all of us, even if at times it seems unobtainable."

Some of this language and conceptualization of gay relationships as "marriage-like" can be found in articles in *One*, a 1950s magazine that grew out of the original Mattachine Society in Los Angeles. What is first noticeable is the dearth of articles on the topic of gay marriages. Using the index, I found only four major articles on the subject. In a cover story for the August 1953 issue, Saunders (1953: 11) argued that "even among the most stable and respectable of homosexuals, there are very few who have lived together an appreciable time." He made a case for homosexual marriages as a way of gaining social acceptance, but he (p. 12) also warned that with equal marriage rights come equal limitations: "necessary homosexual monogamy." Clearly, for Saunders, copying heterosexual marriage also meant copying the ideology of what marriage supposedly meant. And part of that 1950s ideology was the assumption that sex and marriage were for procreation, as several letters in the October and November issues of *One* reminded the readers.

Another side of the debate was presented in April 1959, in the context of a society's rapidly changing values and attitudes toward marriage. Sounding a refrain similar to today's, Stoessel (1959:7) claimed that the family as "the basic unit of loyalty" had collapsed, but for him that was not such a bad thing: "Often marriage has served as a legal sanction for possessing another human being, or for being possessed. At times its rights have resembled property rights." So why marry? The freedom of not having to marry, he argued, allowed homosexuals to seek other reasons for association and to experiment with other forms of relationships.

Stoessel (1959: 7) concluded, "One can only hope that homosexuals will not spend their part of freedom on getting a crack at the old marital system with its ownership and jealous rights, traits that ought to be disappearing into man's ancient and primitive past." But Baker (1959), in a response to a letter from a reader of her column, praised permanent gay marriages and discussed how some homosexual couples have adopted and reared children. Wetmore and Arlec (1956), writing in the *Mattachine Review,* similarly sung the virtues of their nine-year "moral and spiritual union."

In 1963, an article entitled "Let's Push Homophile Marriage" presented gay marriage as "new, a modern concept" and a way of life that was "much, much superior" to the lonely, promiscuous single life of the homosexual (Lloyd, 1963: 5). Letters in later issues about this article included a rebuke for copying heterosexual life (August 1963) and one arguing that since marriage is a sacred rite, if gay marriage were allowed, the heterosexual world could accuse homosexuals of making a mockery of the institution (September 1963). To assimilate our lives to the heterosexual culture or to transform the institutions to fit our lives remains a heated debate thirty years later (see Kirk & Madsen, 1989; Sullivan, 1995).

What is most telling, however, is the relative absence of much discussion about the topic during the pre-Stonewall years. The call was not to reshape the institution of marriage or to challenge the existing laws and religious ceremonies, but to get homosexuals to adjust to the conventions of society to be accepted. Robert Wood (1960: 198–199), a Congregationalist minister from Spring Valley, New York, made perhaps one of the first published cases in this period for religiously and legally recognizing homosexual marriages:

> I am not now discussing a legal marriage between a man and a woman, both of whom are homosexuals, but, rather, a union between two members of the same sex. . . . [W]e must not lose sight of the validity of a union between two men or two women who are truly in love and who really want to spend the rest of their lives together. . . . It follows, then, that if he is seeking a home life, a lifelong, life-sharing relationship with one person, there is no reason why such a relationship should not be considered a marriage. If we are to treat him like everyone else in our parish or community or office, why put his union in a distinct classification?

But a political dimension to gay marriages had not yet emerged, since a political concept of gay identity was only starting to develop. Part of the process of creating identity was an attempt to get gays and lesbians to see themselves not in pathological individualistic terms, but as people who, when organized into some collective sense of identity, could have a happy and successful life. Seeing the possibility of romantic relationships as committed, marriage-like unions was one of those attempts: "you have a bond as firm as that of a great many legal marriages" (Cory, 1951: 238).

A growing public awareness of gay identity and politics emerged more rapidly after the Stonewall rebellion in 1969. And with it came an increase in media attention to gay and lesbian lives and relationships, especially gay marriages. A front-page, two-part feature on "The Boom in Gay Marriages" in the *San Francisco Chronicle* in July 1970 (Grieg, 1970) reported several attempts around the country (including Louisville, Minneapolis, and Los Angeles) by gay and lesbian couples to get legal marriage licenses. Claiming that San Francisco was "in the forefront of the 'odd couple' situation," Grieg (1970: 16) quoted Martin Mongan, county clerk, as saying he was tolerant and would not stand in the way of same-sex couples seeking a license: "Why, one of these days a man may come in here with a sheep or dog he may want to marry. This is a sophisticated city, and I'm prepared for anything."

The second part of the article introduced some of the possible benefits of legal gay marriages, including joint tax returns, adoption, insurance benefits, and a greater acceptability of homosexuality by society and the church. What was emerging in the coverage of gay marriages was no longer simply a recognition that gays and lesbians could have committed relationships, but also a growing understanding of the political and legal aspects of the issue.

Some of this was fueled by Rita Hauser, American representative to the United Nations Human Rights Commission, in a speech before an American Bar Association panel in August 1970, in which she said that laws banning marriage between persons of the same sex were probably unconstitutional. President Nixon's press secretary, Ronald Ziegler, was forced to respond, saying Nixon "doesn't think that people of the same sex should marry. . . . [He] hasn't been for it, he's not for it, and he won't be for it" (quoted in Tucker, 1970: 1).

Throughout the early 1970s, newspapers and magazines continued to report on attempts by lesbians and gays to marry legally. The August 22, 1971 *San Francisco Examiner and Chronicle* (Ellsworth-Jones, 1971) claimed that homosexual marriages were commonplace and the *New York Post* (Trecher, 1971) found some gay people who objected to the notion on the grounds that legal marriage would give the state power to regulate sex and would be just aping heterosexual customs.

In an article in *The Advocate*, Cole (1972: 6) wrote, "Gay marriages have been discovered by the major American news media in recent weeks. . . . The tone of such reports still tends to be arch, but underneath the archness can be discerned for the first time a serious effort to understand." By April 1974, even *Pageant* magazine featured three pages of photos of "the first U.S. homosexual wedding" in San Diego, headlined "The Bride was Male."

One of the most famous cases of the era was the wedding of Anthony Sullivan of Australia and Richard Adams of California in Boulder, Colorado, on April 21, 1975. This drew national attention by raising the issue of immigration of a same-sex spouse of an American citizen. In a ruling from the U.S. Department of Justice denying the visa petition, the Los Angeles district director wrote on November 24, 1975 (copy on file in the International Gay and Lesbian Archives, Los Angeles), "You have failed to establish that a bona fide marital relationship can exist between two faggots." This was rewritten, on December 2, 1975, after an uproar over the language, to read, "A marriage between two males is invalid for immigration purposes and cannot be considered a bona fide marital relationship since neither party to the marriage can perform the female functions in marriage."

Meanwhile, religious ceremonies had begun in Troy Perry's Metropolitan Community Church (MCC) in Los Angeles. A July 7, 1970 article in the *Hollywood Citizen News* (Stumbo, 1970) reported that thirty-six ceremonies between people of the same sex had been performed at Perry's church. Cole (1972: 1) reported that "Despite widespread derision even in the gay world, many homosexuals continue to seek church weddings and to press with more and more determination for legal sanction of their unions." By the mid-1970s, the concept of homosexual marriage primarily referred to attempts to recognize gay couples in a religious or legal ceremony, not just to call for gay people to gain respectability among heterosexuals or to acknowledge that they could indeed couple like heterosexuals.

Academic research in the early to mid-1970s reflected some of these concepts about gay marriages. Warren (1974: 71), in her ethnography of a middle-class, urban gay community, wrote about gay couples: "Their relationship is sometimes described as 'marriage'. . . . More recently, another meaning has been added—gay marriage-ceremony marriage, which of course is rare in the secret community." Jensen (1974) referred to lesbian couples as "quasi-marital unions" and described one partner as the "husband." She claimed (1974: 361) that homosexuals use "heterosexual courtship and marital norms as models."

Saghir and Robins (1973: 72) found that "most homosexual men express a desire to establish homosexual 'marriages'" but that 83 percent of their male sample and 72 percent of their female sample did not usually assume distinct male and female roles in their relationships. When Jay and Young (1979) asked their male respondents if they considered themselves "'married' to another man," 25 percent of those with lovers said "yes" and 3 percent said they had been in a ceremony. Almost 46 percent strongly or somewhat favored gay marriages, 32 percent were neutral, and 21 percent somewhat or strongly opposed them. (By 1994–1995, 46 percent of lesbians and 30 percent of gay men who responded to *Advocate* questionnaires said they "exchanged rings or had a commitment ceremony" [Lever, 1995]).

One indicator of the interest in gay marriages is an analysis of the index to *The Advocate* (Ridinger, 1987) and its references to gay marriage. From 1967 to 1970, there were no entries for gay marriage, but there were fifteen in 1971, twenty-two in 1972, and ten in 1973, the peak years for articles on the topic, most of them focusing on the attempts to get marriage licenses in the cases noted above. Between 1974 and 1977, there were twenty-six and from 1978 to 1982, there were only four. Many of the articles in the late 1970s focused on religious ceremonies, often conducted by the MCC, rather than on attempts by gays and lesbians to get legal marriage licenses. The message was typically not to try to mimic heterosexual marriages with legal licenses, but to create our own ceremonies in our own institutions, even if the event followed traditional heterosexual unions. Then an interesting and telling shift occurred.

Beginning in 1983, *The Advocate* introduced a new category in its indexing: Domestic Partners and Domestic Partner Legislation. In 1983, only three entries were listed under gay marriage and thirteen under domestic partners and domestic partner legislation. (The first domestic partner ordinance was enacted in 1982 [Whitacre, 1993]). In 1988, the category for gay marriage was dropped. The number of entries for the domestic partner categories dramatically increased: from seventeen in 1984 to forty-eight in 1991. Many of these entries were for a feature *The Advocate* introduced in the mid-1980s that highlighted couples coping with domesticity and sexuality in the time of AIDS.

But the introduction of domestic partner language and concepts almost exclusively focused on recognition of spousal-type benefits, such as health and life insurance; bereavement time off from work; inheritance issues; legal contracts; housing; guardianship; domestic violence issues; getting acknowledged in obituaries; hospital visitation rights; and recognition of relationships for frequent flier programs, automobile association memberships, and other discount cards. Most of these seemed directly related to concerns about the death or impending death of a partner, usually related to AIDS.

Although the emphasis in the past decade has shifted toward a more legalistic domestic partner concept, the concept of gay marriages has not totally disappeared. Butler (1990) and Sherman (1992) both present stories of numerous lesbian and gay couples who held public ceremonies, usually in a religious context. At the National March on Washington in October 1987, a massive group wedding ceremony, with an estimated two thousand couples, was performed in front of the Internal Revenue Service building, and in March 1996, 165 lesbian and gay couples were symbolically joined in a San Francisco City Hall ceremony presided over by the mayor.

Recent books by Sullivan (1995) and Eskridge (1996) argue for recognition of legal civil gay marriages on the grounds that the concept of domestic partnerships is too vague about who qualifies as a partner. And the Supreme Court of Hawaii is ruling on the first major case on same-gender marriages, a case that is resulting in a serious national debate on equal rights for gays and lesbians. "Defense of Marriage" bills were passed in Congress in the fall of 1996 to preserve marriage for only heterosexual couples.

Stoddard (1989) and Ettelbrick (1989) have presented competing contemporary arguments on the issue of gay marriage in *Out/Look* (reprinted in Sherman [1992]). For Stoddard (p. 10), the right to marry should be the top agenda item because "marriage is . . . the political issue that most fully tests the dedication of people who are *not* gay to full equality for gay people, and also the issue most likely to lead ultimately to a world free from discrimination against lesbians and gay men." On the other hand, Ettelbrick (p. 14) argues that marriage will not liberate gays and lesbians since it runs contrary to "the affirmation of gay identity and culture; and the validation of many forms of relationships." She feels that the state should not regulate primary relationships and that gays and lesbians should be recognized for creating different forms of relationships and families, not because they would conform to the dominant culture's definitions. Ettelbrick (p. 17) concludes, "Only when we de-institutionalize marriage and bridge the economic and privilege gap between the married and the unmarried will each of us have a true choice."

When the topic is debated, the focus is on whether gay marriage results in gays and lesbians copying, and conforming to, heterosexual institutions or whether domestic partner legislation forces the legal and political system to recognize broader definitions of personal relationships. In either case, the issues of what to do with gay and lesbian couples and how to incorporate the diversity of personal relationships into the larger social system seem to have emerged more forcefully in the AIDS decades.

Coupling: Some Survey Findings

But has the actual number of couples changed dramatically over the years, or just the amount of media attention to the topic of coupling? In the data in Table 3.1 from a variety of surveys (which are limited by the absence of similarly worded questions over the decades and by differences resulting from nonrepresentative sampling), approximately 40 to 50 percent of gay men—both before and during AIDS—responded that they were involved with another man and about two-thirds of them were living with that man.

The median duration of relationships before AIDS varied from 2.9 years (Harry & DeVall, 1978) to 3.5 years (Blumstein & Schwartz, 1983) to 5 years (McWhirter & Mattison, 1984), and between 2 and 3 years in the Bell and Weinberg (1978) survey. These figures are not much different from the 3.7 years in a marketing survey conducted by Overlooked Opinions (1992) in the AIDS years.

Among lesbians, there has been remarkable consistency in the few

Table 3.1. Gay men: Percentage in relationships

Year data collected	In a relationship	Living together (of those in a relationship)	Source
1969–70	33%		Weinberg & Williams (1974)
1970	51% (Whites)	56% (W)	Bell & Weinberg (1978)
	58% (Blacks)	50% (B)	
1975	40%	23%	Harry & DeVall (1978)
1977	46%	47%	Jay & Young (1979)
1978–79	50%	65%	Harry (1984)
Late 1970s	41%	59%	Spada (1979)
1986	44%	64%	McKirnan & Peterson (1989)
Late 1980s	40%		Hays et al. (1990)
1988–1989	50%		Doll et al. (1991)
1988		79%	Out/Look (1989)
1989	36%		Kanouse et al. (1991)
1989	41%		Out/Look (1990)
1991	55%	65%	Overlooked Opinions (1992)
1994	44%	75%	Lever (1994)

surveys available. As Table 3.2 shows, close to three-fourths are in relationships and living together. The median duration of lesbian relationships has ranged from between 2 and 3 years (Bell & Weinberg, 1978) to 2.2 years (Blumstein & Schwartz, 1983) to 3.5 years today (Overlooked Opinions, 1992). The 1959 survey of *The Ladder* subscribers (Armon, 1959) reported a mean between 4 and 5 years.

Without other longitudinal data and more diverse sampling (i.e., non-White, non-middle-class lesbians and gay men), it is difficult to arrive at generalized conclusions. But these data do suggest that the discourse of the 1980s about more gay men "settling down" may, in fact, be just symbolic talk. It is also possible that the people who control the discourse in the gay media are part of the aging cohort of White, middle-class gay men who came out in the 1970s and might have "settled down" anyway, regardless of AIDS (Gorman [1992] and Murray [1996] make similar arguments).

Certainly age is related to changes in relationships, as some pre-AIDS research on gay men suggests. Saghir and Robins (1973: 56) found that "Establishing long lasting affairs was age related. . . . 41% had had long lasting relationships during the age period of 20 and 29 and about one-half (48%) had similar relationships during the age period of 30 and 39." Harry and DeVall (1978) reported that 35 percent of the 18- to 29-year-olds in their sample and 46 percent of the 30- to 39-year olds have a lover. In another sample, however, Harry (1984) found lower percentages involved with a lover in the older age categories: 56 percent of the 25- to 29-year-olds, 54 percent of those in their 30s, 43 percent of the 40- to 44-year-olds, and 45 percent of those between 45 and 54.

Writer Michael Bronski (quoted in Miller, 1989: 143) disputes the notion that AIDS was "suddenly causing gay men to discover the joys of being in a couple": many gay men in the 1970s and earlier wanted

Table 3.2. Lesbians: Percentage in relationships

Year data collected	In a relationship	Living together (of those in a relationship)	Source
1959	72%		Armon (1959)
1970	70% (Black)	64% (B)	Bell & Weinberg (1978)
	72% (White)	67% (W)	
1988		66%	*Out/Look* (1989)
1989	69%		*Out/Look* (1990)
1991	71%	75%	Overlooked Opinions (1992)
1995	67%	79%	Lever (1995)

to couple as much as gay men did in the 1980s, just as there is still a great desire for sexual freedom, as there was before AIDS. He states, "To imply that there was only wholesale sexual license in the seventies and that now, wholesale coupling is the correct, healthier response is ridiculous."

A 1988 survey of readers of *Out/Look* ("Questions For Couples: The Results," 1989), a lesbian and gay quarterly now out of print, lends some support to this perspective. Gay and lesbian couples were asked about the role of AIDS in forming their relationships and in continuing their relationship. Of four hundred responses, 90 percent of the women and 73 percent of the men said AIDS was not a factor in getting into a relationship, although 27 percent of the women and 45 percent of the men said it was relevant in continuing the relationship.

In short, the data do not indicate a greater percentage of gay men coupling or a lower percentage of lesbians leading a single life; the surveys do not describe the nature or content of the relationships. What may have changed from the years before AIDS is the way gays and lesbians talk about their relationships. Is there now just more rhetoric that gay couples are like heterosexual marriages, with more discussions about monogamy, child-raising, and other ideologies associated with "traditional family values?"

Sex and Monogamy

One way to assess this question is to look at sexual practices among those both in and out of relationships. Although the percentage of those in relationships may be about the same, are those in couples engaging in fewer "extramarital" relationships? Is monogamy, which Sadownick (1985) said characterized his relationship, characteristic of other couples' relationships in the AIDS years? Or is it just a claim increasingly made to make one appear more desirable in an era of AIDS?

Again, comparable data over time have not been collected: survey questions were not always worded the same way and the sampling was often limited to White, middle-class gay men and lesbians. In addition, the reliability of data on sexual behavior needs to be kept in mind when interpreting them, especially in years when admission of certain sexual acts and nonmonogamy may be considered more taboo and when such concepts as "monogamy," "sexual partner," and "sex act" are ambiguous (Bolton, 1992b).

It is also important to remember that monogamy rates change over the duration of a relationship and by age, as Saghir and Robins (1973) and Blumstein and Schwartz (1983) demonstrated. Since the median years of these relationships are between three and four, the monogamy rates reflect the early stages of the relationships and, thus, are not reliable predictors of monogamy over a longer period. As Table 3.3 shows, though, recent data on sexual behavior suggest some possible changes during the AIDS decades.

There are some indications that an increase in claiming monogamy, particularly among mostly White, middle-class gay male samples, has occurred among those in relationships. But whether actual behavior has changed is not easily assessed. Patton (1990: 47) argues that a change in the "mythology of promiscuity" has occurred and that non-monogamous gay men with lovers "now talked more publicly of their long-term relationships, while often retaining the same number of partners."

What about gay men and lesbians not in committed relationships? Has there been an increase in abstinence or claims of previous monogamous relationships? Have gay men been moving away from recreational sex, as some writers in the more popular gay press have intimated (such as Marks, 1988 and Miller, 1989)? Has the number of sexual partners decreased in response to the AIDS pandemic? Are gay men becoming less sexual and "promiscuous" as lesbian sexuality more visibly increases and becomes commercialized? Or is this just part of the changing discourse on sexuality as it starts to mimic the ideological rhetoric of heterosexuality and "traditional family values"?

In his review of research on the number of sexual partners among gay men, Bolton (1992a) states that although the numbers of partners declined somewhat during the AIDS years, they were still "high" and,

Table 3.3. Percentage claiming monogomy in relationship

Year data collected	Gay men	Lesbians	Source
Early 1970s	25–75%		Saghir & Robins (1973)
1975	24%		Harry & DeVall (1978)
Late 1970s	4.5%		McWhirter & Mattison (1984)
1978–1979	22%		Harry (1984)
1978–1979	18%	66%	Blumstein & Schwartz (1983)
Late 1980s	57%		Hays et al. (1990)
1989	60%		Kanouse et al. (1991)
1989	53%	88%	Out/Look (1989)
1991	58%	81%	Overlooked Opinions (1992)
1994–1995	52%	87%	Lever (1994, 1995)

furthermore, the rates of abstinence did not significantly increase. Despite the ambiguity of questionnaire wording, vague definitions of sexual partners and contacts, and limitations in sampling, several studies are illustrative of these trends during the AIDS years. Calzavara et al. (1991), Doll et al. (1991), Hays et al. (1990), McKirnan and Peterson (1989), McKusick et al. (1990), and Stall et al. (1992), demonstrate some reductions in sexual partners, although the numbers remain large and abstinence has not significantly increased during the AIDS years.

These studies also show that risky sexual practices have been reduced during the AIDS era, especially in urban areas and among older gay men. Stall et al. (1992: 686) report the highest rates of abstinence among those over forty: "Cohort differences in sexual activity are exemplified by the changes in prevalence of sexual activity and the meaning of sex that occurred among the generation that came of age in America during the 1950s, 1960s, 1970s and 1980s. These same kinds of intergenerational differences may also exist within the gay male community." In short, as Bolton (1992a: 183) concludes, "What is quite clear in the data is that most gay men made changes in specific sexual practices more readily than they reduced the number of their partners." It is thus reasonable to conclude that gay men probably talked more about monogamy and sexual partner reduction than actually practiced them.

Unfortunately, survey data on lesbian sexual behavior have not been collected as systematically. What data do exist, especially in the pre-AIDS years, from Bell and Weinberg (1978), Blumstein and Schwartz (1983), and Saghir and Robins (1973), show that lesbians have fewer sexual partners and lower rates of sexual frequency than heterosexual or gay male couples. Although more current data from *Advocate* readers (a generally higher income and education sample) also suggest this, findings show that lesbians are having more "high-quality sex . . . than are most American women" (Lever, 1995: 24).

In the AIDS years, arguments have been made that lesbians—given the relatively low risk of HIV transmission through female-to-female sex—are becoming more sexual or are, at least, talking more about sex (Van Gelder, 1992). But changes and debates about women's sexuality were already under way just as AIDS emerged. Until the antipornography feminist attacks, many women were involved in an active sexual movement. The appearance of *On Our Backs* and *Bad Attitude*, lesbian erotic magazines, as well as other lesbian S & M publications and an important conference in 1982 at Barnard College entitled "Towards a Politics of Sexuality" (Vance, 1984) illustrate some of the early changes. Throughout the past decades, Loulan's (1984, 1987) books on lesbian sexual passion and Susie Bright's (1990, 1992) writings on lesbian sexuality have also been widely distributed. Lesbian-produced sex videos are more available since the mid-1980s, from the first lesbian-made lesbian sex video in 1985, *Private Pleasures and Shadows,* to over twenty on the market in the early 1990s (Roxxie, 1992).

Lesbian sexuality literature did not, of course, begin to appear in the 1980s, nor was it directly related to AIDS. Pat Califia was writing about lesbian sex in the 1970s; indeed, her book, *Sapphistry: The Book of Lesbian Sexuality,* was first published in 1980 and is now in its third edition. And for some lesbians, non-monogamous sexuality has always been a political statement, as Krestan and Bepko (1980: 285) argued some time ago: "Within the gay community it has become politically suspect in some quarters for two women to choose a monogamous relationship. This 'aping of heterosexual structure' violates the more radical principles of the women's movement."

This trend toward more open discussion and recognition of lesbian sexuality and the diversity of lesbian lives is evident in *The Lesbian News,* a Los Angeles monthly newspaper. The cover story in July 1992 issue, for example, "Inside a Sex Club," describes the events of "Ozone," the women-only night at The Zone, a sex club in West Hollywood that has since closed. With subheadlines of "She likes to get handcuffed, spanked," "Where you can explore sexuality," and "Monogamy is not for everyone," the article details the lowering of inhibitions traditionally associated with women's sexuality (Wilde, 1992).

The advertisements in the same issue also illustrate more sexually explicit attractions, such as "Hot star-spangled go-go's" at Girl Bar; women's night at the traditionally all-male Studio One Backlot; "Liberated Go-Go Girls" and "Bikinis, Beach Balls and Babes" at Club Ms.; and "Hottest Women," accompanied by a photo of a seductive woman holding a metal chain at Girl Bar. The schedule of events for Lesbian Visibility Week lists all-day seminars on lesbian sex with such titles as "Lesbian S/M 101" and "Lesbian Sex/Lesbian Passion." The only other all-day seminar is on "cultural and political" topics. Comparison with earlier issues of *The Lesbian News* indicates that these are more openly discussed aspects of lesbian subculture and they represent a newer form of marketing. The commercialization of lesbian sexuality and culture and the emergence of more venues for sexual interaction—long since established in gay male communities—for women seem to have grown significantly in the late 1980s and early 1990s in urban areas. The annual "Dinah Shore" weekend in Palm Springs now boasts that it is the nation's largest lesbian event.

But these changes in the discourse on lesbian sexuality and its commercialization are not directly related to AIDS or the perception that lesbians are relatively more likely to be HIV negative. Social changes in the 1970s affecting women's sexuality in general probably have had as significant an impact on contemporary lesbian sexuality and its expression. It is important that further work be done studying these changes, especially among lesbians of color and more working-class communities.

Conclusions

The main goal of this chapter was to uncover the impact AIDS has had on lesbians' and gay men's interpersonal relationships from the years before Stonewall, during the liberation years of the 1970s, and into the decades of AIDS. In general, there is little evidence supporting the claims of increases in coupling and settling down into domesticity that characterized many of the popular gay and mainstream media reports on gay men. Although there is research supporting a decrease in number of sexual partners and an increase in claims about monogamy, there is stronger evidence that what changed most as a result of AIDS was the discourse used to describe interpersonal romantic, sexual, friendship, and familial relationships. For lesbians, discussions about sexuality and passion became more open and less tied into stereotypical images of female sexuality.

How much of what has been discussed can be linked to the appearance of AIDS is, of course, difficult to demonstrate conclusively. By analyzing the discourse and images used over the decades with respect to family, friends, and romantic relationships, however, it becomes clear that a significant alteration has occurred in the AIDS decades. The change has evolved from language that attempted to show how gays and lesbians really were just like heterosexuals with the same type of romantic and relationship needs, and not just defined in sexual terms. Describing relationships as marriage-like, the early literature bought into the ideologies of a middle-class, ideal monogamous relationship and recommended mimicking it to gain respectability.

Then, as the liberation movements started to organize gays and lesbians around a shared identity, the discourse focused on more sociopolitical images of a family of oppressed brothers and sisters, made up of friends, lovers, and sexual partners. These images often clashed with a bourgeois sensibility and respectability held by many at the time.

Early attempts by a few to get legal recognition of gay relationships through marriage licensees met with some resistance and accusations of buying into an oppressive heterosexual institution. Although some continued to seek recognition of gay unions, primarily in religious ceremonies, many argued for an alternative family structure. Thus the extension of kinship terminology to friends and lovers was a shift that captured the move from homosexual individuals to a collective gay community and family.

With the appearance of AIDS and increased need for legal, emotional, and financial support, the concept of family changed. As gay men turned to each other for support, with many lesbians contributing to the care of AIDS patients and others taking over leadership roles in gay organizations (see Schneider & Stoller, 1995), and with more lesbian baby boomers turning to parenting roles, images and discourse about gay families turned away from the more political collective form to those of individual relationships. Simultaneously, a movement developed to recognize legally lesbian and gay relationships as domestic partners. AIDS drew attention to the lack of legal rights in gay relationships and the failure of spousal benefits in health, bereavement leaves, and inheritance to include gay and lesbian relationships.

Whatever the language used, irrespective of the images projected, a central implication emerges: how important it is to create social structures of our own, with our own relationships, institutions, and ideologies. Given the saliency of friends and families to mental and physical well-being, and the political and economic power of identity-based communities, understanding the nature and function of interpersonal relationships becomes ever more important.

There are also important implications in studying the language and images of relationships in the time of AIDS. Too many of the safer-sex guidelines and popular press (gay and nongay) stories communicate erroneous and potentially harmful information about sexual partners, monogamy, promiscuity, and coupling (Bolton, 1992a; Murray, 1996). One finding that emerges from the AIDS research about friendships and relationships is particularly relevant, however. To those who attach themselves to gay and lesbian communities of friends and lovers, their lives may be saved by them. As Joseph et al. (1991: 295) found in their research on gay identity and AIDS, "men who are securely incorporated in their network, who have mastered skills of negotiation and social interaction with their peers, and who place a lower importance on sexual activity as part of their gay identity, would find it easier to change risky sexual behavior." And this might just be the key lesson learned about the importance of gay and lesbian relationships in the changing times of HIV/AIDS.

References

Altman, Dennis. (1982). *The Homosexualization of America*. Boston: Beacon Press.

Armon, Virginia. (1959). "The Bilitis Study." *Homophile Studies*, 2(4), 113–124.

Baker, Blanche. (1959). *One*, 7: 23–25.

Barnhart, Elizabeth. (1975). "Friends and Lovers in a Lesbian Counterculture Community." In Nona Glazer-Malbin (Ed.), *Old Family/New Family* (pp. 90–115). New York: Van Nostrand.

Bell, Alan, & Martin Weinberg. (1978). *Homosexualities: A Study of Diversity Among Men and Women*. New York: Simon and Schuster.

Blumstein, Philip, & Pepper Schwartz. (1983). *American Couples*. New York: Morrow.

Bolton, Ralph. (1992a). "AIDS and Promiscuity: Muddles in the Models of HIV Prevention." *Medical Anthropology*, 14, 145–223.

Bolton, Ralph. (1992b). "Mapping Terra Incognita: Sex Research for AIDS Prevention—An Urgent Agenda for the 1990s." In Gilbert Herdt & Shirley Lindenbaum (Eds.), *The Time of AIDS: Social Analysis, Theory, and Method* (pp. 124–158). Newbury Park, CA: Sage Publications.

"The Bride was Male." (1974). *Pageant*, April, 20–23.

Bright, Susie. (1990). *Susie Sexpert's Lesbian Sex World*. Pittsburgh: Cleis Press.

———. (1992). *Sexual Reality: A Virtual Sex World Reader*. Pittsburgh: Cleis Press.

Burke, Phyllis. (1993). *Family Values: Two Moms and Their Son*. New York: Random House.

Butler, Becky (Ed.). 1990. *Ceremonies of the Heart: Celebrating Lesbian Unions*. Seattle: Seal Press.

Califia, Pat. (1980). *Sapphistry: The Book of Lesbian Sexuality*. Tallahassee: Naiad Press.

Calzavara, Liviana M., R. Coates, K. Johnson, S. Read, V. Farewell, M. Fanning, F. Shepherd, & D. MacFadden. (1991). "Sexual Behaviour Changes in a Cohort of Male Sexual Contacts of Men with HIV Disease: A Three-Year Overview." *Canadian Journal of Public Health*, 82, 150–156.

Chauncey, George. (1994). *Gay New York: Gender, Urban Culture, and the Making of the Gay Male World, 1890–1940*. New York: Basic Books.

Clunis, D. Merilee, & G. Dorsey. (1988). *Lesbian Couples*. Seattle: Seal Press.

Cole, Rob. (1972). " 'Marriage' is an Evil that Most Men Welcome." *The Advocate*, 29 March, 1.

Cory, Donald Webster. (1951). *The Homosexual in America*. New York: Paperback Library Inc.

Crawford, Sally. (1987). "Lesbian Families: Psychosocial Stress and the Family-Building Process." In Boston Lesbian Psychologies Collective (Ed.), *Lesbian Psychologies: Explorations and Challenges* (pp. 195–214). Urbana: University of Illinois Press.

Crowley, Mart. (1968). *The Boys in the Band*. New York: Dell.

D'Emilio, John. (1983). *Sexual Politics, Sexual Communities*. Chicago: University of Chicago Press.

Doll, Lynda, R. Byers, G. Bolan, J. Douglas, P. Moss, P. Weller, D. Joy, B. Bartholow, & J. Harrison. (1991). "Homosexual Men who Engage in High-Risk Sexual Behavior: A Multicenter Comparison." *Sexually Transmitted Diseases*, 18, 170–175.

Doty, Robert. (1963). "Growth of Overt Homosexuality Provokes Wide Concern." *New York Times* (Western edition), 27 December.

Ellsworth-Jones, Will. (1971). "Gay Nuptial Rites Get to Be Routine." *San Francisco Examiner and Chronicle,* 22 August.

Eskridge Jr., William. (1996). *The Case for Same Sex Marriage.* New York: Free Press.

Ettelbrick, Paula. (1989). "Since When Is Marriage a Path to Liberation?" *Out/Look, 2,* 9, 14–17.

Goldsby, Jackie. (1989). "All About Yves." *Out/Look, 2,* 34–35.

Gorman, E. Michael. (1992). "The Pursuit of the Wish: An Anthropological Perspective on Gay Male Subculture in Los Angeles." In Gilbert Herdt (Ed.), *Gay Culture in America* (pp. 87–106). Boston: Beacon Press.

Grieg, Michael. (1970). "The Boom in Gay Marriages" and "Gay Married Life." *San Francisco Chronicle,* 14, 15 July, 1.

Hall, Marny. (1978). "Lesbian Families: Cultural and Clinical Issues." *Social Work, 23,* 380–385.

Harry, Joseph. (1984). *Gay Couples.* New York: Praeger.

Harry, Joseph, & William DeVall. (1978). *The Social Organization of Gay Males.* New York: Praeger.

Harvard Law Review Editors. (1989). *Sexual Orientation and the Law.* Cambridge, MA: Harvard University Press.

Hauser, Richard. (1962). *The Homosexual Society.* London: The Bodley Head.

Hayden, Corinne. (1995). "Gender, Genetics, and Generation: Reformulating Biology in Lesbian Kinship." *Cultural Anthropology, 10,* 41–63.

Hays, Robert, Susan Kegeles, & Thomas Coates. (1990). "High HIV Risk-Taking Among Young Gay Men." *AIDS, 4,* 901–907.

Hooker, Evelyn. (1959). "A Preliminary Analysis of Group Behaviour of Homosexuals." *Homophile Studies, 2,* 26–32.

———. (1965). "Male Homosexuals and Their Worlds." Pp. 83–107 in *Sexual Inversion,* Judd Marmor (ed.). New York: Basic Books.

Jay, Karla, & Allen Young. (1979). *The Gay Report.* New York: Summit.

Jensen, Mehri Samandari. (1974). "Role Differentiation in Female Homosexual Quasi-Marital Unions." *Journal of Marriage and the Family* 36: 360–367.

Joseph, K. Michael, S. Maurice Adib, Jill Joseph, & Margalit Tal. (1991). "Gay Identity and Risky Sexual Behavior Related to the AIDS Threat." *Journal of Community Health, 16,* 287–297.

Kanouse, David, Sandra Berry, Michael Gorman, Elizabeth Yano, & Sally Carson. (1991). *Response to the AIDS Epidemic: A Survey of Homosexual and Bisexual Men in Los Angeles County.* Santa Monica: RAND.

Kirk, Marshall, & Hunter Madsen. (1989). *After the Ball.* New York: Doubleday.

Krestan, Jo-Ann, & Claudia Bepko. (1980). "The Problem of Fusion in the Lesbian Relationship." *Family Process, 19,* 277–289.

Lever, Janet. (1994). "The 1994 Advocate Survey of Sexuality and Relationships: The Men." *The Advocate,* 23 August, 15–24.

———. (1995). "The 1995 Advocate Survey of Sexuality and Relationships: The Women." *The Advocate,* 22 August, 22–30.

Lewin, Ellen. (1993). *Lesbian Mothers: Accounts of Gender in American Culture.* Ithaca: Cornell University Press.

Lloyd, Randy. (1963). "Let's Push Homophile Marriage." *One, 11,* 5–10.

Loulan, JoAnn. (1984). *Lesbian Sex.* San Francisco: Spinsters Book.

———. (1987). *Lesbian Passion: Loving Ourselves and Each Other.* San Francisco: Spinsters Book.

Marks, Robert. (1988). "Coming Out in the Age of AIDS: The Next Generation." *Out/Look, 1,* 66–74.

Marlowe, Kenneth. (1965). *The Male Homosexual.* Los Angeles: Sherbourne Press.

Maxey, Steven. (1986). "Why We Must Redefine 'Family' To Include Gay People." *The Advocate,* 25 November, 9.

McKirnan, David, & Peggy Peterson. (1989). "AIDS-Risk Behavior Among Homosexual Males: The Role of Attitudes and Substance Abuse." *Psychology and Health, 3*, 161–171.

McKusick, Leon, T. Coates, S. Morin, L. Pollack, & C. Hoff. (1990). "Longitudinal Predictors of Reductions in Unprotected Anal Intercourse Among Gay Men in San Francisco: The AIDS Behavioral Research Project." *American Journal of Public Health, 80*, 978–983.

McWhirter, David, & Andrew Mattison. (1984). *The Male Couple.* Englewood Cliffs, NJ: Prentice-Hall.

Miller, Neil. (1989). *In Search of Gay America.* New York: Harper and Row Perennial.

Murray, Stephen O. (1995). *Latin American Male Homosexualities.* Albuquerque: University of New Mexico Press.

———. (1996). *American Gay.* Chicago: University of Chicago Press.

Nardi, Peter M. (1982). "Alcohol Treatment and the Non-Traditional Family Structures of Gays and Lesbians." *Journal of Alcohol and Drug Education, 27*, 83–89.

———. (1990). "AIDS and Obituaries: The Perpetuation of Stigma in the Press." In Douglas Feldman (Ed.), *Culture and AIDS* (pp. 159–168). New York: Praeger.

———. (1992a). "Sex, Friendship, and Gender Roles Among Gay Men." In Peter M. Nardi (Ed.), *Men's Friendships* (pp. 173–185). Newbury Park, CA: Sage.

———. (1992b). "That's What Friends Are For: Friends as Family in the Gay and Lesbian Community." In Ken Plummer (Ed.), *Modern Homosexualities: Fragments of Lesbian and Gay Experience* (pp. 108–120). London: Routledge.

Nardi, Peter M., & Drury Sherrod. (1994). "Friendship in the Lives of Gay Men and Lesbians." *Journal of Social and Personal Relationships, 11*, 185–199.

Nonas, Elisabeth. (1992). "All in the Family." *The Advocate,* 13 August, 49–52.

Overlooked Opinions. (1992). "The Gay Market." Chicago.

Patton, Cindy. (1990). *Inventing AIDS.* New York: Routledge.

Plummer, Douglas. (1963). *Queer People.* New York: Citadel Press.

"Questions For Couples: The Results." (1989). *Out/Look,* summer, 86.

Ridinger, Robert B. Marks. (1987). *An Index to The Advocate.* Los Angeles: Liberation Publications.

Riley, Claire. (1988). "American Kinship: A Lesbian Account." *Feminist Issues, 8*, 75–94.

Rodgers, Bruce. (1972). *Gay Talk [The Queens' Vernacular].* New York: Paragon.

Roxxie. (1992). "Girls on Film: Lesbian Erotica Pushes Past Exploitation." *The Advocate,* 20 October, 59–60.

Sadownick, Douglas. (1985). "AIDS and a New Gay Generation: Finding Love and Commitment in a Marriage of Convenience." *The Advocate,* 29 October, 8.

Saghir, Marcel, & Eli Robins. (1973). *Male and Female Homosexuality: A Comprehensive Investigation.* Baltimore: Williams and Wilkins.

Saunders, E. B. (1953). "Reformer's Choice: Marriage License or Just License?" *One, 1*, 10–12.

Schneider, Beth E., & Nancy E. Stoller (Eds.). (1995). *Women Resisting AIDS: Feminist Strategies of Empowerment.* Philadelphia: Temple University Press.

Seidman, Steven. (1992). *Embattled Eros.* New York: Routledge.

Sherman, Suzanne. (1992). *Lesbian and Gay Marriage: Private Commitments, Public Ceremonies.* Philadelphia: Temple University Press.

Shernoff, Michael. (1984). "Family Therapy for Lesbian and Gay Clients." *Social Work, 29*, 393–396.

Sonenschein, David. (1968). "The Ethnography of Male Homosexual Relationships." *Journal of Sex Research, 4*, 69–83.

Spada, James. (1979). *The Spada Report: The Newest Survey of Gay Male Sexuality.* New York: New American Library.

Stall, Ron, D. Barrett, L. Bye, J. Catania, C. Frutchey, J. Henne, G. Lemp, & J. Paul.

(1992). "A Comparison of Younger and Older Gay Men's HIV Risk-Taking Behaviors: The Communication Technologies 1989 Cross-Sectional Survey." *Journal of Acquired Immune Deficiency Syndromes, 5,* 682–687.

Stearn, Jess. (1961). *The Sixth Man.* Garden City, NY: Doubleday.

Stein, Terry. (1988). "Homosexuality and New Family Forms: Issues in Psychotherapy." *Psychiatric Annals, 18,* 12–20.

Stoddard, Thomas. (1989). "Why Gay People Should Seek the Right to Marry." *Out/ Look, 2,* 9–13.

Stoessel, Hermann. (1959). "The Decline and Fall of Marriage." *One, 7,* 5–8.

Stumbo, Bella. (1970). "36 Legal Homosexual Marriages in LA? Are They or Aren't They?" *Hollywood Citizen News,* 7 July.

Sullivan, Andrew. (1995). *Virtually Normal: An Argument about Homosexuality.* New York: Knopf.

"That's What Friends Are For: The Results." (1990). *Out/Look,* spring, 86.

Trecher, Barbara. (1971). "Gay 'Marriages' Catching On." *New York Post* April 14.

Tucker, Nancy. (1970). "Nixon Nixes Same-Sex Marriages." *The Advocate,* 2–15 September, 1, 22.

Van Gelder, Lindsy. (1992). "Lipstick Liberation." *Los Angeles Times Magazine,* 15 March, 30–34, 54.

Vance, Carole (Ed.). (1984). *Pleasure and Danger: Exploring Female Sexuality.* Boston: Routledge and Kegan Paul.

Vetere, Victoria. (1982). "The Role of Friendship in the Development and Maintenance of Lesbian Love Relationships." *Journal of Homosexuality, 8,* 51–65.

Warren, Carol. (1974). *Identity and Community in the Gay World.* New York: Wiley.

Weinberg, Martin & Colin Williams. (1974). *Male Homosexuals.* New York: Penguin.

Weston, Kath. (1991). *Families We Choose.* New York: Columbia University Press.

Wetmore, Chris & John Arlec. (1956). "Twilight Marriage." *Mattachine Review 2,* 6–12.

Whitacre, Diane. (1993). *Will You be Mine? Domestic Partnership.* San Francisco: Crooked Street Press.

Wilde, S. O. (1992). "Inside a Sex Club." *The Lesbian News* 17 July, 44–45, 62–64.

Wood, Robert. (1960). *Christ and the Homosexual.* New York: Vantage.

FOUR

Spiritual Emergencies and Psycho-Spiritual Treatment Strategies among Gay/ Homosexual Latinos with HIV Disease

LOURDES ARGUELLES AND
ANNE RIVERO

Voices

They come thinking they are being punished by God. They want to be cleansed.
> —Ignacio Aguilar, clinical director, Proyecto Amanecer,
> Bellflower, Southern California

I want to die looking young and looking at palm trees. I was born with my young mother looking at palm trees. It is only reasonable that I should die that way.
> —Ricardo, Cuban PWA, died February 1991

AIDS is the force that pushes us through the opening and into the world that never ends.
> —Rene, Chicano PWA, died July 1987

Dying of AIDS is dying religiously, martyred.
> —Jorge, Nicaraguan PWA

I know I have been hexed. I know who did it and when. That is why I have AIDS.
> —Carlos, Mexican PWA

AIDS has contributed to the change in Afro-Caribbean healing practices in the United States. And so has the increased visibility of gays and lesbians in our communities.
> —Chief Alade, North American Yoruba Society

It is a punishment, and so it is only God who can cure me. I go to church all the time. I'm very afraid to die.
> —Anonymous, Mexican PWA

The time of an HIV-positive diagnosis is a time of great crisis and can be a time to reconnect with *la cultura*.
—David Marquez, former clinical director,
Milagros AIDS Project, East Los Angeles

Introduction

For many men, women, and children diagnosed with a deadly disease, the diagnosis and the subsequent unfolding of an illness process can help precipitate a spiritual emergency or a state of profound psychological transformation that involves the individual's entire being. Spiritual emergencies often take the form of states of consciousness of a non-ordinary nature and involve very intense emotions that may lead to new philosophical insights. These experiences tend to revolve around spiritual themes and can include sequences of psychological death and rebirth, feelings of oneness with the universe, and encounters with several mythological beings (Grof & Grof, 1990). Several investigators (Bragdon, 1988; Grof, 1985, 1988, and 1992; Grof & Grof, 1990; Hood, 1986) have explored the healing potential of spiritual emergencies and have mapped out the kinds of circumstances and psychotherapeutic techniques that tend to make these experiences beneficial for the individual and for those closest to him or her. The investigators have also been careful to differentiate between spiritual emergencies and mental states such as psychosis or other serious pathology. These pioneer researchers have encouraged clinicians to deal with certain states such as visions and recall of past lives as difficult stages in a natural developmental process rather than as evidence of disease. Working in this way, some clinicians have felt the need to establish referral and consultation links with traditional and alternative healers and advisers (Achterberg, 1985; Krippner & Villoldo, 1986; Torrey, 1972). Among the positive results of these linkages has been an expansion of options for individuals seeking assistance in coping with their problems and/or further developing their emotional and spiritual lives.

One critique of consciousness research and the non-pathology-oriented treatment of spiritual emergencies in the United States is that there is negligible impact by this kind of research and clinical work among populations of color. What is often overlooked, however, is that from within these populations certain indigenous traditional and alternative practices have been drawn upon and modified to fit very new circumstances by creative clinicians, researchers, healers, and clients. Such culture-based approaches may parallel in process and effectiveness some of the techniques developed by alternative consciousness researchers.

This chapter is about the various spiritual emergencies faced by some Latino gay/homosexual men living and dying with HIV disease and the psycho-spiritual strategies that they and some of their clinicians, traditional healers, and other helpers have accessed or developed. The types of experiences and struggles reported by clients and clinicians have resulted in a broadening of the term "spiritual emergency" to include less acute manifestations and culture-bound syndromes such that the lines are somewhat less sharply drawn between the Grofs' designations of "spiritual emergence" versus "spiritual emergency" (Grof & Grof, 1990). The chapter also illustrates some changes in conventional mental health treatment and traditional and alternative healing practices in various Latino communities in the context of the AIDS pandemic as gay/homosexual HIV sufferers have become more visible in communities of color. It is a chapter based on many years of clinical and prevention education experiences with people with HIV/AIDS, as well as ongoing conversations with therapists and healers who approach the spiritual emergencies and spiritual searches catalyzed by the experience of AIDS using an eclectic combination of culturally sanctioned healing models and more conventional psychotherapeutic strategies. It is a chapter about work in progress.

Meso-American/Chicano Spirituality-based Treatment Strategies

Upon witnessing the spiritual struggles interwoven in coping with HIV/AIDS, the first thing that struck us was that the degree and type of spiritual emergency escalates in accordance with the types of causal attributions made about the illness. This was illustrated in a substantial sample of HIV-infected Latino men served by the Milagros AIDS Project in East Los Angeles. David Marquez, a clinical social worker and the former clinical director of the project, reports that more than 90 percent of the approximately three hundred HIV-infected Latino men whom the project served between 1988 and 1990 believed that their illness was a punishment from God or that they had been hexed (Marquez, personal communications, 1988–1992). The men, who were primarily recent immigrants from Mexico and Central America, had come to the project for both material and emotional assistance. They were having extreme difficulty dealing with their HIV/AIDS diagnosis, with the symptoms of the disease process, and with the social stigma surrounding AIDS. Their sense of hopelessness and helplessness was exacerbated by their beliefs in hexes, spells, or God's punishment as explanations for their current and anticipated suffering with AIDS. Hexes and spells were associated with the notion that people who were full of envy and hatred had made them sick. God's punishment as a causal explanation for suffering was associated with a rather simple moral causal ontology full of references to transgression and sin with same-sex eroticism as its centerpiece. Many of these men reported having previously sought help from *curanderos* and *curanderas* (Latin American traditional spiritual healers) in their local area and as far away as Tijuana, Mexico, to deal with the fear and guilt that resulted from being hexed or punished by God. The men believed that these healers could dispel hexes and intercede with God. The reported results from these contacts were mixed. A small number of men stated that they had received valuable assistance, though some felt that the local healers were not as effective as those they had known growing up in their countries of origin. The majority, however, reported having felt mistreated because of their homosexual behavior and/or exploited economically. Still others complained that they were unable to find good *curanderos* who were accessible in their area, or that they were too ill or lacking in the resources and documentation necessary for crossing the border into Mexico. These reports are in agreement with prior investigations of *curanderismo* networks, which report a decline of practitioners and of usage in large metropolitan areas, as well as distortions of traditional practices in the hands of transplanted or new practitioners (Edgarton, Karno, & Fernandez, 1970; Padilla, Carlos, & Keefe, 1976).

These immigrant HIV sufferers were left, as a last resort, with community AIDS projects, mental health and social service agencies, and conventional medicine. Given that their illness was experienced as a supernatural/spiritual event, they could not see these secular approaches as very helpful. Compliance with treatment or self-care practices was perceived as useless if the hex or divine punishment was still in place. Thus the first item of the clinical agenda for Marquez and his staff of Latino therapists was to help these clients eliminate the effects of the hexes and the notion of God's punishment as a causal explanation for their HIV/AIDS diagnosis and symptomatology. Unlike many clinicians, Marquez never thought that suppressive medication was the first answer to these men's predicaments. Having grown up in a culture in which attributions made to the direct actions of God and spirits, as well as the practice of hexing, were everyday occurrences, Marquez knew that he had to deal with these men's attributions partially in the context of their received culture. As a gay-identified therapist, however, he also felt the need to ensure that the heterosexual assumptions embedded in some of the cultural practices in these men's lives were not reinforced as their cultural connection was strengthened through a culturally based therapeutic intervention. Marquez also understood that the men no longer lived in the context of an intact Latin American-received culture, but in a setting of overlapping cultures and that the culture crossings in which they and their therapists engaged as a matter of routine had important clinical implications.

Predictably, then, Marquez set out to intervene therapeutically in a culturally based, albeit hybrid and eclectic fashion. He used approaches drawn from a combination of Mexican/Chicano healing practices, conventional clinical techniques, and from his therapeutic experiences assisting gay men cope with emotional and social stresses. In addition to his childhood and adolescent experiences, Marquez had gained familiarity with traditional Mexican/Chicano healing practices in the context of an organization named Calmecac, which means "sacred school" in Nahuatl. This organization, the brainchild of U.S.-trained Mexican psychiatrist and shaman apprentice Arnaldo Solis, drew together in the late 1970s and throughout the 1980s some of the best known Chicano clinicians in the Los Angeles area to study and to experiment with a variety of traditional healing practices in the context of their conventional therapeutic work with Latinos. At least two of the members of this small group were openly gay, and it seems that their sexual orientation was not construed as problematic. Solis would become well known for his work with gay Latinos with AIDS in the San Francisco Bay Area. Calmecac, which operated between 1978 and 1990, represented a setting of alternative Latino consciousness research and spiritual emergency clinical practice that partially transformed, and in turn was transformed by, the rapid growth of the HIV epidemic in the Latino community.

Among the therapeutic healing practices effectively utilized by Marquez, and partially developed within the Calmecac collective, was the practice of *conocimiento* (knowing or becoming acquainted with). This exercise was designed to reconnect the client with his received culture and his ancestors by helping him remember where he came from and allowing him to share that personal history within a group therapy context. Another practice was that of encouraging the client to seek ancestor guidance and assistance with the illness. Such connection with deceased ancestors is carried out in the Mexican tradition within the context of the celebration of the Days of the Dead and the building and maintenance of altars both in the home and in work settings. In a riveting video exploration of the meanings of the Days of the Dead for contemporary Mexicans and Chicanos on both sides of the border, Portillo and Munoz (1989) documented the transformations of this celebration and altar-making tradition among the gay Latino community in the San Francisco area. The theme of AIDS and the photographs of lovers and friends lost to the disease, as well as the use of such modern items as neon statues and VCRs in the altars in the Portillo-Munoz video, vividly and publicly illustrate some of the types of practices employed by Marquez and his staff and clients in the privacy of the Milagros AIDS Project.

Rene, a former client of the first author, related his feelings when he saw his friend Ramon put the photograph of his deceased lover in an altar made for the November celebration of the dead in the Logan Heights Latino district of San Diego.

> I felt very strange because in my family's altars we only had pictures of the "blood family" like dead parents, grandparents, and so on. But when Ramon said that our lovers and our friends who had died of AIDS were the "true blood brothers" it made sense. I feel very good thinking that one day many of my friends will have me in their altars and that I will be invited to come back and help them with their problems. I need to prepare in this life to do just that. I need to recenter. AIDS and my friends have given my life a spiritual focus. At first it was difficult because I had to go on living as before, working and shopping while knowing that I am dying. But the altar reminds me that the change is real. It reminds me of where I will be next year, in the spirit world.

A year after Rene's death, Ramon contacted the first author to invite her to visit the altar he had prepared for the Days of the Dead celebrations and mentioned that Rene's picture was in a place of honor.

Marquez reports that the majority of his clients were able to deal more constructively with their illness after months of culturally based therapeutic interventions. These interventions included, in addition to *conocimientos* and altar-making practices, *limpias* (cleansings of body, mind, and spirit), as well as group therapy, in which issues of internal and external homophobia were carefully addressed. He reports that the men began to take better care of their bodies through conventional medical care and with the assistance of *sobadores* (traditional masseuses), *yerberos* (herbalists), and acupuncturists. He reports, however, that a few who had made considerable progress in cognitively restructuring their views of the etiology of HIV infection away from attributing it to hexing or punishment, or who had alternatively dealt with the purported hexing through a *limpia,* or cleansing, tended to regress in their therapeutic progress and in their ability to cope emotionally and physically with their illness when they joined Christian fundamentalist churches. These churches were not tolerant of their sexual orientation and overtly or covertly emphasized the view of AIDS as punishment of God for having transgressed morally. In some studies, membership in these and other institutionalized religions have been found to be highly correlated with fear of death among people with AIDS (Templer, Cappelletty, & Kauffman, 1990–1991).

Asked why he thought the men had joined fundamentalist Christian churches, Marquez stated that though the work at the Milagros project gave them a sense of reintegration with their culture and involved them in spiritual practices, it seemed that the men saw their involvement with the fundamentalist churches as a natural progression in their spiritual development in the absence of other institutional structures. Marquez added that the role of these churches in outreach and material assistance to the most disenfranchised groups of the population, and the concomitant decline in influence of the Roman Catholic Church among Latinos, cannot be overlooked.

Another clinician working to help heal the misattributions of AIDS and other physical and mental disorders to hexing and punishment is Ignacio Aguilar, the director of a Latino mental health project called *Amanecer* (Dawn), located in the heavily Latino area of Bellflower. In addition to being a clinical social worker, Aguilar is reputedly an accomplished *curandero.* His approach differs somewhat from that of Marquez in that he seems less direct in his views on sexuality and in his dealings with internal and external homophobia. In his work the guilt and self-blame, specific or nonspecific, appears to be simply material to be worked through. He approaches the clinical agenda for persons with AIDS, including gay/homosexual men, with a focus on the primary task of assisting in the cleansing of body, mind, and soul, and he adjusts his cleansing methodology according to the geographical and cultural origin of the client. He has found that for the majority of Mexican clients water, signifying purity, is a good cleansing agent. Caribbean clients, primarily Cubans, need to be cleansed using the *santos/orishas* or spiritual beings represented as Catholic saints who in fact mask African spirits or deities in Afro-Cuban *santeria* (Afro-Cuban syncretic religion) tradition (Cabrera, 1980; Canizares, 1993; Sanchez, 1978; Sandoval, 1975). This is more challenging for Aguilar who is not an official practitioner of *santeria*. Aguilar has observed in people living with AIDS or with other terminal or severe chronic illnesses a pattern consisting of a series of crises that he believes are related to strong spiritual longings that have been repressed (Aguilar, personal communications, 1992). These spiritual longings may lead people to search for their "root" spiritualities or spiritual practices with which they became familiar as children but with which they lost contact due to migration, culture blending, or other factors. Others may become attracted to traditional and alternative spiritual traditions when they feel that everything else has failed them. They look for spiritual homes where they can find comfort and answers to the questions arising in the spiritual emergencies that manifest during their times of crisis. Aguilar has also noted that some Latino parents who have remained involved in *curanderismo* practices throughout their lives may bring in their children in an effort to reconnect them with spiritual work and their culture.

Afro-Caribbean Influenced Psychospiritual Treatment

In the western United States (with the possible exception of Los Angeles) finding a clinician and/or spiritual mentor who can help them reconnect with spiritual roots can be much more difficult for Latinos of other than Mexican or Central American backgrounds. Ricardo, a Cuban who died of AIDS complications in 1991, commented on the difficulties of Caribbean gay men in securing psycho-spiritual assistance at a time of emotional and spiritual crisis. He noted that most of the nonconventional healing performed in the San Francisco Bay Area was derived from Mexican and Central American origins, as seems to be the case in Southern California. Though he found *curanderismo* and other Meso American-based syncretic practices interesting and at times sought assistance from various *curanderos*, Ricardo felt that he needed someone experienced in African-oriented spiritual practices to assist him with the overwhelming influx of experiences that he judged to be spiritual.

Talks with Ricardo revealed a dramatic change in his view of himself and the world, such that things that had seemed very important before his AIDS diagnosis no longer seemed so. He also became aware of a free-floating terror that no one could assuage and that he interpreted as a premonition. He reported believing that beings he had never seen but intuited were *orishas* who would come to visit him and tell him about other worlds better than the one he was about to leave. His dreams had mostly to do with his lost homeland and one of its sacred trees, the royal palm. For him, the *curanderismo* tradition was too Christian, too alien, and too bland. The Christian influences in the practices of the *curanderos* bothered him as a gay man, given the homophobia embedded in Christianity both historically and in contemporary settings. He felt at times that *curanderismo* was more Christian than pre-Columbian. He explained that though the *santos* of the Afro-Caribbean traditions to which he felt he belonged were borrowed from the Christian tradition, they actually represented African *orishas*, who often had two genders. As such, the *orishas* engaged in sexual relations with both sexes and danced, played, and laughed. He felt that gay men such as he, as well as transgendered people, could identify with these spiritual beings much better than with the serious and austere saints and the celibate Christ of the Christian traditions. He also felt that more openly gay people were involved in the practice of *santeria* than of *curanderismo*, although he recognized that homophobia was by no means absent in the "houses" of *santeria* (Ricardo, personal communications, 1988–1990). Though the *curanderismo* that Ricardo found in California did draw upon certain Native American traditions and influences, it did not seem to include any influences from certain native groups that considered sacred those individuals and practices involved with gender-blending or same-sex eroticism (Guerra, 1971; Lame Deer & Erdoes, 1973; Williams, 1986).

Had Ricardo been living in the East Coast area, access to the African-based healing he was seeking would have been much easier. One such source is Chief Alade, born Mercer Ashby of a family originally from Barbados. He describes himself as a bisexual chief in the North American Yoruba Society, and his practice is based in Manhattan but extends as far as the Carolinas and Florida. His practice partner, a lesbian clinical psychologist who prefers to remain anonymous, has also recently been confirmed as a chief in the North American Yoruba tradition. Together they have constituted a house called *Abale-Alade-Onisegun* (royal community that deals with medicine), where a great number of gay men, lesbians, and bisexual men and women, whom Alade and his partner consider their godchildren, have found spiritual sanctuary and assistance with their problems.

The AIDS pandemic in the United States and in Africa, according to Chief Alade and his partner, has brought about considerable change in his practice of traditional African religion and healing and in the types of practitioners with whom he works. The chief believes that the four most important changes are the increase in the number of referrals of people with HIV disease to traditional healers, a partial resolution of long-standing rivalries among such healers, the restoration of long-suppressed androgynous or transgendered *orishas* to their rightful importance, and the adaptation and further development of ancient "blood rituals" for the treatment of AIDS (Ashby, personal communication, 1992).

Chief Alade reports that in the last five years, with the rise in the perceived and actual threat of AIDS in communities of color, the number of referrals by conventional clinicians to traditional healers has increased exponentially. The number of clinicians, including his partner, who have sought out apprenticeships in traditional healing, or who have begun to incorporate the philosophies and practices of African religions into their conventional mental health practice, has also greatly increased. A new generation of Afro-Caribbean healers in the United States has also become more interested in relationships with conventional caregivers. Chief Alade himself maintains close relationships with members of the Black Psychologists Association in New York for mutual consultation purposes. Unlike the *curanderos,* clients, and clinicians of the West Coast to whom we have talked, Chief Alade has not found that the majority of those who come to him with an HIV diagnosis believe that their illness results from a hex or from divine retribution. He believes that this difference in attribution may have to do with the fact that many of the people who reach him already believe that they know what to do to counteract hexing. They are likely to have taken care to remove any ordinary spells or hexes before approaching the chief for "higher order" healing. He reports that the concept of divine retribution is something he does not often encounter. He suggests that this may be so because believers in African traditions do not tend to experience their gods as punitive and condemning in the way that Christians do.

People seek out Chief Alade, or are referred to him, as they would search for a specialist after having exhausted their other resources. Referrals come from traditional, alternative, and conventional practitioners working with a variety of people who have a link to African religions by ancestry, socialization, marriage, or personal choice. According to the chief, this is a significant change from the situation ten years ago, when the Afro-Cuban *santeros* who dominated the African healing scene on the East Coast would isolate practitioners such as he and Oba Adefunmi, the founder of the North American Yoruba Society. The reason for the ostracism was their being too "fundamentalist African" and not having strong connections with the powerful *san-*

teros in Cuba and the diasporic religious practices of Caribbean people.

According to Chief Alade, one consequence of this earlier divisiveness and suppression was that few openly gay or lesbian individuals were able to find a comfortable home in the practices connected with the diasporic African religions. He feels that the overlay of Christianity in Afro-Caribbean *santeria* exacerbated any existing homophobia of *santeros* and practitioners alike. As a result, gays and lesbians involved in these practices tended for the most part to remain in the closet or to be fairly discreet about their sexuality. This reported discomfort with varieties of sexuality on the part of transplanted *santeros* appears to be in contrast to what was observed by the first author within the confines of Cuba in earlier decades (Arguelles, 1993; Arguelles & Rich, 1984).

An additional problem, distinct from the issues of sexuality, was that in earlier times in the East Coast area, most of the ceremonies were conducted in Spanish. The language use excluded from serious practice anyone not fluent in Spanish, including many second-generation Latinos.

More currently Chief Alade has observed changes that he considers very positive. The return to some African fundamentalist spiritual practices, primarily of Yoruba origin; the rise in the numbers of visible gay, lesbian, and bisexual people in communities of color; and the diminished influence of aging homophobic Cuban *santeros* have combined to bring about more cooperation and cross-referrals between various African-oriented healers and between their houses. There has also been a proliferation of bilingual ceremonies giving more access to people of varied linguistic backgrounds. A new generation of gay, lesbian, bisexual, and transgendered people with African roots or connections, some of whom call themselves the New Wave Orishas, are indicative of the trend of cooperation, as well as of a return to some fundamental Yoruba beliefs divested of the homophobic Christian overlay of *santeria* and other Afro-Caribbean diasporic traditions.

Another positive development is the resurrection of some forgotten or neglected *orishas*. An example is the *orisha* Inle, who, as Alade theorizes, may have been neglected due to the influence of Christian homophobia. Inle may not have been totally acceptable to the Christian component of the syncretic Afro-Caribbean spiritual blend because of its clearly androgynous nature. The study of Inle has become extraordinarily important for Chief Alade and those who practice with him in his house. As a medicine *orisha*, Inle has also become very important for people living with HIV. Associated with Archangel Raphael in the Catholic tradition, Inle has become the patron *orisha* of many gay and lesbian Latinos involved in African healing practices. His/her feast on October 24 has become a growing gay religious festival in New York. Also important have been the initiation and confirmation of openly gay, lesbian, and bisexual chiefs, such as Chief Alade and his partner, in various African diasporic healing traditions in the United States. These men and women believe that their sexuality imbues them with special gifts to understand and heal, gifts that may be unavailable to those living exclusively as heterosexuals.

A final important change articulated by Chief Alade is that of the adaptation of certain medicinal rituals involving the use of blood, such as those rituals connected with the *orisha* Ogun, for work with people living with HIV disease. The chief was not at liberty to delineate the details of this and similar rituals or to be specific regarding particular changes or adaptations that have taken place. He did note, however, that the use of Inle in these particular rituals was new and important. These rituals, which have become meaningful among HIV-infected people as part of their spiritual healing practices, involve actual and metaphoric transfer of fresh blood. Chief Alade allays the fears of contagion by assuring that tremendous care is taken to insure that HIV-infected blood is not circulated in the rituals.

In the experience of the authors, as well as of the healers and clinicians with whom we have been dialoguing, the tradition-based healing and spiritual practices mentioned in this chapter do not seem to be pulling HIV-infected Latinos away from conventional medical treatment. On the contrary, it has been observed that the benefits derived from participation in these practices seem to put individuals in a more positive frame of mind and enhance their willingness to accept help from more mainstream medical providers.

There are some problems, however, as well as benefits for those who return to root spiritualities and/or traditional healing practices. The first problem may arise with those few traditional healers who are not educated in, or accepting of, the advantages of conventional medical treatment. They may overtly or covertly discourage clients from seeking the optimal range of treatment. Additional vulnerability to such discouragement may exist in persons already experiencing exclusion from mainstream medicine because of economic deprivation or lack of legal documentation. A more intractable problem arises from the opposite direction, that is, from conventional medical practitioners' ignorance and lack of acceptance of traditional and alternative healing practices. Ricardo shared his experience of this phenomenon. He was aware that his San Francisco Anglo gay physician, with whom he felt extremely comfortable and to whom he was grateful for excellent medical treatment, would have been appalled if he had known that Ricardo was seeking the help of *santeros*. He had in fact heard his doctor make derogatory comments about traditional healers and "folk superstitions." Ricardo would occasionally speculate about trying to switch to a Latino physician who might be more understanding of his faith in traditional beliefs and healing practices, but feared that he might then encounter much more homophobia. He once said, "If you have to be Latino, gay, and with AIDS, don't add another stigma to your life with *santeria* practice."

Psycho-Spiritual Practices and HIV/AIDS Prevention Education

The use of traditional psycho-spiritual practices in work with the Latino population and HIV infection has not been confined to clinicians and traditional healers. The AIDS prevention work of some Latino educators has also been influenced by these spiritualities. Pino and Arguelles (1987) developed a prevention education program framed within Meso American traditional spiritualities for use with recent Mexican immigrant women. The format included the use of opening and closing cleansing ceremonies, as well as suggestions for follow-up spiritual practice. The program drew freely from the work of the Calmecac collective. In addition, the late Daniel Lara (former head of Latino programs at AIDS Project Los Angeles), Yolanda Ronquillo (an AIDS educator formerly with the American Red Cross), and Milagros Davila (San Diego County Public Health Department) are all well known for their use of these spiritual traditions in AIDS prevention education. Educators such as these, who have wanted to integrate spiritual concerns into their work, have reported frustration that these concerns have been often ignored or pushed aside in the context of the despiritualization endemic in mainstream agencies and organizations in which they were working. Despite the resistance in these types of settings, dedicated educators have found ways to make possible some introduction of traditional psycho-spiritual frames of reference into AIDS prevention education targeted to the Latino communities. This has largely taken place through less conventional venues. Within some of the community-based agencies in which a culturalist orientation was more prone to see traditional spirituality as an integral part of Latino culture, it was sometimes possible to find more acceptance for these approaches. AIDS prevention thus became, in the work of some educators, another avenue for reconnecting with root spiritualities as elements of Latino culture that were felt to have healing potential. Introduced in the context of these programs, in which participants were not yet overwhelmed by the emergencies brought about by an HIV diagnosis, some ritual spiritual practices were seen as effective and often pre-conscious means to reduce fear and isolation, premised as they were in views of death as a natural, nonthreatening part of life and on the importance of healing the soul as well as the body.

In introducing or reawakening these concepts, it was found necessary to take great care to not confuse healing of the soul and the resultant inner peace with an otherworldly and fatalistic orientation. Interwoven with the spiritual work was much emphasis on empowerment and the development of knowledge and skills to be utilized by participants in their struggles, both individual and collective, against the pandemic. Spirituality could thus become another tool to help in the work of overcoming fear, numbness, helplessness, fatalism, and individual and collective irresponsibility.

For Latinos struggling with HIV, discovery of or return to root spiritualities has not been their exclusive choice in dealing with spiritual struggles or spiritual emergencies. Some have found comfort or transformation in following other pathways. A few have sought a place, albeit a very marginal one, within the institutional structure of the Roman Catholic Church, although some have sought similar accommodations within the context of other Christian traditions. Others have found their way into specifically gay-oriented churches such as the Metropolitan Community Church or the New Life Ministry. Still other gay Latinos have found resonance with non-Western and New Age spiritualities. In so doing they may have established links to previously alien aspects of Anglo or Asian experience and broadened, enriched, and rebalanced their culture-blending. Indeed, as some have found spiritual healing in a return to cultural roots, others seem to have facilitated transformation by stepping into (for them) radically new realms.

The complex forces of spiritual path selection among HIV-infected gay/homosexual Latinos have yet to be clearly conceptualized, but the importance of the spiritual dimension for this population cannot be overestimated. A recognition of that importance and an understanding of possible options in addressing spiritual crises are critical in the development of an optimal interrelationship between conventional mental health care and alternative or traditional psycho-spiritual interventions. It is hoped that our observations, and those of other clinicians and researchers such as those mentioned here, will add to a growing body of knowledge necessary for implementing the most comprehensive and compassionate responses to the psycho-spiritual needs of gay/homosexual Latinos and gays/homosexuals of other ethnicities and cultures as they struggle with the challenge of HIV.

References

Achterberg, J. (1985). *Imagery in Healing: Shamanism and Modern Medicine*. Boston: Shambhala.

Arguelles, L. (1984). "Crazy Wisdom: Notes from a Cuban Queer." In A. Stein (Ed.), *Beyond the Lesbian Nation* (pp. 196–204). New York: E. P. Dutton.

Arguelles, L., and B. R. Rich. (1984). "Homosexuality, Homophobia, and Revolution: Notes toward an Understanding of the Cuban Lesbian and Gay Male Experience." *Signs*, 9 (4), 51–71.

Arguelles, L., and A. M. Rivero. Forthcoming. "Same-Sex Eroticism and Spirituality: Crosscultural Perspectives."

Bragdon, E. A. (1988). *Sourcebook for Helping People in Spiritual Emergency*. Los Altos, CA: Lightening UP Press.

Cabrera, L. (1980). *Yemaya y Ochun*. Miami: Ediciones Universal.

Canizares, R. (1993). *Walking with the Night: The Afro-Cuban World of Santeria*. Rochester, VT: Destiny Books.

Edgarton, R. B., M. S. Karno, & I. Fernandez. (1970). "Curanderismo in the Metropolis." *American Journal of Psychotherapy* 24, 124–134.

Grof, C. & S. Grof. (1990). *The Stormy Search for Self*. Los Angeles: Jeremy P. Tarcher.

Grof, S. (1992). *The Holotropic Mind: The Three Levels of Human Consciousness and How They Shape Our Lives*. San Francisco: Harper San Francisco.

———. (1988). *The Adventure of Self Discovery*. Albany, NY: State University of New York Press.

———. (1985). *Beyond the Brain: Birth, Death, and Transcendence in Psychotherapy*. Albany, NY: State University of New York Press.

Guerra, Federico. (1971). *The Pre-Columbian Mind*. London: Seminar Press.

Hood, B. L. (1986). "Transpersonal Crises: Understanding Spiritual Emergencies." Ph.D. dissertation, University of Massachusetts, Boston.

Krippner, S., & A. Villoldo. *The Realms of Healing*. 3rd Edition. Berkeley, CA: Celestial Arts.

Lame Deer, J. F., & R. Erdoes. (1973). *Seeker of Visions*. New York: Simon & Schuster.

Padilla, A. M., M. L. Carlos, & S. E. Keefe. (1976). "Mental Health Service Utilization by Mexican-Americans." In M. R. Miranda (Ed.), *Psychotherapy with the Spanish Speaking: Issues in Research and Service Delivery*, Monograph 3. Los Angeles: Spanish Speaking Mental Health Research Center, University of California.

Pino, N. & L. Arguelles. (1987). *Flor de Vida: An AIDS Prevention Education Project*. Los Angeles: California State University.

Portillo, L., & S. Muñoz (Directors & Producers). (1989). *La Ofrenda* (videotape recording). The American Film Institute.

Sanchez, J. (1978). *La Religion de los Orichas*. Hato Rey, Puerto Rico: Coleccion Estudios Afrocaribenos.

Sandoval, M. C. (1975). *La Religion Afro-Cubana*. Madrid: Playor.

Templer, D. I., G. Cappelletty, & I. Kauffman. (1990–91). "Exploration of Death Anxiety as a Function of Religious Variables in Gay Men with and without AIDS." *Omega*, 22 (1), 43–50.

Torrey, E. F. (1973). "What Western Psychotherapists Can Learn from Witchdoctors." *American Journal of Orthopsychiatry*, 42 (1), 69–76.

Williams, W. L. (1986). *The Spirit and the Flesh: Sexual Diversity in American Indian Culture*. Boston: Beacon.

PART TWO

COMMUNITIES

FIVE

Elegy for the Valley of Kings: AIDS and the Leather Community in San Francisco, 1981–1996

GAYLE S. RUBIN

This chapter is an exploration of the impact of AIDS on the gay male leather community in San Francisco. In 1981, the first reports of a new disease affecting urban gay men appeared in the *New York Native* and the *Morbidity and Mortality Weekly Report*.[1] That year also marked the first notable AIDS death of a member of the local leather community. In the summer, a strangely aggressive pneumonia suddenly and mysteriously felled Tony Tavarossi. Tony had been active in the San Francisco leather scene for over two decades and had managed the Why Not, the city's first dedicated leather bar (Figures 5.1 and 5.2).[2] Tony's untimely demise baffled his friends. Later they realized that Tony had died of pneumocystis and had been an early fatality of the disease that would be called AIDS.

The Population

"Leather" is a term for a distinctive subgroup of male homosexuals that began to coalesce into coherent communities by the late 1940s. Leather communities appeared first in the major cities of the United States, but developed in other urban centers and in most industrialized capitalist countries.[3]

The leather subculture is organized around sexual activities and erotic semiotics that distinguish it from the larger and more generalized gay male population. "Leather" serves as a marker for a kind of community, a collection of sexual practices, and a set of values and attitudes. The leather "community" is not unitary or monolithic. In addi-

The material in this essay is based on fieldwork in San Francisco from 1978 to 1996. For a more extensive discussion of many points, see Rubin (1994). As always, many people assisted in the completion of this article. I want to express special thanks to Jay Marston for her constant support, and my immense gratitude to Lin Due for so generously applying her editorial prowess to this piece.

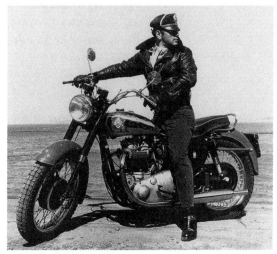

Fig. 5.1. This portrait of Tony Tavarossi was taken in San Francisco in 1960. Courtesy Michael Kelley Photography.

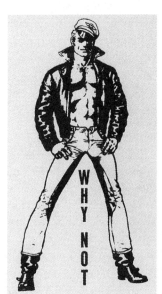

Fig. 5.2. This is the poster of the Why Not, the first San Francisco bar to openly target leatherman patrons. The bar opened in 1961 and closed in 1962, when it was succeeded by the Tool Box.

tion to the common cleavages of class, color, ethnicity, geography, and faction, the apparent homogeneity of "leather" camouflages several major subpopulations divided along lines of sexual practice.[4] Leather can connote brotherhood, masculinity, and independence, as well as certain sexual specializations. It may signal merely a passion for motorcycles. It may indicate an interest in sexual and social interactions among men with masculine personal styles, or announce a preference for some variety of "kinky sex." [5]

By "kinky sex," I mean primarily activities such as sadomasochism (SM), bondage and discipline, and fetishism. Among gay men, the social organization of sexual sadomasochism is generally structured by the idioms of leather, concepts of masculinity, and the institutions of leather communities. Some leathermen consequently consider leather to be fundamentally an expression and symbol of SM (as it is most often spelled in the community). Other members of leather communities have no interest in sadomasochism and consider leather expressive of masculinity, leather fetishism, aggressive coupling, motorcycle clubs, or sentiments of brotherhood, camaraderie, and solidarity. Such men may even resent any association of "leather" with SM.

There are many other sexual specializations located in the leather population, such as interests in rubber, uniforms, or "fistfucking," also known as "handballing" or simply "fisting." Fistfucking refers primarily to the insertion of the hand or arm into the rectum of a partner, although later, as women began to self-consciously embrace the practice, it also came to refer to the use of the entire hand to penetrate the vagina. In contrast to popular stereotypes and misinterpretations of the terminology, fistfucking does not generally consist of ramming a fist into an orifice. Fisting is usually done gradually and slowly, with many techniques to relax the anal sphincter or vaginal opening. In fisting, it is commonly the receiving partner who directs the tempo and force of insertion.[6]

Edgar Gregersen has noted that fisting "may be the only sexual practice invented in the twentieth century. . . ."[7] After its emergence among gay leathermen in the mid-1960s, fisting became so popular that its enthusiasts quickly comprised another major group among leathermen. Fisting has generated considerable cultural and institutional elaboration and "fisters" have become perhaps the third significant subdivision of the leather population along with sadomasochists and men who eroticize masculinity or motorcycles (Figure 5.3).[8]

Virtually all of the erotic desires, practices, and symbols characteristic of the gay male leather community exist elsewhere and find other expressions in different populations and social contexts. Even fistfucking is widely practiced outside the gay male community, and sadomasochism and fetishism are hardly unique to gay men. It has been recognized since early sexology that these are among the most common of the "sexual aberrations" and are frequently found among het-

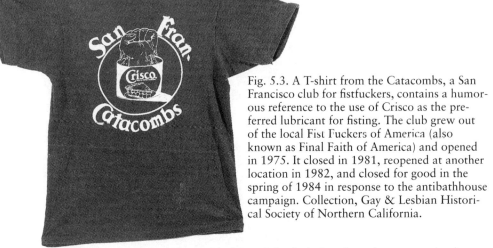

Fig. 5.3. A T-shirt from the Catacombs, a San Francisco club for fistfuckers, contains a humorous reference to the use of Crisco as the preferred lubricant for fisting. The club grew out of the local Fist Fuckers of America (also known as Final Faith of America) and opened in 1975. It closed in 1981, reopened at another location in 1982, and closed for good in the spring of 1984 in response to the antibathhouse campaign. Collection, Gay & Lesbian Historical Society of Northern California.

erosexuals, bisexuals, and lesbians.[9] Such desires have been organized rather differently in both practical and symbolic terms among these different populations.

But there has been a great deal of diffusion among these groups, such that a permutation of "leather" in the gay male sense of "community" has increasingly become a unifying symbol among other populations, such as self-consciously kinky heterosexuals and lesbians.[10] In this broader sense, "leather" has somewhat different valences from its usage among gay "leathermen" or from its specific use as a sexual fetish. In such contexts, "leather" loses its associations with masculinity, but does function as an indicator of community among sadomasochists, bondage aficionados, and fetishists of various genders and sexual orientations.

Gay male leather, with its singular concatenation of desires, experiences, and symbolisms, has been an effective vehicle for establishing communities, identities, institutions, and urban territories. Its sexually demarcated populations are united under the banner of "leather," an identity as "leathermen," and certain expectations of solidarity and sociability.[11]

These groups, although somewhat distinct and occasionally hostile, overlap substantially and are generally comfortable with one another. Individuals within gay leather communities are able to construct a vast array of unique personal styles and erotic careers from the available social and behavioral repertoire. Some specialize sexually or choose a single identification, while others engage in multiple practices and adopt composite leather identities. In gay male leather communities, the different subgroups tend to share core symbolisms as well as institutional structures such as bars, clubs, bathhouses, and territories.

The Site

> This land is too valuable to permit poor people to park on it.
> —Justin Herman, Executive Director, San Francisco
> Redevelopment Agency, 1970[12]

Gay male leather communities have been markedly territorial in major U.S. cities, and in San Francisco leather has been most closely associated with the South of Market neighborhood (Figure 5.4). Market Street is one of the primary corridors of San Francisco transit and traffic. It cuts a sharp diagonal across the city from the Ferry Building to the base of Twin Peaks. The trolley rails along Market Street have long marked a physical and psychological boundary (called the Slot) between the area north of Market, where the local centers of political and

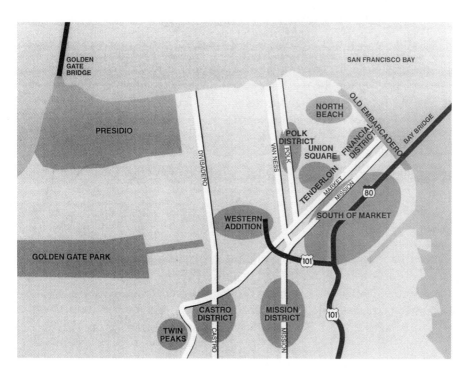

Fig. 5.4. This map of selected San Francisco neighborhoods shows the location of the South of Market area.

commercial power are situated, and the predominantly poor, working-class, and relatively powerless area south of the Slot.[13] South of Market has often been characterized as a blighted area or slum.

The area used to contain a considerable amount of light industry, although most manufacturing has long since departed. It is a district of wholesalers, warehouses, and service businesses for the more expensive retail and corporate areas nearby. The area is full of print shops, photo labs, typesetting companies, and graphics designers. It is the place to find commercial equipment, industrial parts, and many varieties of repairs and supplies. Although the main thoroughfares are mostly commercial, a working-class residential population traditionally occupied the smaller side streets and alleys. South of Market has never been exclusively gay or leather. The gay leather presence there has coexisted with other commercial uses and residential populations.

By the early 1950s, it was evident that the area was ideally positioned for redevelopment. Its convenient proximity to the major downtown area, its comparatively low land values, and its reputation as a slum made South of Market the logical candidate for a massive influx of real estate capital. Much of the conflict over redevelopment in San Francisco has been fought over the area.[14]

The San Francisco Board of Supervisors designated a large part of the area for urban renewal in 1953, following the recommendations in a 1952 report by the Redevelopment Agency. But redevelopment meant displacing much of the residential population as well as exercising the power of eminent domain against entrenched property owners. Controversies and litigation delayed redevelopment, which has taken much longer than its proponents had envisioned.

During the period of legal and political contestation, the old neighborhood was significantly dismantled. Housing was demolished and entire streets disappeared. But construction of office towers and public buildings awaited the outcome of litigation, so the new neighborhood remained largely unrealized. In the interregnum, different kinds of residents and enterprises flowed into the destabilized niche. From the late 1960s through the mid-1970s, there were plenty of vacant buildings, both residential and commercial. Rents and land values were cheap, until speculation and resurgent redevelopment activity began to drive them higher. Street life at night was sparse. The streets seemed to empty when the businesses closed and the daily workforce departed. Parking at night was plentiful.

This combination of factors made South of Market a kind of urban frontier. The area began to attract artists looking for affordable studio space, musicians in search of practice venues where they would not bother neighbors, squatters who took up residence in abandoned factories, and gay leathermen. The blue-collar character of the neighborhood appealed to the aesthetics of leather, and the relative lack of other nighttime activity provided a kind of privacy. Urban nightlife that was stigmatized or considered disreputable could flourish in relative obscurity among the warehouses and deserted streets.

In 1962, the first leather bar opened in the South of Market area. It was the Tool Box, on the corner of Fourth Street and Harrison. The first leather bars on Folsom Street were Febe's and the Ramrod; both opened in 1966 and were quickly followed by others. Since the late 1960s, San Francisco leather bars have been heavily concentrated along Folsom Street, and leather bars and businesses sprouted in the surrounding blocks.

By the late 1970s, South of Market had become one of the most extensively and densely occupied leather neighborhoods in the world. The area contained most (but never all) of the local leather institutions and commercial establishments and still functions as the local leather "capital." [15] As a result, South of Market acquired a number of nicknames indicating its role in the city's gay and sexual geography. Local gay argot designated the area as Folsom Street, the Folsom, the "Miracle Mile," and the "Valley of the Kings." This last appellation conveyed an image of powerful, cocky, independent, and sexy masculinity. It contrasted with Polk Street's "Valley of the Queens," a reference to the older and sometimes more effeminate population of gay men associated with the area, and the Castro's "Valley of the Dolls," an allusion to its hordes of young and beautiful men.

In addition to being a center for leather social life by the late 1970s, South of Market had become one of the most significant local gay neighborhoods, along with Polk Street and the Castro. By then, the Castro was unquestionably the center of local gay politics, but the Folsom had become the sexual center. The same features that made the area attractive to leather bars made it hospitable to other forms of gay sexual commerce. Many of the nonleather gay bathhouses and sex clubs also nestled among the warehouses. Just before the onslaught of AIDS, South of Market had become symbolically and institutionally associated in the gay male community with sex.

The Coming of AIDS and the Fall of the Folsom

The years between 1975 and 1982 were a period of triumphant expansion for the gay male leather community in the South of Market area. But by the mid-1980s, both neighborhood and community were devastated. The AIDS epidemic brought a tsunami of mortality to gay men in San Francisco. The resulting social changes and personal duress provoked crises of belief, outbreaks of superstition, accusations of blame, and desperate strategizing to fight the disease. It was a time of confusion, uncertainty, depression, and fear.

In the Castro, businesses were closing as their owners died. Each week the obituaries announced more losses: singers, record producers, therapists, doctors, bartenders, community activists, dancers, and politicians. An anguished pall hung over the Castro in the mid-1980s, but although the neighborhood suffered through a period of stunned shock, the economic and social reversals did not persist. The Castro recovered quickly and has remained culturally vital, politically active, populous, and prosperous.

By contrast, many of the changes in gay South of Market have been dramatic and enduring. Previously, if one bar or sex club closed, a new one would usually open. There had always been closures, but the systems of leather social life had been stable or expansive since the mid-1960s.[16] When leather bars or sex clubs closed in the mid-1980s, however, new ones did not replace them. Most were succeeded by restaurants, bars, dance clubs, and music halls catering to a predominantly heterosexual clientele. By 1987, the institutional infrastructure of leather had undergone substantial attrition and the neighborhood had become a case study in urban succession. Instead of the hordes of gay men en route to the baths and leathermen on the prowl, the Folsom was suddenly filled with the mostly nongay, nonleather, and evidently heterosexual patrons of the new eateries and other nightspots.[17]

These changes likely account in part for a persistent belief, often expressed within both the gay community and the nongay press over the course of the last decade, that the leather population has been hit harder by AIDS than other groups of gay men. The following statement exemplifies this view:

> Protestations from gay leaders notwithstanding, the AIDS epidemic hit Folsom St. aficionados sooner and much harder than it hit other gays, long ago sending the S and M subculture into a tailspin from which it has never recovered.[18]

There are no demographic studies that could prove or disprove such assertions, nor any hard data demonstrating such differential AIDS mortality among gay sexual subpopulations. Mortality within the leather community has been severe, as has been the overall—and overwhelming—gay male mortality in San Francisco. But the assertion of greater AIDS mortality for leathermen is unsupported and probably unwarranted. So why has the Castro prospered while the South of Market has undergone such profound deterioration as a gay neighborhood? And why does the stereotype persist that leathermen die of AIDS in much greater numbers than ordinary homosexuals?

Although I do not want to underestimate the devastation that has resulted from the sheer loss of life, the effects of AIDS on the leather community have been mediated through complex grids of signification, public policy decisions, and preexisting economic pressures on the South of Market neighborhood. I would argue that the patterns of urban succession in the South of Market area resulted from geographic competition for the area that had long preceded AIDS, and from public policy decisions about disease control, as much as it did from the disease itself. Moreover, rather than destroying the leather community, AIDS has both reinforced some aspects of its social structure and produced changes in others.

Folk Theories of AIDS and the Leather Community

> If anyone had bothered to do a survey they may not be surprised to find that during the early stages of the AIDS epidemic, participants and patrons of the SM/Leather world comprised a greater portion of the deaths in our community. I wonder why. It's hard enough staying alive just being vanilla.
> —Carl Brighton[19]

> I had always thought AIDS was something that happened to people who hung out in leather bars and had 500 sexual contacts a year—I knew I wasn't like that.
> —Gary Walsh, psychotherapist, after his diagnosis[20]

Although the level of change in South of Market led to presumptions of greater mortality among leathermen in comparison to other gay men, prior prejudices about leather sexuality also contributed to the notion that men who hung out in the leather bars were more subject to the disease. Stereotypes that leather sexualities (particularly SM and fisting) were inherently dangerous, unsafe, undesirable, or unhealthy have been easily assimilated into concerns over AIDS-related risks and hazards. Thus leather sexualities have been prominent among the ideological scapegoats for AIDS fear, panic, and loathing.

In the early 1980s, after awareness of AIDS emerged and before HIV was identified, theories of AIDS etiology proliferated, both in the society at large and within the gay community. Terror and uncertainty bred wild ideas of the meanings, locus, and causes of AIDS. In the absence of an identifiable microorganism, speculation about the causes of AIDS was rampant. Like witchcraft accusations, such causal fantasies generally reflected antecedent fears, antagonisms, and superstitions.[21] Accusations focused disproportionately on unpopular behaviors and scorned populations.

Much of this process of assigning causality and significance has been covered elsewhere.[22] Here I want to convey only the atmosphere of the time and discuss the role of antileather prejudice in some of the gay community's indigenous AIDS folklore. *Promiscuity* was a popular target. There were several versions of the promiscuity theory. The most common was that AIDS resulted from "repeated assaults on the immune system" brought about by promiscuity. These repeated exposures to illness and STDs were thought to result in "immune system overload." A variant was that semen might be immunosuppressive, and thus exposure to too many different seminal fluids broke down immunity.[23] The semen explanation appeared in another group of putative causes focused on *substances*. But promiscuity and related explanations were primarily rooted in a critique of gay male *lifestyles*. Blaming gay lifestyles for AIDS was a powerful and chronic theme.

Lifestyle causes blended imperceptibly into *spiritual* flaws, political differences, or failures of understanding. Among the phrases found in the local gay press to account for AIDS in the early 1980s were a failure "to recognize the spirit and soul of another," "failing to recognize femininity," "absence of love," "not loving ourselves enough," "macho posturing," and a "clone" attitude. The following letter to a local gay newspaper illustrates a particularly mean-spirited version:

> When I became involved in the Gay movement some fourteen years ago, we were a diverse group of women and men with a common enemy, the white macho sexist dominated system . . . Somewhere along the way came the macho (cock brain) gay man and our oppressors became ourselves . . .
> I live in the Castro, but:
> I do not belong to a gym,
> I love the Sisters,
> I hate gender classifications,
> I support the recall,
> I do not own a three piece suit,
> My role models are lesbian couples,
> And I'm glad AIDS is making clones look like fools.[24]

In addition to semen, many *substances* were blamed. These included sexual lubricants, such as the Crisco favored by fisters, and poppers (amyl nitrate and butyl nitrate), which were widely used as inhalants for quick, intense highs during sex or dancing.[25] Explanations to how poppers could have caused AIDS or AIDS-related syndromes included the possibility of a contaminated batch or the dubious deduction that because nitrates in food caused cancer, nitrates in inhalants might cause Kaposi's sarcoma. The concerns over poppers resulted in new legal restrictions on their use and availability. Other substances thought to have caused AIDS included methamphetamine (crystal meth), polio vaccine, hepatitis B vaccine, smallpox vaccinations, and even fluoride in city water supplies.

Substance theories inevitably melded into *conspiracies*. Had someone introduced a deadly communicable disease into the gay community? Perhaps right-wingers, the federal government, or the CIA had developed a chemical or biological agent and either accidentally or deliberately infected the urban gay male population; hepatitis B vaccine was frequently cited as the possible means of its introduction. Perhaps AIDS was an unintended accident of the development of agents of biological warfare.

Others proposed that the villains responsible were not outside but *inside* the gay community. An important group of folk theories centered on blaming *subgroups within the gay community*. Usually these were previously despised or stigmatized sexual populations. For example, one article cited pedophiles in a chain of causality involving Haitian monkeys. The article speculated that a group of boy-lovers on holiday in Haiti were having sex with local lads while frolicking monkeys dropped feces on the revelers. It was proposed that a monkey disease might have been transmitted through the droppings to the Haitian boys and their partners among the vacationing boy-lovers, who presumably brought the organism back to the baths of New York.[26]

Although drag queens were also occasionally mentioned, the most popular group to blame for AIDS was "sleazy South of Market leathermen." Two examples are:

> We have been a plague upon ourselves! In the late '50's and early '60's, when I first came out, backroom bars were non-existent, baths far and few between, the S&M scene a small, closed and very secret society. Fist-fucking was almost unheard of and "rimming" almost never done. . . . The leather scene was now being written up by gossip columnists in various big-city newspapers. Even Bloomingdales, in the mid-70's, did a major promotion featuring black leather clothing. In the late 50's almost no one had ever heard of terms such as 'scat,' 'water sports,' fist-fucking, tit clamps, etc. Now, not only does everyone know what these terms mean, but many have actually experienced them as well. . . . [27]

> Clutching our carcinogens and holding butch poses, we treat each
> other's bodies like disposable bottles, stumbling drunk and wasted
> through smoke-filled bars, giving and getting attitude, while a
> cancerous angel of death spreads his black leather wings and pre-
> pares to fly over Folsom and Castro.[28]

Such comments exemplify the way leather sex and leathermen became common scapegoats for AIDS fears and easy targets for AIDS
blame. Leathermen were already disdained, and their sexual practices,
especially SM and fisting, were often feared or disparaged. Thus they
became easy symbols for danger. Moreover, since leathermen were often characterized as more "sexual" than others, it was easy to consider
them more prone to exposure to a disease that appeared to be sexually
transmitted. Even the South of Market neighborhood became a geographic magnet for AIDS-related apprehensions. Its disturbing affiliations with leather sexual activities were intensified by the presence of
so many of the city's baths and sex clubs, leather and nonleather alike.

Sexual practices that already seemed frightening or dangerous for
any reason were quickly and easily amalgamated into the category of
unsafe sex, although "unsafe" in this context was supposed to indicate
only those practices that might transmit AIDS. This confusion of different meanings of sexual safety is poignantly evident in the way fisting
was treated in public discussion and in safe-sex guidelines.

The following paragraph appeared in a 1984 article on practices
thought risky for AIDS, and on why the city of San Francisco should
close the baths and sex clubs to protect gay men from the disease:

> Fisting: A few weeks ago I read a moving account in B.A.R. by a
> man whose friend sat down one day and quietly died as his body
> cavity filled up with blood. I understand that fisting has its plea-
> sures, but its dangers can't be underestimated. There is one thin
> layer of cells in the mucous membrane of the anus which is easily
> perforated. There are a lot of colostomies out there as a result of
> fisting, a specialty of some of the private sex clubs.[29]

Fisting has its risks, particularly due to mechanical damage, and
some injuries occur from the practice. But this description of potential
injury does not contain even a speculative argument for a relationship
between fisting and AIDS, the ostensible subject of the piece. There is
no connection articulated in this text between fisting and issues of
AIDS transmission, risk, and safety; the pertinence of fisting to this
discussion relies entirely on eliding the difference between two quite
distinct forms of "danger." This passage conflates ideas of sex that

is "unsafe" because it may lead to AIDS with sex that is "unsafe" because it may lead to physical trauma. Such confusion of AIDS-dangerous sex with other notions of sexual peril has been especially rife with regard to SM or fisting.

Similar assumptions shaped the role of fisting in guidelines for AIDS risk reduction. The first such guidelines were circulated locally in late 1983. These proposals were based on the educated (but at that time unverified) guess that AIDS was caused by a sexually transmissible microorganism. It is difficult to recapture the level of confusion and ambiguity attending these early efforts at preventing the as-yet unknown organism from spreading.

In general, the safe-sex campaigns were a sex-positive response to the illness. Instead of telling gay men not to have sex at all, the evolving risk-reduction guidelines attempted to instruct gay men on how to have sex while denying the organism a route of transmission. As medical knowledge evolved, so did the guidelines, for the most part.

Fisting was a glaring exception. By 1984, when anal intercourse became the major risk factor associated with AIDS, most guidelines began to recommend wearing condoms for anal sex and listed only unprotected anal intercourse as high-risk behavior. Fisting was still listed as high-risk behavior in many safer-sex guidelines in the late 1980s, long after it had been eliminated as a serious candidate for AIDS transmission. It was probably the assumption of many health professionals that fisting was inherently and grossly "unsafe" regardless of its relationship to AIDS that kept it in on lists of high-risk behaviors. It was not until the early 1990s that most guidelines for AIDS risk reduction either suggested using rubber gloves for fisting or simply eliminated fisting from the category of risky sex.[30]

Antileather prejudices also played critical roles in Randy Shilts's popular but troubling book, *And the Band Played On.* Shilts's book has been subjected to a great deal of well-founded criticism, including the observation that the book is best regarded as a work of fiction rather than journalism.[31]

Shilts frequently expresses squeamishness toward fistfucking, hostility toward leather and S&M, and a confused theory of gay sexual guilt for the spread of AIDS in which bathhouses and leather sex were emblematic of social and sexual disintegration. Although Shilts certainly did not think leather sex practices rather than HIV "caused" AIDS, his work constructs a powerful narrative in which moral flaws of gay male social life appear responsible for the concentration and rapid spread of AIDS among gay men.

In these exemplary passages, Shilts articulates his theory, using aspects of leather culture as signifiers of the fall:

> Slowly, the relational aspects of the sexual interaction dropped away. Intimacy disappeared and, before long, people were wearing outward signs of sexual tasks, hankies and keys, to make their cruising more efficient. . . . Stripped of humanity, sex sought ever-rising levels of physical stimulation in increasingly erotic practices.[32]

> As the focus of sex shifted from passion to technique, Ken learned all the things one could do to wring pleasure from one's body. The sexual practices would become more esoteric; that was the only way to keep it from getting boring. The warehouse district alleys of both Manhattan and San Francisco had throughout the 1970s grown increasingly crowded with bars for the burgeoning numbers of leathermen. . . . By 1980, it was a regular industry.[33]

According to Shilts, an alleged lack of intimacy by gay men was responsible for the spread of a plague. He espouses a morality in which sex for the sake of simple pleasure is characterized as evil and presumes that leather sexual practice is dehumanizing and lacks intimacy. In Shilts's moral history, the emergence of leather communities is explained as a consequence of some ostensible flight from sexual passion to sexual technique. There is no trace of knowledge of the history of leather, nor any acknowledgment of leather as a distinct subculture. Instead, leather communities, territories, and practices are simply used as loaded rhetorical tools.

Contrary to Shilts's stereotypes, leather and SM men often do pursue intimacy through sexual encounters, albeit within the languages of bonding and erotic signification specific to their particular sexual cultures. They are, moreover, as interested in romance and partnership as any other group of men. Shilts interprets and judges leathermen according to his limited framework and makes no attempt to understand others on their own terms.

Shilts's text exemplifies the kinds of prejudices that targeted leathermen, their places of recreation, their sexual practices, or their neighborhoods as scapegoats for the ravages of AIDS.[34] Similar attitudes underpinned the campaigns to close San Francisco's gay baths. These efforts had a profound effect on the leather community and on South of Market as a gay neighborhood.

Closing the Baths: A Classic Sex Panic

> Before there were any openly gay or lesbian leaders, political clubs, books, films, newspapers, businesses, neighborhoods,

churches or legally recognized gay rights, several generations of pioneers spontaneously created gay bathhouses and lesbian and gay bars. . . . gay baths and bars became the first stages of a movement of civil rights for gay people in the United States. . . . Gay bathhouses represent a major success in a century-long political struggle to overcome isolation and develop a sense of community and pride in their sexuality, to gain their right to sexual privacy, to win their right to associate with each other in public, and to create "safety zones" where gay men could be sexual and affectionate with each other with a minimal threat of violence, blackmail, loss of employment, arrest, imprisonment, and humiliation. . . .

As a historian, it is clear to me that yet another government campaign to dismantle gay institutions, even in the well-motivated attempt to stop the spread of AIDS, will only backfire . . . Instead of wasting its time defending its bathhouses, its bars, and its very right to exist, the gay community must be allowed to devote all its resources, including the bathhouses, toward promoting the research, health programs and safe sex educational measures that will save lives.[35]

—Allan Bérubé

Although bathhouse closure may appear tangential to the impact of AIDS on the leather community, the links are strong. Bathhouse closure exemplifies the way in which public policy decisions driven by misplaced passions often had unintended and unanticipated consequences. As was the case with many sexually transmitted diseases, early attempts to explain and combat AIDS often assumed a profoundly moralistic cast that had little intrinsic connection to the exigencies of epidemiological investigation or intervention. Sex prejudice, sex moralism, and sex panic often powered analysis and policy.[36]

Proponents of closure, such as Randy Shilts, argued that their program was an obvious and commonsense measure to save lives. They portrayed the debate about bathhouse closure as pitting public health and the need to save lives against civil rights concerns. This perspective oversimplified and distorted the situation.

And the Band Played On is often treated as a history of the closure debates. Unfortunately, it is a selective, partisan, and polemical account. Through his articles in the San Francisco Chronicle, Shilts aggressively argued for closing the baths.[37] In And the Band Played On, Shilts justifies his position in part by neglecting to report on the contemporaneous development of safer-sex education programs. Safe-sex programs were well under way when the bathhouse debate ignited in the spring of 1984. But there is not a single entry for "safe sex" or "risk reduction" in the index of And the Band Played On. The omissions conveniently allow Shilts to claim that "nothing" was being done and that bathhouse closure was the only available strategy for combating the disease.[38]

Although the safe-sex guidelines had their problems, as with fisting, on the whole safe-sex campaigns were a highly effective response in the early phases of the epidemic. The campaigns worked on the premise that it was not the number of partners a person had, the location where sex acts took place, or the presence or absence of sex toys or fetish gear, that mattered. What mattered was whether the activity provided an opportunity for transmitting a pathogen. Beginning late in 1983, intensive education programs within the gay male community resulted in shifts in sexual practice unprecedented in their scope, speed, and efficacy.[39]

Safe-sex campaigns in San Francisco attempted to use existing gay male institutions, such as the baths, as a means of spreading sex education among gay men. Some of the early programs took place in South of Market leather clubs such as the Cauldron (Figure 5.5). Leather sex clubs such as the Cauldron and the Catacombs were exemplary in their attempts to deal with the crisis, posting information as it became available and encouraging patrons to follow any reasonable suggestions. The baths and sex clubs varied in their willingness to cooperate however. That some of them refused to do so was one of the many factors contributing to the volatile campaign to close the baths.[40]

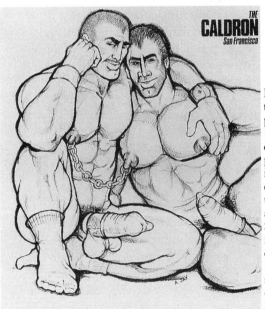

Fig. 5.5. The Cauldron, a sex club that opened in 1980, used an A. Jay poster to promote safe sex from 1983 to 1984, the year it closed because of the antibathhouse campaign. The club owners took a leading role in the safe-sex campaign early in the AIDS epidemic. In 1982 the club had already raised funds for an anti-VD campaign. By 1983 Hal Slate, one of the owners, was promoting sex without fluid exchange at the club and in the local gay press. In 1984 the Cauldron was also the scene of an important public forum on safe sex. Courtesy estate of Al Shapiro.

The antibathhouse approach to dealing with the epidemic emerged during the same period in which safe sex educational tactics were being developed and risk-reduction guidelines were disseminated. The campaign to close the baths was an alternate strategy and based on very different assumptions. Rather than promoting changes in sexual behavior to reduce the risk of transmission, the move to close the baths emphasized reducing the opportunities for gay men to have sex at all.

Allan Brandt, a social historian of syphilis, offers a series of well-crafted considerations for evaluating proposed public health policies for dealing with AIDS.[41] He observes, "In view of the fear and aversion that surround AIDS, there is a clear danger that policies with little or no potential for slowing the epidemic could nevertheless have considerable legal, social, and cultural appeal."[42] Brandt suggests that any policy proposal must be evaluated in terms of its effectiveness, such that "there must be considerable evidence that any particular policy offers substantial benefit," and in terms of its justice, that it is "the least restrictive of all possible positive measures."[43] He also highlights the importance of considering "Who will bear the burdens of any particular intervention? What are the potential unintended consequences of any particular policy?"[44] Although Brandt is primarily addressing draconian proposals that have originated outside the gay community, such as quarantines and compulsory testing, his admonitions should apply as well to proposals that originate within the gay community. In the rush to close the bathhouses, few of these criteria were met.

Bathhouse closure, far from being an obvious public health measure constrained by political pressure, was a cause of political pressure overwhelming public health considerations. Health officials in many cities opposed closure. Even Mervyn Silverman, public health director in San Francisco, had first opposed closing the baths. He relented only after political pressure mounted and kept his job. The health commissioner of New York City opposed closing the gay baths and resigned under pressure.[45] The baths in Los Angeles and many other cities were never closed. It is ironic that although there are still no legal gay bathhouses within the city limits of San Francisco, establishments in nearby municipalities such as Berkeley and San Jose were never closed and have continued to thrive.

It is arguable that what mattered in the long run was changing behavior, not its location. Closing the baths may have actually impeded the progress of safe-sex education. Even in situations in which the ownership did not cooperate, safe sex was spreading, like the epidemic itself, from person to person, through sexual contact, as men would engage each other in discussions of what they were or were not about to do. Wholesale closure eliminated opportunities for sex education along with opportunities for sex. At the baths, the concentrated populations of those at high risk for AIDS provided opportunities for educators to disseminate condoms and written guidelines for AIDS risk reduction.

In contrast, men in the parks were harder to reach with educational materials than those who assembled at the baths. There were no large containers of condoms readily available in the parks. There were no facilities for washing up and there were fewer opportunities for the kinds of leisurely conversations about safe sex that were taking place regularly at the baths and sex clubs. Bathhouse closure may actually have increased, rather than decreased, the rate of exposure.[46]

The social costs of closure were also treated cavalierly. Those who pushed for closure appeared to assume that nothing important or good ever happened in the sex palaces. They placed little value on the baths and clubs and failed to recognize them as important institutions that served many needs within a diverse gay male community.[47] The putative advantages of closing the baths were not balanced with any assessment of the losses involved, and these were considerable.

Calls for closure quickly claimed most of the specialized leather, SM, and fisting sex clubs even before any city actions were taken. The major gay baths had deep pockets and expensive attorneys and could afford a protracted legal fight. By contrast, many of the leather clubs were relatively small operations in which a dedicated owner had invested most of his capital and a great deal of personal commitment. They could not afford prolonged litigation. As the agitation for closure became frantic, most of the men who ran the leather clubs elected to shut down and limit their losses. Closure of clubs such as the Catacombs and the Cauldron meant the deeply felt loss of important leather community institutions.[48]

The wider social and economic fallout from closure of the baths and sex clubs was also substantial. Although the owners of bathhouses were frequently vilified as greedy capitalists (and some undoubtedly were), the debates never grappled with the importance of the baths to gay male social life or the economic impact of closure on the gay economy. Bathhouse closure caused massive destruction of gay social institutions, accumulated capital, and labor.

The time, work, effort, and money put into such places evaporated. Owners lost their investments, equipment was destroyed or scattered, knowledge and technique for managing sexual environments were lost, and many of the small touches that made the old places so appealing vanished. Artwork, music tapes, furniture, sound systems, iron cages, leather slings, wooden bondage racks, video recorders, porn videos, and the many elements of decor—mirrors, disco lights, murals, and a thousand other results of the labors of love—were dismantled, destroyed, or dispersed.

New sexual spaces began to reemerge by the end of the 1980s. These were initially in rented flats and begun on determination and a shoe-string budget. Many were small, some were dirty, most were ill equipped and completely lacking in the accumulation of small improvements that had made the older clubs comfortable and sexy. The newer sex spaces were, with very few exceptions, badly undercapitalized. Some of the clubs lacked even the most basic of the amenities that were taken for granted in the old facilities. The physical plant, the infrastructure of semipublic sex, has been degraded as a result.

This began to change only in 1992, when two clubs opened that permit only safe sex on the premises. Eros and Blowbuddies are well-executed sexual facilities. They have been followed by others, and something of a sex club renaissance is now under way. The infrastructure of gay male commercial sex is being slowly rebuilt. Nonetheless, few of the current facilities can compare with the sex palaces of yesteryear. Nostalgia for those well-developed installations has contributed to calls in the local gay press for removing all of the regulations put in place by the closure campaigns.

Dismantling the regulatory apparatus might hasten the recovery of baths and sex clubs, but some changes that the closure drive brought about are irreversible. Of these, the most relevant to this discussion is that the campaign against the bathhouses accelerated the displacement of the gay and leather communities in the South of Market area.

"South of Market Dies Screaming" (graffiti, 1986)[49]

Once the rough threatening preserve of welders, wholesalers, butcher supply houses, winos, struggling artists and gay men who dressed in black leather motorcycle outfits and metal studs, Soma has suddenly become fashionable. . . . Now the streets are lined with shiny BMWs and Mercedes. . . .
—*New York Times*, 1988[50]

When gay people take over a neighborhood, they call it gentrification. When straight people take over a neighborhood, they call it a renaissance.
—Tom Ammiano, local comic and politician, 1988

By forcing the leather-oriented sex clubs to close, the war against the baths eliminated an important social and economic sector of leather community life. In addition, because so much of the gay commercial sex establishment was in the South of Market area, closure eviscerated a substantial segment of the nonleather gay economy there. The loss of the bathhouses and sex clubs, which drew gay customers and employed gay men in the neighborhood, weakened the gay presence in the area. The combination of abrupt bathhouse closure and preexisting damage from urban renewal were significant factors in the startling collapse of gay South of Market in the mid-1980s.

The visible changes in the neighborhood occasioned dozens of articles in the local and even national press celebrating the area's sudden respectability and trendy "renaissance." [51] Virtually all the commentary cited AIDS as the cause of South of Market's population shifts. But these changes had been under way for some time, or were brought about less by the disease than by ill-conceived measures for fighting it.

Adding to the pressure was the physical position of the neighborhood. The Castro is far away from centers of retail power, finance, and redevelopment. The proximity the leather neighborhood enjoyed to downtown San Francisco, once a convenience, had now become a menace.

Redevelopment had been making inroads into South of Market since the 1950s, but it suddenly accelerated in the late 1970s. As Chester Hartman observes, South of Market redevelopment "spanned the political lives of five mayors—George Christopher, John Shelley, Joseph Alioto, George Moscone, and Dianne Feinstein." [52] Moscone was elected in 1975 and was more closely allied with neighborhood and antidevelopment constituencies than the other two more prodevelopment candidates, John Barbagelata and Feinstein. The Moscone administration was "more oriented to neighborhood concern and consequences of downtown growth," and his appointments to the Planning Commission reflected these priorities. [53]

Feinstein became mayor when Dan White assassinated Moscone in 1978. That tragedy significantly altered San Francisco's politics and geography. Feinstein's friendlier stance toward development was reflected in an unprecedented building boom and in a marked increase in the pace of "urban renewal" in the South of Market area. Among White's legacies is some responsibility for the radical Manhattanization of San Francisco in the 1980s.

The sudden escalation of redevelopment led to a land rush. In 1981 the San Francisco Planning and Urban Research Association (SPUR) released a report on South of Market development and held a conference to promote its findings. The flier for the conference shows Mayor Feinstein about to fire a starter's pistol for the developers preparing to sprint across Market Street in quest of the "South of Market Pot O'

Gold." Sticking out from under the "Pot O' Gold" is the hand of someone crushed beneath it, an apt image for the fate of the old neighborhood (Figure 5.6).

Leather bars in old Victorian houses were not suited to compete
with new, high-investment, high-rise, high-rent buildings or even the
midlevel eateries and other enterprises that would service them. Long
before AIDS was a factor, conversion to straighter, more respectable,
more expensive bars and restaurants was well underway South of Market. AIDS enhanced changes already in progress.

Redevelopment is now rapidly encircling the Folsom. At the northeast corner is the Moscone Center and the Yerba Buena complex,
which includes two new museums and a performance center.[54] More
large civic projects and many private developments are planned. An
ever expanding area around Yerba Buena was being repainted, remod-
eled, refurbished, rebuilt, or simply torn down to make room for construction. What remains of the leather bar area is within a few blocks
of Yerba Buena.

At the southeast corner is a growing retail complex which now includes Toys "R" Us, the Bed and Bath Superstore, Trader Joe's, and an

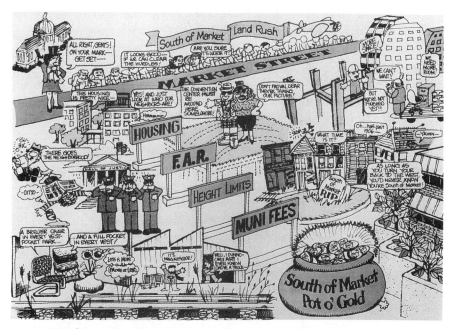

Fig. 5.6. This flier promoted the 1981 "South of Market: San Francisco's Last Frontier" conference sponsored by the San Francisco Planning and Urban Research Association. Courtesy SPUR:
San Francisco Planning and Urban Research Association.

entire city block devoted to a huge Price-Costco warehouse store. The back of the Price-Costco parking lot faces two of the remaining leather bars, the Lone Star and the SF Eagle. Shoppers laden with carts of paper towels and a year's supply of Windex are not a promising mix with gay men dressed in leather. The potential for conflict and violence along these ruptured territorial membranes is immense. In October 1995, three men attacked and severely beat a patron leaving the Lone Star. He dragged himself over to the Eagle to obtain assistance, and his assailants were soon apprehended in front of a nearby music club.[55] It is difficult to imagine how these businesses can continue to coexist. The differences of scale between Price-Costco and the leather bars in size, capital investment, and mayoral benediction are extreme. It is quite evident that if anything gives, it will not be Price-Costco.

The intersection of Folsom and Eleventh Street is a vivid example of neighborhood change. At the height of leather occupation, the intersection was a major stop on a circuit traveled between the various bars, baths, and eating places. There were leather bars on two of the corners and the intersection formed a corridor between the bars located farther south or west, such as the Ambush, Arena, and the Eagle, and bars farther east, such as the Brig and the Ramrod.

Once the heart of the Miracle Mile, Eleventh and Folsom has now become a barrier to gay male leather traffic. One corner site became a rock-and-roll dance club, the other a bar featuring local bands. Several other music clubs and restaurants opened within a block; the intersection is now a major thoroughfare of San Francisco nightlife. On weekend nights, hordes of revelers throng the area. Their presence draws hungry panhandlers, and city policies have also driven much of the homeless population out of the major tourist neighborhoods and into adjoining areas such as South of Market. Street crime has increased as both affluent club patrons and the vulnerable poor are targeted by a variety of scammers, shake-down artists, muggers, and thieves. The police cars that endlessly prowl Eleventh and Folsom are evidence of how highly charged this strip of real estate has become.

To get between the remaining leather bars, a gay man has to navigate through crowds that can be hostile and dangerous. In 1987 a young heterosexual tourist was assaulted and murdered near the corner after he was apparently mistaken for a homosexual.[56] It is deeply ironic that contrary to stereotyped expectations, the displacement of those "threatening men in black motorcycle outfits" by a predominantly heterosexual street population has made this neighborhood considerably less safe than it used to be.

The depth and breadth of such changes are not due to AIDS. They have been fueled by the redevelopment process and expedited by the damage the neighborhood gay economy sustained following the closing of the baths. It was for these reasons that the South of Market gay presence underwent so much more attrition than did the Castro's. Because the territorial succession was dramatic, visible, and seemingly abrupt, it was misread as indicating higher levels of AIDS mortality among the population of gay men who socialized and lived there.

The Shock of AIDS

> Duke Armstrong, Chuck Arnett, Ike Barnes, Frank Benoit, David Britt, Robert Chesley, Cirby, Barry Cundiff, Rich Demarest, Robert Douty, Claude DuVall, Dirk Dykstra, Michel Foucault, Johnie Garcia, Louis Gaspar, Jack Green, Jerry Green, Richard Hamilton, Peter Hartmann, Jim Heady, Fred Heramb, Joe Hollinger, Peter Jacklin, A. Jay, Mark Joplin, Albert Krause, Ken Lackey, James Leuer, David Lewis, Zach Long, David Lourea, Mack MacKinnon, Steve Maidhof, Geoff Mains, Robert Mapplethorpe, Paul Martin, August Mesenbrink, Stephen Mistler, Skip Navarrete, John Preston, Robert Pruzan, Mario Purami, Rick Redewill, Michel de la Roche, John Rowberry, David Salsbury, Robert Scott, Hal Slate, Cynthia Slater, Scott Smitherum, Alexis Sorel, Jim Stajduhar, Tony Tavarossi, Coulter Thomas, Jim Ed Thompson, Terry Thompson, Patrick Toner, Jerry Vallaire, Michael Valerio, Gary "Ram" Wagman, Gene Weber, Louis Weingarden, Randy West, Warren West, Kurt Woodhil.

This list of AIDS casualties includes individuals who were deeply involved in the leather community and others whose sole affiliation was that they partied on Folsom Street. It includes artists, artisans, musicians, photographers, producers, bar and sex club owners, founders and officers of motorcycle and social clubs, craftsmen, tailors, shop owners, physicians, therapists, visionaries, electricians, educators, editors, lovers, bodybuilders, titleholders, mystics, gallery owners, caregivers, friends, politicians, and activists. These names touch on almost every aspect of leather society. Few communities can withstand this kind of mortality, or can bear the way AIDS has torn at the fabric of social life. Nonetheless, gay male leather in San Francisco has survived and adapted to serious challenges no one could have foreseen.

The loss of so many individuals created a crisis of leadership. Many positions of power and responsibility were suddenly vacated because of waves of AIDS mortality. Individuals whose talent, money, or work created the institutional structure and inimitable style of the leather community are gone. Many fine players, with great technical expertise, took their knowledge with them to the grave. There are survivors, of course, but not enough to fill every need or position. Recruitment of leadership and individuals willing to take on community responsibilities has been an AIDS-related challenge.

Yet the sheer level of mortality has also severely strained the mechanisms for socializing and integrating new members of the community. Formerly the transmission of cultural norms and expectations was largely accomplished through interpersonal contact such as mentoring, friendship, and sexual liaisons. Now many of the experienced men who would have welcomed and educated newcomers are gone. Consequently, men currently coming into leather often get much of their education from books and classes rather than from personal contact.

AIDS has hit with particular ferocity men in the age group between thirty and fifty. Older men have been less affected, and younger men have grown up in an era of safer sex. These demographics have left a gap between the group that formed the leather community in the 1940s and 1950s and whose leather styles and attitudes are more classic, and a group of new wave, postpunk, postmodern youngsters. A perceived split between "old leather" and "new leather" has resulted. This ostensible split is complex and a flashpoint onto which many social and political frictions have been mapped, but it is at least partially due to AIDS-related disruptions in the machinery of socialization.

AIDS has unquestionably contributed to substantial erosion among some leather institutions, particularly the gay motorcycle clubs and fraternal organizations. The gay bike clubs were, along with the leather bars, among the earliest and most enduring foundations of leather social life since their inception in the mid-1950s.[57] In the early days of leather, the bike clubs organized most social events. Their country runs and city events made much of the leather social calendar well into the early 1980s. But many major clubs and the events they sponsored did not survive into the 1990s. Some clubs have formally disbanded and many are simply not functioning. The Warlocks, one of San Francisco's two oldest motorcycle clubs, is among those that no longer exist, and important events, such as the CMC Carnival, have also vanished.[58]

The Efflorescence of the Title System

Although some of the older institutional forms are floundering, new ones are thriving. AIDS support organizations and the events that raise money for them are omnipresent. Virtually every public event in the gay male leather community raises money for AIDS. Much of leather social life now occurs at AIDS fund-raisers, and many of those are the hundreds of contests held to confer leather "titles." [59]

An example is the AIDS Emergency Fund (AEF), a pet charity of the San Francisco leather community. It was founded by leathermen who were inspired by the bike clubs, which maintained a fund to help out members who were injured, ill, or otherwise in need of assistance. Similarly the AEF gives direct grants and financial help to people with AIDS. Fund-raisers for the AEF are ubiquitous, and the proceeds of many title contests flow into the coffers of the AEF.

The contests feature entertainment and usually have a mechanism to extract money from the crowd, such as auctions of leather goods and services. Some auction items are contributed by individuals or businesses and some come from leather "estates." For example, one wealthy leatherman who died left his money to his undergraduate college. But his leather estate—piles of leather pants, chaps, harnesses, equipment, sex toys, erotic art, bike club pins, and miscellaneous memorabilia—was sold at three different auctions to raise money for the AEF.

These auctions not only raise much-needed funds for charities, but also help preserve the community's material culture and historically significant artifacts from destruction and dispersal. A great deal of important memorabilia has been destroyed by embarrassed families or lost by careless heirs. The auction system has been an effective method to redistribute such items in the community.

The twin needs for AIDS fund-raising and recruitment of new leadership probably account for the rapid expansion and augmented prestige of the leather title system. The present title era was inaugurated only in 1979, when the International Mr. Leather Contest was first held in Chicago. International Mr. Leather (IML) was initially conceived as a male beauty pageant and an excuse to party. The winner was supposed to embody some version of idealized, masculine, leather sex appeal. IML was successful and became an annual celebration.

Cities began to hold local leather title contests to choose candidates to compete in Chicago. Individual bars, clubs and businesses began to sponsor candidates, and a city such as San Francisco might send several contestants. Within the decade, title contests had sprung up everywhere; San Francisco alone boasts dozens of titles.

Another major title grew out of *Drummer* magazine. Mr. Drummer has now become International Mr. Drummer. Unlike IML contestants, contestants for International Mr. Drummer have to qualify by winning one of the many regional Mr. Drummer contests. Consequently the Drummer title has spawned a system of regional satellite titles. The proliferation of titles over the last decade has become sufficiently notable to incite community commentary and humor. Jokes about "Mr. Bum Fuck Leather" express a certain bemusement at the ever-increasing segmentation of titles for ever-smaller units of the community.

For the first few years of International Mr. Leather, the contest was treated as a social event and the winners were considered glamorous icons who were expected to do little but show up and look gorgeous. Titleholder careers typically included a big photo spread in one of the leather-oriented magazines, or perhaps a new profession as a model or actor in porn movies.

This all began to change in the mid-1980s. Some of the titleholders began to take their positions more seriously and to use their celebrity to promote various causes. Patrick Toner, International Mr. Leather 1985, exploited his title to raise money for AIDS charities and organizations. By 1986, anger at government neglect of AIDS, right-wing restrictions on AIDS educational materials, and an increased targeting of SM erotica by obscenity prosecutions were causing the leather community to become more politically mobilized. Scott Tucker, a veteran gay activist, won the 1986 International Mr. Leather title in part by giving a very political speech that articulated such concerns.

The AIDS activism and political savvy of those mid-1980s International Mr. Leather titleholders began to alter expectations about the kind of person who should occupy the role, and what was expected of those who did. Increasingly, both major and local titleholders were expected to perform community service and function in some leadership capacity. Thus the character of title holders began to shift, as well as public perceptions of the significance of titles. No longer just hunks and sex symbols, the titleholders began to be spoken of as "leaders."

The emergence of female titleholders also facilitated the politicization of titles. SM women had been staging small-scale Ms. Leather title contests in the San Francisco area since 1981. In 1987 these sporadic contests became more formalized with the incorporation of International Ms. Leather (IMsL). The individual who ran the early International Ms. Leather corporation decided that the titleholder should be a "spokesperson" for leatherwomen. So that title contest, from its inception, was promoted as anointing leadership.

The notion of the titleholders as the community leadership is problematic. To some degree, the emphasis on the title system eclipses other forms of leadership. Despite the depredations of AIDS, there are still other systems of leather community leadership. There are people who become leaders in the old-fashioned way: they put in their time. These are the people who run organizations, who are elected officers, who have done community work for many years, or who own and run businesses that provide community space, services, publications, or products. Many of these individuals will never stand up on stage in a jockstrap (or G-string). For the most part and with some significant exceptions, the title system selects for the young, the pretty, and the stage performers.

But the title system does efficiently recruit people into community service work. A major difference between old-style methods of conferring leadership and the title system is speed. Within the title system, a person can be designated a leader in a weekend. The speedy ascent of titleholders to positions of leadership has advantages for a community seeking to replace fallen soldiers. But it has the disadvantage of sometimes elevating the incompetent or the inappropriate. Although most titleholders are dedicated, talented, intelligent individuals with true leadership capabilities, some titleholders have been inexperienced and lacking basic knowledge of the community they are supposed to "lead." Tucker commented on these advantages and limitations of the title system:

> You have certain judges and each of them have their own ideas about what's sexy, what's intelligent, what is really leather. So there's too much of an accidental element, I think, in titleholding and contests to be truly representative. It's not a democracy. It's theater. And sometimes a winner is going to have leadership skills and sometimes not. I think it's expecting too much of a titleholder, necessarily to be a community leader. . . . Really, it is a sort of role. It's a theatrical role and you are expected to give something back, like your time, at the very least, and do some fundraising and do some public speaking.[60]

Despite its limitations, however, the title system has made many positive contributions to the leather community. Title contests and events to which titleholders lend their glamour have raised fabulous sums of money for various community projects. The title system provides an easy way to communicate quickly new community priorities or to mobilize energy for other worthy goals, such as the preservation of leather history or support for important court cases bearing on the legality of SM sex or leather erotica.

The title system has also helped facilitate a growing integration of the leather communities on a national and international level. It has been one of the mechanisms for the dissemination of political information throughout leather populations. National titleholders are invited to participate in regional contests. They bring political education, make contacts, and create networks that have drawn many members of the less-metropolitan leather communities into national events and organizations. The title system has created mechanisms for solidarity, celebration, and integration in a community ravaged by disaster and mortality.

As the title system has expanded in numbers and influence, however, it has also increased its own demands on community resources. Although the title system raises money, it consumes resources prodigiously. Vast amounts of money are spent producing the contests, on transportation to and from contests, on hotel rooms, on leather outfits and stage sets. Sometimes when I contemplate the title system, I cannot help but recall the way communities under stress sometimes generate luxuriant new social forms whose importance fades when the crisis subsides. The title system is a visible manifestation of large-scale shifts in leather social structure over the last decade. How much significance it will retain once AIDS no longer menaces the population remains to be seen.

The Resilience of Leather: Changes and Continuities in the Leather Community

Against all odds and expectations, the San Francisco gay male leather community has weathered AIDS, sex panics, and urban renewal. The structures of leather social life have undergone substantial change. But the community and its culture endure. Although the leather territory has shrunk and continues to be imperiled by aggressive redevelopment, the Folsom is still the central focal point for local leather and remains a magnet for leather tourists.

That territorial occupation, however, is now intermittent in both temporal and spatial senses. Where there used to be leathermen thronging the Folsom every day, such hordes now appear only for major leather holidays and festivities. Two street fairs are among the most critical of these in maintaining the Folsom's leather ambience. In 1984 a group of community organizers and housing activists decided to start a South of Market street fair. The Folsom Street Fair was intended to make a political statement that South of Market, far from being an empty slum in need of urban renewal, was already occupied. The fair, it was thought, would bring together and display all the disparate elements of a vital and viable neighborhood. Thus the fair has never been an exclusively gay event or leather event. Nonetheless, the founders included leathermen, and given the strong presence of leather in the area, it has always had substantial leather participation.

Like most San Francisco street fairs, the Folsom Street Fair has entertainment, sales booths, and opportunities for political organizing, fund-raising, and education. Although most commercial booths feature generic street fair merchandise such as polished rocks and mediocre ceramics, the fair is also a showcase for services and crafts directed at leather consumers. These include piercers, artists, makers of bondage furniture, whip-makers, and purveyors of other SM equipment. SM clubs hold small-scale rummage sales to raise funds, and various community service organizations hand out literature and sign up members. Last but hardly least, the Folsom Street Fair has become an occasion for the leather community to come out in full dress and in force.

A second South of Market street fair was started in 1985 on Ringold Alley. It was called Up Your Alley, or the Ringold Alley Fair. In 1987 the fair moved to Dore Alley between Harrison and Folsom. A single nonprofit organization now runs both the Folsom Street and Dore Alley fairs. These fairs have become important social and economic events for the leather population.

In the early stages of the AIDS epidemic, the disease affected the leather economy largely by draining investment and capital. During the mid-1980s, it discouraged investment in the gay economy, especially in businesses that were sexually related. Many individuals made decisions to put their money elsewhere. They retired, sold their South of Market buildings, terminated their leases, and moved to the country or the suburbs. AIDS-related capital flight took money out of the gay and leather economy.[61]

Illness and medical expenses also consumed large amounts of money and continue to do so. Fund-raising to help the sick has gone on for so many years that many organizations now struggle to raise funds. Capital has also devolved through inheritance. Often when couples who have accumulated some assets have both died, their estates have passed on to family heirs outside the gay community. Some inheritance and insurance money has come back into the gay or leather economies through surviving lovers and other bequests. Some individuals have left money to fund gay or leather institutions, but these are uncommon.

Patterns of investment have shifted in the age of AIDS: businesses that facilitate direct sexual contact are less numerous than previously and enterprises promoting sexual fantasy have burgeoned. Phone sex, computer sex, and print publishing have all been growth industries. As AIDS has loosened its psychological grip or created investment opportunities, capital has begun to flow back into gay and leather economies. Businesses in the Castro are booming and leather businesses are again proliferating in the South of Market area.

The neighborhood now houses two major leather publishing empires, the Desmodus group, whose lead magazine is *Drummer,* and the Brush Creek organization, whose major titles include *Bear, International Leatherman,* and *PowerPlay.* Moreover, most of the local nonleather gay media now have their offices in the South of Market area. Several large South of Market leather shops have not only survived, but have expanded into substantial retail and mail order emporia. Some of the old leather bars have remained and a few new ones have opened, as have others in the Castro and Mission districts. All of these businesses help retain a leather presence by providing employment and attracting customers.

Nonetheless, the leather occupation is thinner and more spatially dispersed. The leather bars and businesses are interspersed among the yuppitoria—the music halls, upscale restaurants, and big-box warehouse stores. Leathermen on the street must navigate among or around these straighter crowds. They must contend with a much more mixed commercial environment and variegated street life than they formerly enjoyed. The intermingling of gay or leather sites with straight or mainstream undertakings has meant a loss of the very privacy that once drew leathermen to the South of Market area. The leather community once shunned this kind of exposure, but coexisting has become an adaptive necessity.

This is ironic in that overall the leather community has become more privatized. Many of the visible public spaces have closed due to AIDS, redevelopment, or city regulation. The sex scene in particular is less conspicuous than it was before AIDS and the bathhouse closure debates. In the immediate aftermath of the bathhouse crisis, the sex world reverted to an older, pre-Stonewall model. The clubs became more discreet and less accessible to the uninformed public, crusading media, and a potentially irate populace. Although there are occasional flare-ups of police repression or city regulation, these tend to be less frequent when the sex is underground, out of sight, and out of the headlines.

Safer sex is now a norm. Virtually all the existing sex clubs and private party groups require observance of safe-sex procedures. Primarily this means use of condoms, strong prohibitions against unprotected anal intercourse, and policies with regard to unprotected oral sex, although these are inconsistent. There are acrimonious differences of opinion over whether fellatio transmits HIV. Nevertheless, the conflict is usually over *what* is safe, not over the principle of safer sex, particularly with regard to "public" sex play. "Public" in this context refers to sex in places where there are more than a few participants, but few of these places are truly public.

Although AIDS has made the leather community smaller, it has also made it tighter and more socially integrated. Suffering and the sense of common struggle have drawn people together. Leather society is certainly more gender-integrated than it was even ten years ago, and it is more nationally confederated and politically cohesive.

In the late 1970s, gay male leather was still largely a bastion of determined, sexualized, separatist masculinity. Although they could not be legally excluded, women were not commonly found in leather bars. Many leather bars were openly hostile toward female customers, although a few welcomed women. Technically private, the sexual spaces could enforce even more restrictive policies.

This had already begun to change in San Francisco before AIDS, and a few women had been accepted in some previously all-male arenas. AIDS further eroded those gender barriers and further encouraged developing notions of leather solidarity and community that incorporate men, women, and transpeople who may be heterosexual, bisexual, lesbian, or homosexual, but who share some common interests in SM, fetishism, or kinky sex. "Leather" has much broader connotations than it once did.

As the epidemic hit, leatherwomen became involved in a wide variety of AIDS work and activism. Their contributions to personal support, fund-raising, institution-building, and political activism have been appreciated by men who have often felt beleaguered and bereft. Although AIDS support work fulfilled some traditional expectations men have of women, AIDS activism has also been an example of women moving along traditional gender routes into less gender-typed positions.

The title system has also been a force toward gender integration. The male and female titleholders make courtesy calls and are invited to one another's events. When a female titleholder is on stage as a major celebrity at a mostly male event, the other women in the audience seem less foreign, and the same dynamic has held for men at women's events.

In addition, the various major titles, male and female, are treated as roughly equal even though the women represent a much smaller economic and population base. These rough equivalencies of titleholder visibility and status are sometimes read as equalities of communities. Seeing men and women together on stage has sometimes increased the expectations of seeing men and women together as officers, on boards of directors, and even in some of the social clubs. There are, of course, still gender-segregated areas of the community, but women are now visible participants in most public events. Much of the leather leadership has supported the creation of space for the genders to mingle and work together. National political organizing has been a critical arena in which leather gender segregation has been significantly attenuated.

Besides AIDS, several troubling political developments have brought about unprecedented political cooperation among various leather constituencies. Since the late 1970s, feminist antipornography activism has singled out SM erotica as its privileged target. Early feminist anti-porn literature reframed concepts of obscenity to conflate images of sexual violence with representations of kinky sex. These assumptions about SM sex had been assimilated into mainstream, right-wing, and legal discourses by the mid-1980s. Many leaders of leather and SM communities accurately forecast that such ideas would result in new legal restrictions against SM and leather media.[62]

These predictions materialized with the 1985 Fraser Report in Canada, the 1986 Attorney General's Commission on Pornography (the Meese Commission) in the United States, in Senator Jesse Helms's 1989 amendment restricting funding for the National Endowment for the Arts, and the 1993 *Butler* decision by the Canadian Supreme Court.[63] Such state actions have all led to the suppression or prosecution of SM imagery. In addition, fifteen gay men in England's 1990 *Spanner* case were convicted of felonies and given prison sentences for consensual acts committed in private and with each other. The men were arrested and found guilty on the evidence of a videotape made for private use. The defendants lost an appeal to the Law Lords and are now pursuing an appeal to the European Court.[64]

Such cases, court decisions, and legislation have all made it apparent that SM and leatherpeople are disproportionately targeted by cultural anxieties about sexuality. SM and leather behavior and imagery have become increasingly criminalized over the last decade.[65] The need to defend their interests and safety has encouraged leatherfolk to build national and even international SM and leather political coalitions. Organizations such as the National Leather Association and the SM/

Leather Contingents in the major national gay rights marches have brought together gay leathermen, kinky heterosexuals and bisexuals, SM lesbians, and transgendered sadomasochists into nationally integrated organizations. San Francisco has been an epicenter of such national organizing.

San Francisco leather had already been active in creating a community more integrated by gender and sexual orientation. The mixed-gender, mixed-orientation play parties at the Catacombs (and, later, the Shotwell Meeting House) helped facilitate friendships between gay men, lesbians, heterosexuals, and bisexuals.[66] Informal diplomatic relations between the discrete leather populations were formalized in the mid-1980s, when appointed representatives of various community segments would meet regularly to exchange information and news.[67] Such contacts led to the formation of an SM Community Contingent, which first marched in the 1986 San Francisco Gay Freedom Day Parade (Figure 5.7).

Many San Franciscans took the lessons from their experiences of local mixed parties, diplomacy, and political unity into the context of

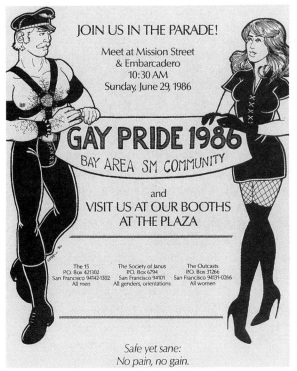

Fig. 5.7. Dirk Dykstra created this flier for the Bay Area SM Community marching contingent in the 1986 San Francisco Gay Pride Parade.

national organizing. San Francisco leather activists have been very active in mobilizing a leather political constituency that crosses boundaries of gender, sexual orientation, and kink of choice.

Resurgent Leather

The resilience of leather in San Francisco is now most evident every year in late September, during Leather Pride Week. Leather Pride Week began almost accidentally, when *Drummer* publisher Tony DeBlase decided to upgrade the Mr. Drummer title. Previously the Mr. Drummer contest had been considerably less prestigious than the International Mr. Leather Contest in Chicago. In 1988 DeBlase decided to move the date of the Mr. Drummer contest to coincide with the Folsom Street Fair, held on the last Sunday of September. As he recounts:

> I decided to move the contest . . . I looked around for where else to put the contest, to put it with another event, so that people would have more than just the contest to come to San Francisco for. You know, IML has made its name, not because it's a Chicago contest, but because it attracts people from all over the world. . . . I wanted to be able to try and do the same thing, to . . . make a major event to bring people in for. It seemed to me the other thing I could tie to was the Folsom Street Fair . . . Since the contestants arrived on Wednesday night, and they had things going Wednesday night, Thursday night, and Friday night, I started calling it Leather Pride Week in San Francisco . . . at that time it consisted of the Mr. Drummer events, Alan Selby's Fetish and Fantasy and the Folsom Street Fair . . . People saw the name, and other people said, Well, I'm going to do something for Leather Pride Week too.[68]

Each year more satellite events accumulate around the main anchors of the *Drummer* contest and the culminating Folsom Street Fair. Each year more leather pride flags adorn the city and more visitors come. Leather Pride Week in San Francisco has become a major attraction for international leather tourism. The Folsom Street Fair has become one of the largest public events in California, evidently exceeded only by San Francisco Gay Pride and the Rose parades.[69]

The leather pride concept spread rapidly, and there are now leather pride celebrations in many other cities. But there is nothing else quite like leather week in San Francisco: a nonstop round of conferences, parties, art shows, performances, the *Drummer* title events, fundraisers, networking, and retail frenzy. The Folsom Street Fair is now the culminating event: that one day, Folsom Street again belongs to the leatherfolk.

Yet in the long run, South of Market is probably lost, despite the stubborn vitality of a few remaining strongholds. AIDS did not destroy the Folsom, but redevelopment is an implacable force. The redevelopment juggernaut is powered by capital and political strength that dwarfs anything possessed by the leather community. But the community has shown itself to command robust social reserves, surprising economic vigor, and adaptability. If the leather community must leave South of Market, it will find some other urban niche.

The gay male leather population has been a major force in establishing national political organizations and forging alliances with other constituencies of kinky folk. It has developed new forms of leadership to replace its depleted troops. Although many of the old institutions have shriveled, others have been sustained.

Despite the losses of key individuals to AIDS, the gay male leather community has continued as a viable and evolving social form. It is now smaller and more private than it was during the 1970s and 1980s. In some ways, it has returned to the structural adaptations developed when it arose as an alternative subculture during the 1940s and 1950s. Along with other black-clad rebels such as beatniks and bikers, gay leather was one of the many richly inventive countercultural formations that nurtured social and sexual possibilities far removed from the sanitized visions of postwar suburban America.

Gay male leather occupies urban space that is less visible than it once did. Many extraordinary, irreplaceable individuals have died and their absence is deeply felt. Nevertheless, the community lives. It will survive scapegoating, ill-conceived public policy, the possible loss of its neighborhood, and the disease itself. The gay male leather community continues to show how unlikely groups of people find ways to exist and even flourish along the margins of dominant systems of social, political, and moral power.

Notes

1. Kinsella (1989).

2. Fritcher (1991), Rubin (1991).

3. For early observations of San Francisco's leather bars, see Achilles (1967); for discussions of the relationship between urban size and gay bar specialization, see Harry (1974) and Harry and DeVall (1978).

4. Leathers (1980).

5. "Leather" is in effect a "key symbol," as described in Ortner (1973).

6. Hamilton (n.d.); Mains (1988, 1989); Herrman (1991); Rubin (1991).

7. Gregersen (1983: 56–57). David Halperin recently called my attention to a similar observation recounted by Edmund White: "At the baths everyone seemed to be lying face down on the cot beside a can of Crisco; fistfucking, as one French *savant* has

pointed out, is our century's only brand-new contribution to the sexual armamentarium" (White, 1980: 245).

8. For example, see Paul Mariah's 1968 ode to fisting, "The Figa," in Mariah (1978).

9. Krafft-Ebing (1899); Ellis (1942, 1947); Freud (1966 [1905]).

10. Obviously, associations of various kinds of black leather (such as boot, garment, or glove leather) with sadomasochism and fetishism predate the post–World War II biker styles adopted by gay leathermen. Leather is a sexually and symbolically charged substance for sadomasochists and fetishists of many persuasions, such as heterosexuals. But the symbolic and social role of such leather differs for heterosexual sadomasochists. For a longer discussion of this point, see Rubin, 1994. For the more recent use of leather as a marker of community among SM lesbians or SM communities with mixed genders and orientations, see Califia (1987) and Truscott (1990). For writings on the sociology of sadomasochism, see Gebhard (1976); Martin Weinberg, Williams, and Moser (1984); Thomas Weinberg (1987); and Thomas Weinberg & Levi Kamel (1983).

11. For further discussion of gay male leather, see Baldwin (1993a); Bean (1994); Mains (1984); Rubin (1984a, 1989, 1991, 1994); Mark Thompson (1991); and Vollmer (1981).

12. Hartman (1974: 19).

13. Averbach (1973); Clark, 1987.

14. Hartman (1974, 1984); DeLeon (1992); San Francisco Redevelopment Agency (1952); R/UDAT (1984).

15. Jay 1976; Cook 1977; Rubin 1984a, 1994; Mark Thompson 1982.

16. Both Hooker (1967) and Achilles (1967) discuss the concept of a "gay bar system" that may be stable although individual bars are not.

17. Bean (1988); Rubin (1989, 1994).

18. "The Death of Leather" (1985).

19. Brighton (1994: 8).

20. Shilts (1984c: 22).

21. A classic discussion of this process can be found in Evans-Pritchard (1976).

22. Triechler (1988); Berube (1988); Crimp (1988a, 1988b); Bolton (1992); Farmer (1992); Fee and Fox (1988, 1992); Nardi (1988); Herdt and Lindenbaum (1992); Murray and Payne (1988, 1989); Patton (1985, 1990); Watney (1987).

23. Excellent and exhaustive dissections of the promiscuity discourse can be found in Bolton (1992); Crimp (1988b); Murray and Payne (1988).

24. Starkey (1983).

25. Lauritsen and Wilson (1986).

26. Waddell (1984).

27. Knapp (1983).

28. Evans (1982).

29. Robinson (1984).

30. A longer discussion of AIDS safe-sex guidelines and fisting can be found in Rubin (1991).

31. See, for example, Crimp (1988b); Murray and Payne (1988); Murray (1989); Bolton (1992).

32. Shilts (1987: 89).

33. Shilts (1987: 46).

34. For further details of Shilts' antileather attitudes and rhetoric, note the following in Shilts (1987): the squeamish description of fisting (23–24); a hostile description of a leatherman (46); a disgusted account of the Ambush, a popular leather bar that also functioned as a kind of South of Market community center (86).

35. Berube (1984c). See also Berube (1984a, 1984b, 1984c, 1996).

36. See Brandt (1985).

37. Shilts (1984a, 1984b, 1984d, 1984e); Schweikhart (1984).

38. Shilts (1987). Note that in contrast to safe sex, index entries for bathhouses are among the most numerous for any topic. Only numbers of entries for the Centers for Disease Control, blood donors, Marcus Conant, Don Francis, Bill Kraus, and the National Institutes of Health come close to those for bathhouses.

39. My argument here about safe-sex campaigns as relatively sex-positive, politically progressive, and effective responses is about the early years of the epidemic, particularly 1983–1985. There is a growing literature about the political and practical shortcomings of safe-sex education, particularly as it has become increasingly institutionalized. For this discussion, see Patton (1990, 1996), Rofes (1996), and Odets (1995).

40. Excellent accounts of the fight over closing the bathhouses can be found in Murray and Payne (1988), Kinsella (1989), and Murray (1989). For a very partisan account, see Shilts (1987). Fitzgerald (1987) is flawed by similar assumptions and prejudices about gay male sexuality. A less egregious but still problematic rendition appears in Bayer (1989).

41. Brandt (1988).

42. Brandt (1988: 165).

43. Brandt (1988: 164).

44. Brandt (1988: 163).

45. See "N.Y. Health Chief Resigns" (1985). According to this article, Commissioner David Sencer is said to have notified Mayor Koch that he feared that "closing the gay bathhouses would increase the spread of the disease by making it harder to reach homosexuals for education." A month before the resignation, the *New York Times* editorialized against closing the baths ("Morality, AIDS, and the Bathhouses," 1985).

46. See two excellent discussions of these and other issues raised in the bathhouse closure debates in Murray (1989); and Bolton, Vincke, and Mak (1994).

47. Berube (1984a, 1984b, 1984c, 1984d, 1996); Styles (1979); Martin Weinberg and Williams, (1975).

48. See Rubin (1991) for a more detailed account. See also Fritscher (1978) and Mains (1984), for additional material on the Catacombs.

49. "South of Market Dies Screaming" was spray-painted, along with a skull and crossbones, on one of the freeway abutments on Second Street between Harrison and Bryant, in 1986.

50. "Off-Beat Rough Toward Chic Very Fine" (1988).

51. See also Saroyan (1989).

52. Hartman (1984: 24).

53. Hartman (1984: xvii).

54. The Moscone Center opened in 1981, the same year Tony Tavarossi died. AIDS and redevelopment hit South of Market in tandem.

55. Conkin (1996).

56. *San Francisco Chronicle*, "East Coast Student Slain on S.F. Street," July 14, 1987, p. 4; "$10,000 Reward Offered in Killing of Visiting Student," July 15, 1987, p. 4; "S.F. Man Held in Slaying of Student Tourist," July 16, 1987, p. 1.

57. Baldwin (1993a); Rubin (1984a, 1994); Mark Thompson (1991); Bean (1994).

58. "The CMC Carnival" (1977).

59. See Baldwin (1993b).

60. Tucker interview (1991: 46–47).

61. There was also some AIDS related out-migration that went against the usual direction of gay and leather migration. At least since the 1950s, the dominant tendency is for such sexual migrants to seek the big cities. But in the early 1980s, there were gay men and leathermen who left the cities for smaller towns and rural areas to escape AIDS or live in calmer circumstances.

62. For early antiporn feminism, see Lederer (1980); for discussions of pornography and feminism, see Snitow (1983), Vance (1984), Burstyn (1985), Segal and McIntosh

(1992), Assiter and Carole (1993), Duggan and Hunter (1995), Feminist Anti-Censorship Taskforce (1992 [1986]), Rubin (1984, 1993a); for the role of SM imagery in antiporn rhetoric, see Rubin (1982 [1981], 1993b, 1993c) for the spread of anti-SM assumptions into mainstream and state discourse, see also Vance (1986a, 1986b, 1989, 1990a, 1990b, 1990c, 1990d, 1993).

63. Special Committee (1985); Attorney General's Commission (1986); Vance (1986a, 1986b, 1989, 1990a, 1990b, 1990c, 1990d, 1993); Rubin (1993b, 1993c); *R v. Butler* (1992); Califia and Fuller (1995); Fuller and Blackley (1995).

64. *R v. Brown* (1993); Bill Thompson (1994); Law Commission (1995); Hamilton (1992); "Sado-masochists Jailed for 'Degrading' Acts" (1990); "S&M is Illegal in England" (1992); Wockner (1991a, 1991b); Woods (1992); see also *People v. Samuels* (1967).

65. See my comments on the criminalization of SM in Rubin (1993a, 1993b).

66. Rubin (1991); Truscott (1991).

67. Norwood (1986) was a report to this informal local summit, called KISS/M, an acronym made by combining "Keep It Simple Stupid" and "SM."

68. DeBlase interview (1993: 152–155).

69. Don Thompson (1994).

References

Books and Articles
Achilles, Nancy. (1967). "The Development of the Homosexual Bar as an Institution." In John Gagnon and William Simon (Eds.), *Sexual Deviance* (pp. 228–244). New York: Harper and Row.
Assiter, Alison, & Carole, Avedon. (1993). *Bad Girls and Dirty Pictures: The Challenge to Reclaim Feminism*. London: Pluto.
Averbach, Alvin. (1973). "San Francisco's South of Market District, 1858–1958: The Emergence of a Skid Row." *California Historical Quarterly,* 52 (3), 196–223.
Baldwin, Guy. (1993a). *Ties That Bind: The SM/Leather/Fetish Erotic Style*. Los Angeles: Daedalus.
———. 1993b. *The Leather Contest Guide: A Handbook for Promoters, Contestants, Judges, and Titleholders*. Los Angeles: Daedalus.
Bayer, Ronald. (1989). *Private Acts, Social Consequences: AIDS and the Politics of Public Health*. New York: The Free Press.
Bean, Joseph W. (1988). "Changing Times South of Market." *Advocate* (California supplement), March 29, pp. 4–7.
———. (1994). *Leathersex: A Guide for the Curious Outsider and the Serious Player*. Los Angeles: Daedalus.
Bérubé, Allan. (1984a). Documents on the gay baths in San Francisco, the closure debate, and the court papers. Compilations for the San Francisco Lesbian and Gay History Project.
———. (1984b). "Don't Save Us from Our Sexuality: Placing the Bathhouse Controversy in Historical Perspective." *Coming Up!,* April.
———. (1984c). "The History of Gay Bathhouses." Declaration submitted in support of San Francisco bathhouse patrons to the Superior Court of California, November 5.
———. (1984d). "The History of the Baths." *Coming Up!,* December.
———. (1985). "Social History of Gay Male 'Bars': Saloons, Taverns, Restaurants, Night Clubs, Cabarets, Bars: Readings, 1870–1984, United States." For the San Francisco Gay Men's History Study Group.
———. (1988). "Caught in the Storm: AIDS and the Meaning of Natural Disaster." *Outlook,* Fall.

———. (1996). "The History of the Bathhouses." In Dangerous Bedfellows (Eds.), *Policing Public Sex: Queer Politics and the Future of AIDS Activism* (pp. 187–220). Boston: South End Press.

Bolton, Ralph. (1992). "AIDS and Promiscuity: Muddles in the Models of HIV Prevention." *Medical Anthropology*, 14, 145–223.

Bolton, Ralph, Vincke, John, & Mak, Rudolf. (1994). "Gay Baths Revisited: An Empirical Analysis." *GLQ: A Journal of Lesbian and Gay Studies*, 1 (2), 255–273.

Brandt, Allan M. (1985). *No Magic Bullet: A Social History of Venereal Disease in the United States since 1880*. Oxford: Oxford University Press.

———. (1988). "AIDS: From Social History to Social Policy." In Elizabeth Fee and Daniel M. Fox (Eds.), *AIDS: The Burdens of History*. (pp. 147–171). Berkeley: University of California Press.

Brighton, Carl. (1994). "Claims He Loves Leather, But . . .". Letter to the editor, *Bay Area Reporter*, 19 May, 8.

Burstyn, Varda. (1985). *Women Against Censorship*. Vancouver: Douglas and McIntyre.

Califia, Pat. 1987 (1982). "A Personal View of the Lesbian S/M Community and Movement in San Francisco." In Samois (Ed.), *Coming to Power* (pp. 243–281). Boston: Alyson.

Califia, Pat, & Fuller, Janine. (1995). *Forbidden Passages: Writings Banned in Canada*. Pittsburgh: Cleis.

Clark, Thomas R. (1987). "Labor and Progressivism 'South of the Slot': The Voting Behavior of the San Francisco Working Class, 1912–1916." *California History: The Magazine of the California Historical Society*, 66 (3), 196–207, 235–36.

"The CMC Carnival." (1977). *Drummer*, pp. 20, 74–77.

Conkin, Dennis. (1996). "SoMa Bashing Trial Begins." *Bay Area Reporter*, October 24, p. 2.

Cook, Joe. (1977). "Famous Dungeons of San Francisco." *Drummer*, pp. 17, 8–11.

"Criminalizing Gay Sex." (1992). *The Pink Paper*, February 23, p. 9.

Crimp, Douglas (Ed.) (1988a). *AIDS: Cultural Analysis, Cultural Activism*. Cambridge, Massachusetts: MIT Press.

———. (1988b). "How to Have Promiscuity in an Epidemic." In Douglas Crimp (Ed.), *AIDS: Cultural Analysis, Cultural Activism* (pp. 237–271). Cambridge, Massachusetts: MIT Press.

"The Death of Leather." (1985). *San Francisco Focus*, November.

DeBlase, Anthony F. (1993). "Leather Concordance." Manuscript.

———. (1996). *Leather History Timeline*. Third Edition. May 10. Chicago: Leather Archives and Museum.

Deleon, Richard Edward. (1992). *Left Coast City: Progressive Politics in San Francisco, 1975–1991*. Lawrence: University Press of Kansas.

D'Emilio, John. (1983). *Sexual Politics, Sexual Communities: The Making of a Homosexual Minority in the United States, 1940–1970*. Chicago: University of Chicago Press.

———. (1989). "Gay Politics and Community in San Francisco since World War II." In Martin Bauml Duberman, Martha Vicinus, and George Chauncey Jr. (Eds.), *Hidden from History: Reclaiming the Gay and Lesbian Past* (pp. 456–473). New York: New American Library.

———. (1992). *Making Trouble: Essays on Gay History, Politics, and the University*. New York: Routledge.

D'Emilio, John, & Freedman, Estelle B. (Eds.) (1988). *Intimate Matters: A History of Sexuality in America*. New York: Harper and Row.

Duberman, Martin Bauml, Vicinus, Martha, & Chauncey, George Jr. (Eds.). (1989). *Hidden from History: Reclaiming the Gay and Lesbian Past*. New York: New American Library.

Duggan, Lisa, & Hunter, Nan. (1995). *Sex Wars.* New York: Routledge.

Ellis, Havelock. (1942). *Studies in the Psychology of Sex.* Vol. 1. New York: Random House.

———. (1937). *Studies in the Psychology of Sex.* Vol. 2. New York: Random House.

Evans, Arthur. (1982). Letter to the editor, *Bay Area Reporter,* November 24, p. 6.

Evans-Pritchard, E. E. (1976). *Witchcraft, Oracles, and Magic among the Azande.* Oxford: Clarendon Press.

Farmer, Paul. (1992). *AIDS and Accusation: Haiti and the Geography of Blame.* Berkeley: University of California Press.

Fee, Elizabeth, & Fox, Daniel M. (Eds.). (1988). *AIDS: The Burdens of History.* Berkeley: University of California Press.

———. (1992). *AIDS: The Making of a Chronic Disease.* Berkeley: University of California Press.

Feldman, Douglas A., & Johnson, Thomas M. (Eds.). (1986). *The Social Dimensions of AIDS: Method and Theory.* New York: Praeger.

Feminist Anti-Censorship Taskforce. (1992 [1986]). *Caught Looking: Feminism, Pornography, and Censorship.* East Haven, CT: Long River Books.

Fitzgerald, Frances. (1987). *Cities on a Hill: A Journey through Contemporary American Cultures.* London: Picador.

Freud, Sigmund. (1966 [1905]). "The Sexual Aberrations." In *The Basic Writings of Sigmund Freud.* New York: Modern Library.

Fritscher, Jack. (1978). "Upstairs over a Vacant Lot . . . The Catacombs." *Drummer,* 23, pp. 8–11.

———. (1991). "Artist Chuck Arnett: His Life/Our Times." In Mark Thompson (Ed.), *Leatherfolk.* Boston: Alyson.

Fuller, Janine, & Blackley, Stuart. (1995). *Restricted Entry: Censorship on Trial.* Vancouver: Press Gang.

Gagnon, John, & Simon, William. (1967). *Sexual Deviance.* New York: Harper and Row.

Garber, Eric. (1990). "A Historical Directory of Lesbian and Gay Establishments in the San Francisco Bay Area."

Gebhard, Paul H. (1976 [1969]). "Fetishism and Sadomasochism." In Martin S. Weinberg (Ed.), *Sex Research: Studies from the Kinsey Institute.* New York: Oxford University Press.

Gorman, E. Michael. (1986). "The AIDS Epidemic in San Francisco: Epidemiological and Anthropological Perspectives." In Craig R. Janes, Ron Stall, & Sandra M. Gifford (Eds.), *Anthropology and Epidemiology: Interdisciplinary Approaches to the Study of Health and Disease.* Boston: D. Reidel Publishing.

Gregersen, Edgar. (1969). "The Sadomasochistic Scene." Talk delivered at the annual meeting of the American Anthropological Association. New Orleans.

———. (1983). *Sexual Practices: The Story of Human Sexuality.* New York: Franklin Watts.

Hamilton, Angus. (1992). "Criminalizing Gay Sex." *The Pink Paper,* February 23, p. 9.

Hamilton, Art. (n.d.). *The Fist Fucker's Manual.* New York: Mark Distributors.

Harry, Joseph. (1974). "Urbanization and the Gay Life." *Journal of Sex Research,* 10 (3), pp. 238–247.

Harry, Joseph, & DeVall, William B. (1978). *The Social Organization of Gay Males.* New York: Praeger.

Hartman, Chester. (1974). *Yerba Buena: Land Grab and Community Resistance in San Francisco.* San Francisco: Glide Publications.

———. (1984). *The Transformation of San Francisco.* Totowa, NJ: Rowman & Allanheld.

Herdt, Gilbert. (1992). *Gay Culture in America: Essays from the Field.* Boston: Beacon Press.

Herdt, Gilbert, & Lindenbaum, Shirley. (Eds.). (1992). *The Time of AIDS: Social Analysis, Theory, and Method*. Newbury Park, CA: Sage.

Hernandez, Marcus. (1989). "Mr. Marcus: A New Gay Leather Bar Opens South of Market." *Bay Area Reporter*, September 14, p. 38.

———. (1990a). "Mr. Marcus." *Bay Area Reporter*, February 1.

———. (1990b). "Mr. Marcus: Something Old, Something New." *Bay Area Reporter*, August 18, pp. 55–57.

———. (1990c). "Mr. Marcus: Heading into the New Year, But First . . ." *Bay Area Reporter*, December 20, p. 61.

———. (1991). "Mr. Marcus: Southern Scandals." *Bay Area Reporter*, April 4, pp. 19–20.

Herrman, Bert. (1991). *Trust: The Hand Book; A Guide to the Sensual and Spiritual Art of Handballing*. San Francisco: Alamo Square Press.

Hooker, Evelyn. (1967). "The Homosexual Community." In John Gagnon & William Simon (Eds.). *Sexual Deviance*. New York: Harper and Row.

Jay, A. (1976). "Folsom Street: San Francisco's Leather Lane." *QQ*, September/October, pp. 25–27, 44–47.

Kinsella, James. (1989). *Covering the Plague: AIDS and the American Media*. New Brunswick, NJ: Rutgers University Press.

Knapp, Don. (1983). "A 20 Year Cycle." *Bay Area Reporter*, March 10, p. 13.

Krafft-Ebing, R. von. (1899). *Psychopathia Sexualis*. Philadelphia: F. A. Davis Company.

Lauritsen, John, & Wilson, Hank. (1986). *Death Rush: Poppers and AIDS*. New York: Pagan Press.

Leathers, Rick. (1980). "Two Nations—One Territory: S&M vs. Leather." *DungeonMaster*, 5, July, pp. 1–2.

Lederer, Laura (Ed.) (1980). *Take Back the Night: Women on Pornography*. New York: Morrow.

Mains, Geoff. (1984). *Urban Aboriginals: A Celebration of Leathersexuality*. San Francisco: Gay Sunshine Press.

———. (1988). "View from a Sling." *Drummer* 121.

———. (1989). *Gentle Warriors*. Stamford, CT: Knights Press.

Mariah, Paul. (1978). *This Light Will Spread: Selected Poems 1960–1975*. South San Francisco: ManRoot.

Mendenhall, George. (1981). "Police Misconduct Increases: Trouble in Ringold Alley." *Bay Area Reporter*, November 24, pp. 1, 5.

"Morality, AIDS, and the Bathhouses," (1985). *New York Times*. November 19, 18.

Murray, Stephen O. (1979). "The Institutional Elaboration of a Quasi-Ethnic Community." *International Review of Modern Sociology*, July–December.

———. (1989). "'Scientific Evidence' and Moralism in the San Francisco Bathhouse Closure." San Francisco: Instituto Obregon.

———. (1992a). "Components of Gay Community in San Francisco." In Gilbert Herdt (Ed.), *Gay Culture in America: Essays from the Field*. Boston: Beacon.

Murray, Stephen O., & Payne, Kenneth W. (1988). "Medical Policy without Scientific Evidence: The Promiscuity Paradigm and AIDS." *California Sociologist*, 11 (1/2), 13–54.

———. 1989. "The Social Classification of AIDS in American Epidemiology." *Medical Anthropology*, 10, 115–128.

Nardi, Peter M. (Ed.). (1988). *California Sociologist*, 11(1–2) (special issue).

"N.Y. Health Chief Resigns in Dispute over AIDS." (1985). *San Francisco Chronicle*, December 5, p. 31.

Norwood, Jim. (1986). "A Preliminary Examination of Sexual Behavioral Changes in San Francisco's S/M Community Five Years after the Onset of AIDS." Paper presented to KISS/M, San Francisco.

Odets, Walt. (1995). *In the Shadow of the Epidemic: Being HIV-Negative in the Age of AIDS*. Durham: Duke University Press.

"Off-Beat Rough Toward Chic Very Fine." (1988). *New York Times,* September 15.

Ortner, Sherry B. (1973). "On Key Symbols." *American Anthropologist,* 75, 1338–1346.

Patton, Cindy. (1985). *Sex and Germs: The Politics of AIDS.* Boston: South End Press.

———. (1990). *Inventing AIDS.* New York: Routledge.

———. (1996). *Fatal Advice: How Safe-Sex Education Went Wrong.* Durham: Duke University Press.

Robinson, Frank. (1984). "A Horror Story and a Challenge." *Coming Up!,* April, p. 10.

Rofes, Eric. (1996). *Reviving the Tribe: Regenerating Gay Men's Sexuality and Culture in the Ongoing Epidemic.* New York: Harrington Park Press.

Root-Bernstein, Robert. (1993). *Rethinking AIDS: The Tragic Cost of Premature Consensus.* New York: The Free Press.

Rubin, Gayle S. (1982 [1981]), "The Leather Menace." In Samois, ed. *Coming to Power.* Boston: Alyson.

———. (1984a). "The Valley of the Kings." *Sentinel USA,* September 14.

———. (1984b). "The Valley of the Kings: Sexual Identity and Community Formation." Paper presented at the annual meeting of the American Anthropological Association, Denver.

———. (1984c). "Thinking Sex." In Carole Vance (Ed.), *Pleasure and Danger.* New York: Routledge and Kegan Paul.

———. (1989). "Requiem for the Valley of the Kings." *Southern Oracle,* fall.

———. (1990). "The Catacombs: Temple of the Butthole." *Drummer,* 139, May, pp. 28–34.

———. (1991). "The Catacombs: A Temple of the Butthole." In Mark Thomson (Ed.), *Leatherfolk* (pp.) Boston: Alyson.

———. (1993a). "Misguided, Dangerous, and Wrong: An Analysis of Anti-Pornography Politics." In Allison Assiter & Avedon Carol (Eds.), *Bad Girls and Dirty Pictures: The Challenge to Radical Feminism.* London: Pluto.

———. (1993b). Afterword to "Thinking Sex." In Linda S. Kauffman (Ed.), *American Feminist Thought at Century's End: A Reader.* Cambridge, MA: Blackwell.

———. (1993c). Postscript to "Thinking Sex." In Henry Abelove, Michele Aina Barale, & David M. Halperin (Eds.), *The Lesbian and Gay Studies Reader.* New York: Routledge.

———. (1994). *The Valley of the Kings: Leathermen in San Francisco, 1960–1990.* Doctoral dissertation, Department of Anthropology, University of Michigan.

R/UDAT (Regional/Urban Design Assistance Team). (1984). *South of Market Analysis.* San Francisco: Urban Planning and Design Committee of the American Institute of Architects.

"Sado-masochists Jailed for 'Degrading' Sex Acts." (1990). *The Guardian,* December.

Samois. (1979). *What Color Is Your Handkerchief?* Berkeley, CA: Author.

———. (1982 [1981]). *Coming to Power.* Boston: Alyson.

"S&M Is Illegal in England." (1992). *Growing Pains,* May, 1–2.

San Francisco Redevelopment Agency. (1952). *The Feasibility of Redevelopment in the South of Market Area.* June 1.

Saroyan, Wayne A. (1989). "Glory Days South of Market." *San Francisco Chronicle,* January 1, review section, p. 6.

Segal, Lynne & McIntosh, Mary. (1992). *Sex Exposed: Sexuality and the Pornography Debate.* London: Virago.

Schweikhart, Gary. (1984). "Shilts Responds to Critics." *The Sentinel,* March 29, pp. 1, 3–4.

Shilts, Randy. (1984a). "Gay Campaign to Ban Sex in Bathhouses." *San Francisco Chronicle,* March 28, pp. 1, 20.

———. (1984b). "Politics and Bathhouses: Local Complexities." *San Francisco Chronicle,* January 15, This World section, pp. 15–16.

———. (1984c). "Psychologist Gary Walsh Dies." *San Francisco Chronicle*, February 22, p. 22.

———. (1984d). "Silverman Delays on Gay Bathhouses." *San Francisco Chronicle*, March 31, p. 1, 10.

———. (1984e). "Silverman Feeling Bathhouse Heat." *San Francisco Chronicle*, March 29, p. 2.

———. (1987). *And the Band Played On: Politics, People, and the AIDS Epidemic.* New York: St. Martin's Press.

Smith, Ted. (1983). Letter to the editor. *Bay Area Reporter*, August 18, p. 8.

Snitow, Ann, Stansell, Christine, & Thompson, Sharon. (1983). *Powers of Desire*. New York: Monthly Review.

Starkey, Ray. (1983). *Bay Area Reporter*, April 14, p. 9.

Styles, Joseph. (1979). "Outsider/Insider: Researching Gay Baths." *Urban Life*, 8(2), 135–152.

Thompson, Bill. (1994). *Sadomasochism*. London: Cassell.

Thompson, Don. (1994). "The Greatest Leather Show!" *San Francisco Bay Times*. September 22, p. 50.

Thompson, Mark. (1982). "Folsom Street." *Advocate*, July 8, pp. 28–31, 57.

———. (1991). *Leatherfolk: Radical Sex, People, Politics, and Practice.* Boston: Alyson.

Triechler, Paula. (1988). "AIDS, Homophobia, and Biomedical Discourse: An Epidemic of Signification." In Douglas Crimp (Ed.), *Cultural Analysis, Cultural Activism.*

Truscott, Carol. (1990). "San Francisco: A Reverent, Non-Linear, Necessarily Incomplete History of the S/M Scene." *Sandmutopia Guardian and Dungeon Journal*, p. 8.

Vance, Carole S. (Ed.). (1984). *Pleasure and Danger: Exploring Female Sexuality.* Boston: Routledge & Kegan Paul.

———. (1986a). "Meese Commission: The Porn Police Attack." *Gay Community News*, July 27–August 2, p. 3.

———. (1986b). "Porn in the USA: The Meese Commission on the Road." *The Nation*, August 2–9, pp. 1, 76–82.

———. (1989). "The War on Culture." *Art in America*, December, pp. 39–45.

———. (1990a). "Misunderstanding Obscenity." *Art in America*, May, pp. 49–55.

———. (1990b). "Negotiating Sex and Gender in the Attorney General's Commission on Pornography." In Faye Ginsburg & Anna L. Tsing (Eds.), *Uncertain Terms: Negotiating Gender in American Culture.* Boston: Beacon Press.

———. (1990c). "Reagan's Revenge: Restructuring the NEA." *Art in America*, November, pp. 49–55.

———. (1990d). "The Pleasures of Looking: The Attorney General's Commission on Pornography vs. Visual Images." In Carole Squiers (Ed.), *The Critical Image: Essays in Contemporary Photography.* Seattle: Bay Press.

———. (1993). "Feminist Fundamentalism: Women Against Images." *Art in America*, September, pp. 35–39.

Vollmer, Timothy. (1981). *Male Images: The Politics of Gender.* Senior honors thesis, Department of Anthropology, University of California.

Waddell, Tom. (1984). "The Simian Connection: A Possible Link to AIDS." *Coming Up!* April, p. 12.

Watney, Simon. (1987). *Policing Desire: Pornography, AIDS, and the Media.* Minneapolis: University of Minnesota Press.

Weeks, Jeffrey. (1981). *Sex, Politics, and Society: The Regulation of Sexuality since 1800.* London: Longman.

Weinberg, Martin. (1976). *Sex Research: Studies from the Kinsey Institute.* New York: Oxford University Press.

Weinberg, Martin, & Williams, Colin. (1974). *Male Homosexuals: Their Problems and Adaptations.* New York: Oxford University Press.

————. (1975). "Gay Baths and the Social Organization of Impersonal Sex." *Social Problems,* 23(2), 124–136.

Weinberg, Martin S., Williams, Colin J., & Moser, Charles. (1984). "The Social Constituents of Sadomasochism." *Social Problems,* 31(4), 379–89.

Weinberg, Thomas. (1987). "Sadomasochism in the United States: A Review of the Recent Sociological Literature." *Journal of Sex Research,* 23(1), 50–69.

Weinberg, Thomas, & Levi Kamel, G. W. (1983). *S and M: Studies in Sadomasochism.* Buffalo: Prometheus Books.

White, Edmund. (1980). *States of Desire.* New York: Bantam.

Wockner, Rex. (1991a). "London S/M Gays Fight Oppression." *Bay Area Reporter,* February 21, p. 20.

————. (1991b). "SM Crackdown in London." *Bay Area Reporter,* January 24, p. 16.

Woods, Chris. (1992), "SM Sex Was a Crime, Court Rules." *Capital Gay,* February 21.

Government Reports
Attorney General's Commission on Pornography. (1986). *Final Report.* Washington, DC: U.S. Department of Justice.

Law Commission. (1995). *Consent in the Criminal Law: Consultation Paper 139.* London: HMSO.

Special Committee on Pornography and Prostitution. (1985). *Pornography and Prostitution in Canada.* Ottawa: Canadian Government Publishing Center.

Interviews (conducted by the author)
Tony DeBlase (1993).
Scott Tucker (1991).

Legal Cases
People v. Samuels, 250 Cal. App. 2d 501; 58 Cal. Rptr. 439 (1967).
R v. Butler 8CRR(2)1(SCC) (1992).
R v. Brown and other Appeals 2 All ER 75 (1993).

Owning an Epidemic: the Impact of AIDS on Small-City Lesbian and Gay Communities

BETH E. SCHNEIDER

Like most of the history of the contemporary lesbian and gay movement and politics, the stories told, the activism described, the models promoted, and the problems delineated about the impact of HIV/AIDS on lesbian/gay communities in the United States are stories of the crisis in San Francisco, Los Angeles, New York. (See, among others, Altman, 1987; Kramer, 1989; Petrow, 1990; Patton, 1990; Kayal, 1993). This is not wholly unreasonable. These cities represent the sites of our largest lesbian/gay communities, and the places where the first cases were identified. Although each of these cities has its own story (and they do differ in some essential ways from one another), there are however, few other places that compare to them.[1]

Nevertheless, AIDS is widespread in the United States. Initially a bicoastal disease limited to large metropolitan centers, AIDS has since diffused to other cities, smaller towns, and rural areas. For example, in New York state, AIDS is spreading faster now on a percentage basis in smaller cities than in larger ones ("Rural New York and HIV," 1992). By 1991, 80 percent of all new cases in the United States were outside the major metropolitan areas. And using geographical mapping techniques, Gould (1991) demonstrated corridor effects not just along the Boston-to-Miami route, but from large urban centers to rural areas along high-speed road, rail and air linkages. He estimated that at least one case of HIV existed in 98 percent of the 3,300 counties in the United States.

In addition to large cities that are the primary focus of media portrayals and most lesbian/gay writing, there are a number of small cities

In addition to the participants at the Rancho Santa Fe conference, I wish to thank the members of the 1994 University of California, Santa Barbara AIDS Research Group (Lyn Gesch, Glyn Hughes, Matt Mutchler, Joe Rollins, and Tim Wun) for their careful reading and many suggestions.

with relatively large AIDS caseloads for populations with fewer than fifty thousand residents, among which are several recognized gay resorts and gay-friendly cities such as Key West, Florida; West Hollywood, California; Laguna Beach, California; Palm Springs, California; and North Fort Myers, Florida; with a significant number of Black homosexual men with AIDS.

In this chapter, I am interested in the extent to which lesbian/gay communities take "ownership" of AIDS. By "ownership," I mean if and how people identified as lesbian, gay or bisexual treat AIDS as a community problem, consider work on AIDS prevention and service provision part of lesbian/gay political activity, and devote time, money, and organizational resources to confronting the multifaceted aspects of the illness.

More specifically, I explore a variety of approaches to the problem of AIDS by lesbian and gay people and organizations in small cities and rural areas not known as gay-friendly. To the extent possible, I examine the similarities and differences between the problems and politics of the epicenters and these other locales. I begin with a summary of the conclusions drawn by lesbian and gay activists, journalists and scholars on the impact of AIDS in the lesbian/gay community, noting (1) that the focus is almost always either New York or San Francisco; (2) that considerable energy is invested in debates about the politics of AIDS organizations; and (3) that much of this writing takes the notion of community for granted and tends to ignore the possibility of multiple community responses to AIDS. Then I examine what has been written about AIDS outside the epicenters, taking special note of "coming home" stories and their meaning for understanding the impact of AIDS in small cities and towns.

Next I present four case studies. I constructed two cases using at least one method—participant observation, interviews, and media analysis. In the two other cases, I borrowed from stories told by others in previously published work (Hackney, 1991; Miller, 1989). The sketches of these four sites during the years between 1985 and 1991 reveal several strategies utilized by gay men and lesbians in small cities and towns when confronting the problem of HIV/AIDS.

What becomes clear is that some features of the response to AIDS closely resemble those of the larger cities in the early years of the epidemic. Other aspects seem uniquely structured by complex interconnections between a city's size, regional location, extent of urbanism, number of AIDS cases, distance from the epicenters, and more political factors such as the presence of an intensely organized Christian fundamentalist populace and the degree of visibility and extent of cultural infrastructure of lesbian/gay communities. The cases focus on Bismarck, North Dakota; Gainesville, Florida; Lexington, Kentucky; and Santa Barbara, California. Examination of these four cases reveals a pattern of increasing ownership of AIDS by individuals in the gay and lesbian community and by its institutions. But even when the conditions seem least favorable for "ownership," the community resources sparse, and government agencies the major players, gay and lesbian people have been at the hub of AIDS-related activity.

The Epicenter Experience

Central to the writing about the experience of AIDS in the epicenters in the late 1980s are descriptions of escalating disaster (Berube, 1988; Foster, 1988; Kramer, 1989). One example, from among many, reads:

> This rapid growth in the incidence of AIDS cases sends shock waves through the communities most severely affected. Quickly people in these areas and risk groups come to know personally someone who is sick and, soon thereafter, several people. . . . This phenomenon was seen first and most dramatically in some of the gay communities of New York and San Francisco . . . where young gay men "buried" thirty or more friends in just a few years' time (Drucker, 1991:46–47).

Certainly early in the epidemic the loss of large numbers of men in a relatively short time preoccupied most participants and observers (Kramer, 1989; Levine, 1992). But very quickly, additional dynamics were noticed and analyzed.

In addition to the deaths, AIDS was understood in the first several years to have taken tremendous sacrifices of survivors' money, time, and careers, diverted people from doing gay and lesbian political work, and drained financial resources from gay organizations (Altman, 1987; Cruikshank, 1992). The tendency to focus on sacrifice and diversion has not disappeared; it is part of an ongoing and heated dialogue in major media and in many lesbian and gay organizations about the potential and actual impact of AIDS on the marginalization and underfunding of gay rights and sexual liberation issues and on the direction and pace of community development (Rist, 1989; Rofes, 1989; Vaid, 1995; Winnow, 1989).

Emerging at the same time as this litany of problems was the emphasis on the positive consequences of the epidemic. Beginning with speeches at the 1987 Lesbian and Gay March in Washington, some argued that AIDS demonstrated the need for an active and vibrant lesbian and gay movement. It mobilized the community around a single threat, involving those who had not been politically active before as volunteers or financial supporters or activists (Kayal, 1993; Omoto & Crain, 1995), and unified lesbians and gay men in cooperative efforts previously unseen in many cities and in national political arenas (Schneider, 1992). Lesbian and gay leadership increased in visibility and power. AIDS also stimulated personal transformations for gay men, especially for those whose identity centered on sex (Adam, 1992). As Miller (1989:135) observed, AIDS created

> a new basis for community among gay men . . . a community founded on caring. And AIDS was bringing individuals into organized gay life who had never been involved before. . . . the new breed of AIDS activists were not only to be found in New York and Boston and San Francisco. They were also in small towns and mid-size cities and among gays of color.

Many people, HIV infected or not, felt it was time to come out of the closet. Lesbian/gay community-based service organizations were sustained and a new politics emerged, focused on working directly and collaboratively with government (Foster, 1988; Petrow, 1990; Altman, 1994). AIDS propelled the political lobbying efforts of the gay and lesbian community at all levels of government (Altman, 1987; Vaid, 1995).

Institutional growth is one very important outcome of the crisis. New media and organizations of all types—social, cultural, political—emerged. Of crucial relevance to the analysis here is the prideful assertion (and it surely is something to be proud of) that hundreds of organizations have sprung up to assist people with AIDS. Altman (1994), a decade into the epidemic, argues forcefully that these organizations could not have existed without the extensive political organizing in the 1970s by lesbian and gay-identified people. The Gay Men's Health Crisis (GMHC), the first freestanding AIDS service organization, reported on its programs as a model for others to follow (Katoff et al., 1991); in both western Europe and the United States, AIDS organizations emulated GMHC's work (Altman, 1994). The San Francisco experience, with its decentralized, but vast specialization of health and community organizations for people with AIDS and its collaboration of public health officials and the affected communities, was considered the exemplar of a municipal response to AIDS service provision and prevention for the country (Petrow, 1990; Fernandez, 1991).

Yet at the same time, considerable controversy in the large cities has developed about the politics of the AIDS service organizations, most of which were created or transformed from other organizations by the very single-minded efforts of members of the gay and lesbian community in the early years of the epidemic. AIDS educational and social service organizations (e.g., Gay Men's Health Crisis, Shanti, San Francisco AIDS Foundation, AIDS Project Los Angeles, AIDS Action Council, Whitman-Walker Clinic, among many others) marshaled the energy of politically aware volunteers to provide caregiving for people with AIDS (Kobasa, 1991; Kayal, 1993). Over the last decade, these organizations have become enormous, bureaucratic, and wealthy, with volunteers playing relatively less of a leadership role, professional staff more of one. Often the most powerful organization in a major city with roots in the gay community is an AIDS social service organization with a budget in the millions and thousands of volunteers (Altman, 1994; King, 1993). Nationally, organizational practice and public relations strategies vary in how much they identify as gay community organizations.

It is this question of organizational identity and culture that has been so contentious. Many AIDS activists have raised crucial issues about the relationship of AIDS organizations to lesbian and gay communities (Callen, 1990; Kramer, 1989; Patton 1990; Rofes, 1989). In their writings, they observe that many of these organizations publicly claim they are not gay organizations at all, although they were founded by gay and lesbian activists and the majority of the staff and their volunteers are gay men and lesbians. This substantial participation is minimized for public relations purposes. Many have lost direct and obvious public links to the grassroots as they became increasingly reliant on government funds. For some, there is a purposeful "degaying" of the organizational culture and identity in the interests of seeking broader support and funding, often through the continual assertion that "AIDS is not a gay disease" (King, 1993). Some critics see the loss of a political agenda accompanying these decisions ("hiding behind their 501C3 tax exemption") and point to the obvious contradictions between these actions and the movement agenda of ending homophobia, coming out in all contexts, and taking credit for doing the monumental job of confronting AIDS, especially in the provision of effective AIDS education and prevention.[2]

In sum, most of the writing about the impact of AIDS in the major cities takes for granted the existence of a gay and lesbian community with a developed organizational infrastructure and a history of political struggle, publicly known gay leaders, and multiple organizations already serving a wide range of social, political and service-related needs. The profile assumes that there is cultural freedom for the expression of multiple viewpoints, including debates about AIDS service organizations and their relationship to governmental agencies and to groups of people with AIDS. Lastly, the writing assumes that AIDS has made an enormous difference in the lives of lesbians and gay men through personal loss as well as through the involvement of some community members in political spheres from which they had previously been absent (Altman, 1994; Schneider, 1992).

Outside the Epicenter

> In San Francisco and New York City, the battle against AIDS has been a Verdun, with trench lines everywhere and the dead carried daily off the field. But in much of the rest of America, AIDS came as it did in Kokomo and Swansea, a seemingly random shot from a sniper's rifle. "Why here?" those in the heartland asked themselves, for even as AIDS sprang up in more and more places, it was still entirely unexpected wherever it appeared, the uninvited guest who upends the party. The disease struck, not the many, but a single friend or neighbor (Kirp, 1989:17).

In their documentation of the reactions to HIV-positive schoolchildren and their families in numerous small towns and large cities, Kirp et al. (1989) demonstrate both the acceptance as well as the hostility generated by the disease. In grappling with the problem of AIDS, communities had to struggle over how they would understand AIDS, whether as a gay disease or something else, and in these struggles ("dramas of innocence and pollution") confront their deeply embedded cultural ambivalence about homosexuals and homosexuality.

Ambivalence and hostility are common throughout the country, though they are presumed to be far more widespread in nonmetropolitan areas. This belief supports the myth that all the lesbians and gay men from small cities and towns have moved to bigger cities. And certainly many have done so to seek greater employment opportunities and avoid the constraints of small-town life. Although there are a few small towns that are unusual, such as the resort or college communities of Northampton, Key West, or Provincetown, all known for their gay-friendliness, most small cities and towns are not so solicitous. Though these locales vary widely in how much diversity is tolerated, in most lesbians and gays are hesitant to come out (though a considerable number do) and they are far less organized in ways that give them continual visibility. When possible, they travel to large cities for sex, relationships, and gay culture.

Yet despite potential and actual work discrimination, harassment, silence, and social oppression, there are lesbian and gay communities in many unlikely places; small cities often have chapters of ACT-UP or Queer Nation, and many places have support groups, Metropolitan Community Churches, or gay and lesbian centers. Spiro and Lane (1992) found people in very small towns throughout the country who refuse to separate their rural identity from their lesbian or gay one, who see themselves as representing a "proud Queer presence." Fostering the growth of lesbian/gay communities in these places are factors such as the existence of colleges or universities, active feminist organizations, a gay bar, and proximity to large cities. These institutional factors are also crucial considerations in the ways in which these communities deal with AIDS.

Not only are there many lesbian and gay people firmly committed to living in these areas (Miller, 1989; Poole, 1992), but now the disease has created patterns of migration to hometowns (see Verghese, 1993, for an example of a small community facing the problem of the return of its sick sons; see also Davis & Stapleton, 1991). In conversations with gay men in rural Minnesota, Miller (1989) found that some are staying in rural areas when they might have moved to the cities and others are moving back to rural areas because of AIDS; they claim they are safer, that there are fewer opportunities for sexual contact. The decision to stay or the decision to return frequently brings about a reconciliation with families. Sometimes gay men can no longer tolerate the devastation of their social networks in New York or San Francisco. At other times they return to die in a familiar place at the home of their biological family. For example, a longtime volunteer at GMHC, Gary Cathey moved from New York to his family's farm in Minden, a town of fifteen thousand located east of Shreveport, Louisiana, where he worked with his father and managed the family's ranch (Bull, 1992).

> I felt helpless in the face of the epidemic in New York. . . . When the numbers began to expand exponentially and many of my friends started dying, it was just too much to take. . . . I went home to get away from the epidemic.

But restless there, he founded the Shreveport chapter of ACT-UP in a political district that had paid little attention to AIDS.

The Cathey story is not so unusual as it might seem. The gay press is full of obituaries of young men who left San Francisco or Los

Angeles and, for example, "died peacefully at the home where he grew up in Leola, Pa., after a valiant struggle with AIDS." Though in rural America, "the fear of being found out" (as gay, as a person with AIDS) "is almost as great as the fear of the disease itself" (Poole, 1992:36), those who return to their hometowns often force a confrontation with their family and with the community, especially since there is little anonymity in the smallest of towns. As Poole demonstrates in his essay on Montana, a state with no city larger than eighty thousand, people fluctuate between the denial of AIDS and acceptance of it, especially if they know the person. Many of the sons who return have come from the major cities, know what kinds of care is conceivable, and organize AIDS care networks, when none exist, as was done with the Yellowstone AIDS Project. They work with volunteers to deal with the "courtesy stigma" attendant upon this activity. They agitate to improve the often limited and certainly unspecialized care available in rural areas (Hackney, 1991; Poole, 1992).

In small cities and rural areas, lesbian and gay people, and lesbian and gay groups (when they exist) have confronted AIDS through a variety of different means. In some of the states with low incidence of AIDS cases, the social organization around both gay/lesbians and AIDS is minimal, and the environment suggests a high potential for HIV transmission due to a combination of high alcohol usage, a very closeted majority, and the use of roadside cruise areas as major sites for sex. In other places, there are thriving projects, such as the one started by a group of lesbians through the Mississippi Gay and Lesbian Alliance, which bought a home for men who returned to Jackson from the cities after a diagnosis but whose families would not take them in.

The four case studies offered here allow for an examination of how gay people in small cities grapple with the problem of AIDS and the varieties of political and organizational strategies they take in confronting this epidemic. In these cases, cities with populations under three hundred thousand are the focus, with three closer to one hundred thousand residents. None are suburbs. Each story is constructed using different combinations of available materials from among interviews, media reports, or participant observation. Two rely heavily on the published work of others. As a consequence of this opportunistic case selection, the stories read differently, as the authors or the informants tended to emphasize slightly different points. Even so, each case purposely spans approximately the same period of time, from the mid-1980s to 1991, one in which the need for AIDS organizations, and much of the controversial politics surrounding them, were intensely experienced everywhere in the United States.[3]

In looking at these cases, I attempt to account for the primary social, cultural or political features that shape a community's response to AIDS. Whenever possible, I compare the experience described in each of these cases to one another and to what is known about the epicenters' experience. Major dimensions that structure community responses include geographic locale, the proportion of the population with HIV/AIDS, size, organizational development, and political influence of the lesbian/gay community at the time of the onset of AIDS; prior relations with, and reliance on, local governmental support; and the presence of the organized religious right.

The Cases

Bismarck, North Dakota

In rural states and small cities in the mid-1980s, AIDS was considered a remote danger, a disease of the big cities, of New York and San Francisco. In North Dakota in 1987, most health officials believed that those infected likely acquired HIV from sexual contacts outside the state. There were very few drug users, and estimates of male homosexual and bisexual populations in North Dakota were around 5 percent of the total population. Health educators assumed that most gay men leave the state; most believe that those who remain are married men who live in rural areas with their wives and children, but travel on weekends for sex to larger places like Fargo, North Dakota, or Minneapolis.

In 1987, there were seven cases of AIDS reported in North Dakota; by March 1992, there were twenty-five, the fewest reported cases of any state. Nevertheless, working from lessons observed in the large cities, health and political leaders planned a campaign to build public support and state financing for tough prevention and education measures to keep North Dakota's incidence very low. As one said, "We are in a position to learn from the tragedies in New York and California" (Schmidt, 1987).

The plan, delineated in a 131-page report in 1987, included comprehensive education in public schools; mandatory testing of prisoners, prostitutes, and marriage license applicants; and privacy guarantees through new laws guarding patient confidentiality and prohibition of discrimination, a package of measures more liberal than might be expected from a conservative, relatively homogenous, and highly rural state (51.2 percent rural). One spot was explicitly set aside on the state's AIDS Task Force for a gay representative.

Because there were, and are, so few cases, the state's chief epidemiologist refused to release information usually made public, such as the age group, geographical spread or sex of the cases. He feared any such information would provide clues to the identity of the persons involved. As will become clear, this same effort to protect individuals from possible local harassment and hostility occurred in Kentucky.

Miller's (1989) description of Bismarck (population 44,485) animates the North Dakota story. At mid-decade, Bismarck had no AIDS organization or gay bar; there was no community center that served as a source for health education about AIDS and no gay/lesbian group, as there was in other small cities, such as Fargo. Under these circumstances, gay men related to AIDS by taking certain precautions (such as the avoidance of sex when they went to Minneapolis for the weekend!). But they did not practice safer sex and they persisted in the belief that they were safe in rural areas. When men they knew died, the deaths were rarely acknowledged.

According to Miller's (1989) informants, the situation was changed by one man, Darrel, who set up a library of gay books in his home after testing positive. He also replaced the one gay community representative on the task force who stepped down. His attentiveness to the need for AIDS information among people who were gay resulted in the formation of a group, The Coalition, with multiple purposes, among which were weekend "get-togethers" with meetings, workshops, and some social events. This group, whose attendance never reached beyond thirty-five, offered support, education, and safe-sex programs for the gay community and educated social workers about HIV. In North Dakota, it was primarily married gay men who were the targets of The Coalition's efforts. Darrel, among others, recognized that the homosexual activities of men in the state were underground and acted to structure educational and testing programs for that population.

In Bismarck, no existing community group addressed the problem of AIDS; no resources of an already existing organization were drawn on to confront the problem of AIDS. The Coalition was a collection of lesbian/gay people motivated by AIDS to organize themselves. It centered on one person, someone willing to be public about his status and to travel throughout the state. One person, an HIV-positive man, fashioned a lesbian/gay community in his basement, where meetings were held and the library was located. Miller (1989:94) observed:

> If it could be said that AIDS was having any kind of positive effect in North Dakota, it was that The Coalition was creating a sense of community for the first time in years. There had never been a gay bar in Bismarck, and although there was a gay and lesbian group there in the late seventies . . . it was short-lived. Until The Coalition was formed, Bismarck gay men and lesbians were just a disparate group of people, many of whom had little contact with one another.

The existence of AIDS generated whatever community there was in Bismarck. As in other small towns, one person was often enough political leadership. There was little need for an AIDS service organization during that period; volunteers were unnecessary. A social group of both lesbians and gay men owned the prevention aspect of the issue for the community. In such a context, political conflicts over the primacy of AIDS versus other gay issues were pretty much inconceivable.

Bismarck represents small cities without a lesbian/gay infrastructure. In this rural context, AIDS provided a vehicle for some mobilization, and the community it generated seems to have centered in those years on AIDS, not lesbian/gay interests. But as with virtually every other locale—in the epicenters or not—it was the community that took primary, if not exclusive, responsibility for providing safe-sex education to gay men.

Gainesville, Florida

The Gainesville case is framed by dimensions quite different from Bismarck's. Gainesville is a city of eighty-five thousand, including thirty-five thousand students of the University of Florida. Located in a state ranking third in the total national number of AIDS cases, and with an infection rate of 1 in 100, twice the national average, Gainesville's per-population AIDS cases were quite low compared to those in other Florida cities. In the late 1980s and the first years of the 1990s, there were gay and lesbian groups on the campus, engaged in struggles to retain their rights to meet and be funded, and a small gay community in the town. Neither the campus group nor the town one had as its primary focus AIDS-related work, though the gay and lesbian switchboard in town provided some AIDS information. An AIDS Institute, run by the university and headed by a prominent researcher, was set up in a private hospital.

It was the North Central Florida AIDS Network (NCFAN) that was the primary provider of AIDS education and services. This operation began in Alachua County, Gainesville's location. In the early 1990s it served all of North Central Florida's Health and Rehabilitative Services District (HRS III), a total of fourteen counties, some of the most rural in Florida. From January 1980 through June 30, 1992, the district reported 460 diagnosed AIDS cases; of these, 133 were diagnosed in Alachua County.

NCFAN developed on its own and was not the result of work by an already existing lesbian or gay organization. No lesbian or gay organization existed in 1985 from which an AIDS organization might have emerged. But some founding members were members of the lesbian/gay community, all were friends who, as a group of health professionals and significant others of HIV-positive people, recognized the need for more education for the entire community and better services for those dealing with HIV disease. My informant believed they were motivated by their knowledge that needs were not being met and that HIV was spreading quickly.

This organization relied on the professional expertise of its members in health and social work and their associations with churches, medical facilities, the gay/lesbian community, and counseling centers to develop programs, raise money, and provide resources. They developed support groups, buddy programs, HIV/AIDS education workshops, and a hot line. There was nothing else like it in the area. Later an association developed with the HRS, and the Network expanded its services to cover the entire HRS District III. Since then the state, through HRS, has been contracting with the Network to provide educational services. The association also provided a salary for one part-time office manager. All other positions were, and continue to be, staffed by volunteers.

The Network volunteer staff came from many parts of the Gainesville community. It was primarily White, approximately 50% homosexual, and approximately 40% female. The men involved were mostly gay; most of the women were heterosexual. Lesbians from the local community were only minimally involved in Network programs. My informants claim that the NCFAN had a good relationship with the very small and somewhat closeted lesbian/gay community in town. Local nightclubs held benefits regularly. For a brief period in the early 1990s, an ACT-UP chapter drew more public attention to the seriousness of AIDS, distributed condoms to teenagers, and made local lesbians aware of the lack of attention by the federal government to women's specific symptoms and the lack of education targeted at women in the area.

This level of activity was occurring in this highly rural area with a strong Christian fundamentalist religious presence. The NCFAN was forced to deal regularly with the identification of AIDS as a "gay problem." Church outreach was very difficult. At the same time, most people in Gainesville, including the lesbian- and gay-identified, did not consider NCFAN a lesbian/gay organization. My sense is that the lesbian/gay community never saw this Network, a major component of a multicounty governmental health entity, as its own organization, though lesbians and gay people were an integral part of the volunteer base. In a move prompted by the local ACT-UP and by national politics, the county hired a lesbian for the staff to demonstrate its commitment to AIDS education for the lesbian/gay community. Even so, the agency seemed to have gone out of its way to degay AIDS as did many other AIDS service organizations in the United States and Britain: through the continual assertion that AIDS is "not a gay disease" and that the organization desires to serve everyone (King, 1994).

The Gainesville experience is not unusual. On the one hand, AIDS fed on the already existing hate and generated some additional backlash in that very conservative area. Local politicians and the powerful Christian right used the epidemic to paint both lesbians and gay men as public health risks. AIDS also contributed to the defeat of a measure to include sexual orientation in the local antidiscrimination laws. At the same time, AIDS forced the community to confront how marginalized it was and contributed to a rebirth of groups and political action around lesbian/gay issues. Thus the dominant role of the network meant lesbian and gay people were doing AIDS work through a government-supported entity, and the lesbian/gay community did not "own" AIDS through community-based organizations. The nature or the activities around AIDS, and their limits, however, played a crucial role in the dynamics of the community-building and political activity in the 1990s.

Lexington, Kentucky

Hackney (1991) describes the impact of AIDS on community responses in Lexington, Kentucky, a place with approximately 12 percent of the total of 718 cases in the state (1992 data). Like Bismarck, Lexington is located in a rural (50.9 percent urban), low-incidence state. But unlike Bismarck's, the Lexington gay community in the late 1980s was somewhat organized both on and off the local campuses, even while it worked in an environment that encouraged invisibility as the price for tolerance. Unlike Gainesville, Lexington was heavily reliant from the beginning on the initiative of county health authorities and on the willingness of interested nongay social service organizations and public and private medical facilities to grapple with the epidemic. This case study is based on the Hackney analysis.

People were known to be ill in the gay community by 1984, but no mobilization by the lesbian and gay community occurred during that time. Like its counterparts elsewhere in the country, the county health department opened an alternative test site in 1985, but was slow to respond to the epidemic as it was unfolding in the gay community. There was resistance to the perceptions and concerns of the gay community throughout the decade. On its own, the local gay group, Gay and Lesbian Services Organization, held safer-sex workshops on the campus of the University of Kentucky, the gay hot line workers were trained to give AIDS-related information, and some volunteers from the gay community were trained by the hospice organization for the time when they might be needed.

The United Way rejected a request from the Gay and Lesbian Services Organization to fund AIDS prevention in the gay community because it was a "controversial group." Complaints from the gay community about the lack of funds for education resulted in a long series of meetings with the health department. Eventually its administration decided to use federal funds earmarked for states for prevention to hire one educator, the AIDS Coordinator, for one-on-one education when people came to be tested. This decision was unacceptable to gay community activists, who were working from a more collective model of education based in the experiences of the epicenter cities. It was, however, a fairly typical (and politically noncontroversial) expenditure of money in many hundreds of counties throughout the country. No other county money was targeted for education and prevention for the gay community through 1990.

Under pressure from the Episcopal Church, which was given a mandate by its national organization to do something about AIDS, the health department set up an AIDS Crisis Task Force in Lexington, providing a mailbox and a lawyer to handle incorporation papers and tax-exempt status. This task force had three goals: provide education to people with AIDS and their families, to persons judged to be at high risk, and to the "general public"; volunteer to assist people through a buddy program, counseling, and client services; support the "worried well."

In the four years of its existence documented by Hackney (1991), the task force had carried out only the educational function. Money remained unspent, the state review process of educational materials limited what was available to the most tame kind of media, grassroots involvement never materialized, and education remained pitched at the general public rather than at specific groups. Though it developed cooperative educational efforts with the local hospitals, it failed to attract volunteers and its outreach to the African American community was poor. Over the years, it had difficulties sustaining interest, it engaged in no serious fund-raising, and its educational component had no active agenda. In the city itself, there was vocal opposition by the religious right to the use of public monies to assist persons with AIDS. Consequently, the task force, with representatives from many human service and religious groups, was viewed, as it has been in most places without strong AIDS advocacy groups, as an extension of the health department and an information clearinghouse, a very weak representative of people with AIDS.

The lack of support and usefulness of the health department to the lesbian and gay community generated multiple efforts to improve conditions in Lexington. First was the development of a support group of HIV-positive men. Meeting at the county medical facilities, these men became acutely aware of their dependence on the health department for space and of the lack of anonymity involved in meeting in public places. This group eventually chose to meet in an *unadvertised* location, coordinated by a volunteer social worker, a self-help model of organization undertaken by the most affected persons that, in its practice, confirmed their fear and their invisibility.

A second effort was undertaken by the new task force president, a gay man from a larger city who initiated an AIDS awareness program for the local gay men's community in 1987. Disaster accompanied his major campaign to distribute cards with safer-sex messages, condoms, and suggestions for house parties when he notified the press of his condom distribution plan, bringing television cameras to the gay bar at which the campaign was kicked off. Customers fled the scene, the bar owner ejected the project, the task force president lost his credibility. The task force was never again willing to be involved in education efforts in the gay community.

Finally, in 1987, some members of the gay community invited a representative from Cincinnati, known in that region to have a larger, more organized gay community and as a more liberal place, to provide a "Stop AIDS" safer-sex workshop to a cross section of the community. Attendees reaffirmed a commitment to the goal of providing risk reduction and AIDS education in the gay community and plans emerged to form an organization, AIDS Volunteers of Lexington (AVOL), with officers, a board of directors and several goals: education on the epidemic and safer sex, support systems for people with AIDS, and whatever else the membership deemed necessary. This was an AIDS grassroots organization, putting the needs of the community first. The leadership of AVOL undertook fund-raising and volunteer recruitment. Frustrated with the government, the lesbian and gay community was going to take care of its own.

Soon AVOL requested that the Gay and Lesbian Services Organization "assume fiscal and corporate control in order to take advantage of GLSO's tax-exempt status and experience in handling funds" (Hackney, 1992:74). Many projects were undertaken toward the goal of giving the Lexington community the same level of care and education anyone could get in San Francisco: buddy programs, education in bars, emergency funds for limited financial assistance, self-care manuals, training for hospice care, and a residence for AIDS patients. AVOL became the home of the HIV support group and the sponsor of a family group, the latter only after assurances that its meeting location would not be revealed. Eventually the success of AVOL in fund-raising, combined with the continued fear of many members of being associated with homosexuals and homosexuality, prompted its separation from GLSO and its incorporation in 1990 as a new organization.

According to Hackney, much to the chagrin of its leadership, even after AVOL incorporated as its own group, some patients refused assistance because AIDS-related services were perceived to be gay-oriented and undesirable to patients and/or their families. The perception of the AIDS organization as a gay organization posed credibility problems for its funding and with referral sources. This is a very common dynamic even when gay men are a considerable proportion of the population served by the organization. (In Kentucky at that time, men who had sex with men comprised more than 70 percent of the reported cases.) Hackney remarks that "some of the strongest criticism that the local AIDS service groups are 'too gay' seems to be coming from professionals who are gay themselves . . ." who claim that "gays are not trustworthy or competent to handle referrals of non-gays" (1992:80).

The Lexington story illustrates how a lesbian and gay community can come to take charge of its AIDS problem out of frustration with the resistance and fear of governmental organizations, funding sources, and community members themselves. The decision to be a freestanding AIDS service organization, one heavily staffed by lesbian and gay people and previously nurtured by and fiscally facilitated by the lesbian/gay organization, was a political compromise, fraught with many of the same contradictions that have emerged over the years in the larger metropolitan areas (King, 1993; Rofes, 1990). This case also reveals the consistent reliance in small cities on organizing models and personnel from the epicenters.

Santa Barbara, California

Santa Barbara showed a different pattern of involvement with AIDS by the gay and lesbian community between 1985 and 1992. Santa Barbara represents an instance of the lesbian/gay community and its only organization "owning" AIDS from the beginning of the epidemic and refusing, even under pressure, to relinquish control. Santa Barbara is in the wide corridor between Los Angeles and San Francisco. Both places have been its model for what can be done in a gay/lesbian community. With a population of 87,000, however, Santa Barbara is the largest city in what the state considers a rural county. The university bearing its name is in a different jurisdiction and undergraduate students are not typically part of the Santa Barbara census. Nor were they active in the town community in those years.

Since 1978, the city has been home to a nonprofit organization serving some of the needs of lesbians and gay men. That organization, legally incorporated as Western Addiction Services (WAS), provided counseling for community members with drug and alcohol problems and served as a resource center and hot line for information and referrals for lesbians and gay men. It ran on a modest budget, with a contract from the county for the counseling and some donations. There were three paid staff members and never enough money. During the early 1980s, the project undertook a number of activities to enhance its reach and relevance in the gay community: a Gay Pride Banquet and Dance, and newsletter, Pride Weeks in conjunction with the Metropolitan Community Church and a gay business and professional organization. Western Addiction Services appeared on the letterhead and its officers and executive director signed all the contracts, bank agreements, and other legal papers under that name. Informally, the operation was called the Center; if someone were being precise, it was the Gay and Lesbian Resource Center.

From the beginning of Santa Barbara's response to AIDS, the sole AIDS service provider in the county was a program of Western Addiction Services. This project, the AIDS Counseling and Assistance Program (AIDSCAP), was begun through the efforts of the WAS executive director in conjunction with an openly gay county health educator who had skills in writing grant applications. The latter, who previously had made his home in Seattle and San Francisco, was already aware of the problem in the larger cities and determined to have his new city do a credible job in dealing with people with AIDS. Both were also convinced that in such a closeted town, no one else was going to undertake this work. Both saw this as a problem of gay men, a problem that belonged to the community.

AIDSCAP grew. The original contract with the state of California covered a paid staff of three, and over time, the increase in clients meant an increase in volunteers. By the late 1980s, there were the equivalent of five people working for the project, 150 volunteers, and 35 clients. Most of the staff was heterosexual, and about one-half of the men volunteering were gay. Through those early years, all but one of the clients was gay. As it developed, an increasing proportion of the time of the entire agency staff and virtually all the money contributed to the organization as a whole went to AIDS service provision. Each of the several executive directors during that period, in conjunction with a sizable number of gay/lesbian community activists involved with the University AIDS Education Task Force or the county's AIDS Task Force, spent considerable time struggling with the county over its lack of funding for prevention education for bisexual and gay men; AIDS-CAP funds were for services only. The effort to secure such monies did not prove fruitful until 1991, but the fight served to link further the politics of AIDS to the gay community.

Paradoxically, the more AIDSCAP seemed a viable project, the more status accrued to the parent organization. Increasing demands were placed on WAS to provide additional programs to a wider range of gay and lesbian people in the community; some argued that too much time was being devoted to AIDS. At the same time, many people who had become active in the community because of AIDS began to talk about wanting to separate AIDSCAP from this gay-identified group to increase its funding base among the closeted gay men of a local wealthy enclave and make its appeal broader for potential nongay clients.

In 1990, the community of lesbian and gay people who had some relationship to the center and/or to AIDSCAP suffered through a major dispute. Some members of the Board of Directors wanted to get rid of the old legal name, Western Addiction Services; it hardly reflected what the bulk of agency time or staff was devoted to, and it had no meaning in the community. No one used it except on occasion when writing checks. Instead, those members wanted to use "Gay and Lesbian Resource Center" as a name that reflected what the organization was and as a way for the primarily gay-identified organization to be more visible. Some argued that the gay and lesbian community should be proud of its work dealing with AIDS and should get credit for providing these services when no one else would; that the services were good; and that nongay clients were welcome to use them. Others whose major concern was AIDS service provision hated this plan; they believed that the change would further conflate AIDS with lesbian and gay politics, alienate rich donors, and discourage clients who were not gay men from getting access to the services. Members of both the board and the staff of the organization were in considerable anguish over this decision. Months of meetings ensued. Eventually, the board held a community meeting to announce it was voting to change the name to the Gay and Lesbian Resource Center and to affirm that AIDSCAP would continue to be its project. No staff members or volunteers abandoned the project; one board member resigned.

In the two years after that decision, the AIDSCAP project and the gay and lesbian programming grew tremendously. More money was donated to the agency overall, thousands took part in an AIDS walk, and more Latino and African American clients, both men and women who were not gay, were served. The budget continued to be heavily dominated by funds for AIDS services, but many members of the community were inspired enough by the board's decision to generate what was for such a small town an unusually large number of non-AIDS-related projects independent of Resource Center control. There were no plans to release the AIDS service component. The Center continued to insist that AIDS is everyone's disease and continued to serve any person needing assistance; most of the members with any historical sense continued to affirm the origins of its AIDS project. In many ways, the Center in those years was using its link to AIDS to try to undermine homophobia in major institutions in the community. It was the Center, along with a small ACT-UP chapter, that convinced the city and then the county to pass AIDS antidiscrimination ordinances. This required that increasing numbers of community members come out. This particular strategy resembled neither that of the other small cities presented here nor the profile of the AIDS service organizations in large cities. Even though the Center's work continued, the dual aspect of the organization's efforts subjected it to multiple, contradictory political pressures from both inside and outside the lesbian/gay community. It was, and still is, living within a rhetorical and cultural context in which claims that it is doing too much or doing too little about AIDS are justifiable, and virtually no one is satisfied with its work on lesbian/gay issues.[4]

Conclusion

"Ownership" of AIDS is not a simple matter. This examination of the stories/histories of the relationship of lesbian and gay people in small cities demonstrates the complexity and variety of the possible responses. The dramatic experience of escalating disaster occurs much more slowly in small cities and towns than in the large cities. Knowledge of AIDS cases accumulates over a longer period of time, and the likelihood that persons with AIDS will remain closeted seems greater.

Nevertheless, self-identified lesbians and gays position themselves to be part of whatever organizational and governmental response occurs. But whether and how AIDS is "owned" cannot be predicted without moving beyond the personal effort to a serious consideration of a wide range of factors, such as the presence of a visible lesbian/gay organization, the existence of facilitating institutions such as colleges and feminist organizations, and the kind of county or state public health response to the epidemic. These stories suggest that smaller places are much more likely than larger ones to be reliant on government funds or agencies. They are less likely to have the breadth and depth of private donors who could fund AIDS prevention education and, consequently, provide targeted AIDS education for the gay population.

And yet lesbian and gay individuals and/or groups did provide that education, seeing it as a commitment and responsibility of kinship and fellowship, and as a right gay men deserved. The commitment to AIDS is not surprising. In the United States, gay and lesbian communities of all sizes and in every part of the country are linked to each other through media, conferences, and professional and social organizations of all types, and at major events such as Pride Marches and Gay Games. Models of AIDS activism and AIDS service provision from the AIDS epicenters are readily available to those at the periphery. Even controversies with major relevance at the core can find their way to the smaller contexts.

With regard to AIDS, additional linkages are available. In the four cases, the smaller cities relied on materials and programs of more major metropolitan areas (not necessarily New York or San Francisco, but Minneapolis and Cincinnati) to assist with their AIDS prevention programs. The breadth of services of Shanti and Gay Men's Health Crisis is yearned for and, to the extent possible given certain features of their locales, frequently offered.

An issue that is shared by all places grappling with AIDS is the perception of AIDS as a gay disease or the perception of an AIDS organization as gay-oriented (Patton, 1996). This is a major issue in the large cities, one that has fueled the debate about the degaying of AIDS. But it is similarly a problem in the smaller cities. In Gainesville, Lexington, and Santa Barbara, how much to hide the gay participation, leadership, or ownership of AIDS in an organization serving people with AIDS is no less a controversial matter, one that gets resolved differently depending on the history of the organization involved (state-initiated, gay-initiated AIDS organization, or lesbian/gay). The struggle may be less intense than those in the overheated political atmosphere of New York or San Francisco, but as the Santa Barbara example illustrates, the struggle is no less crucial to the survival of the lesbian/gay community.

AIDS has had a major impact on small cities and towns in ways both similar and different from its impact on the epicenter. The need to have a response to AIDS motivated the growth of community in Bismarck; the lack of control over AIDS generated new community activism in Gainesville; the separation of AIDS services from gay services in Lexington raised questions about the power of the community; the overlap of AIDS work and gay work in Santa Barbara and the need to acknowledge the gay ownership sharpened the political profile of the Center in those particular years.

In the larger places, AIDS generated the activism and the organizational growth, but it was not the pivotal factor operating to generate and/or change the nature of lesbian/gay politics and community. In the smaller places, AIDS seems to have made a *disproportionately* greater impact on bringing people out of the closet, creating activists where none existed, and making visible the presence of gay people.

AIDS, coupled with the hostility of the religious right to funding for AIDS education and to gay people generally, has changed the character of lesbian and gay lives. Self-identified gay men and lesbians have individually asserted an "ownership" of the epidemic through volunteering to provide services and AIDS education. Collectively, a profile of the "ownership" of AIDS reveals a less consistent, politically complicated pattern in the small cities and towns. Where an organized gay base was absent, communities had a difficult time establishing AIDS organizations. Nevertheless, as Altman (1994:9) provocatively suggests, there is an important distinction between community-based organizations and AIDS service organizations, with the former implying "political representation and empowerment" for the community being served. In this regard, the smaller cities with their smaller AIDS projects are absolutely and relatively resource poor, but they offer the possibility for more direct engagement by lesbian and gay people.

In one respect, lesbians and gay men have been at the forefront of prevention efforts everywhere in the country. With government funding withheld from gay-positive education, most communities have managed their prevention work on private funds and volunteer time. Though the lessons of San Francisco are repeatedly cited as the model for community action (Petrow, 1990), each city has had to labor to generate its own program for its particular conditions. To the extent that lesbians and gay men are central to these activities—and it is my contention that even in the smallest, least well-organized places they are—lesbian and gay communities "own" AIDS.

Notes

1. The epicenters vary in some fundamental ways. San Francisco has a much higher proportion of cases of HIV/AIDS to the population than New York or Los Angeles, though New York and Los Angeles each has more overall cases. The cities vary in the degree to which the lesbian and gay communities are visible and have economic and political power. The profile of the epidemic is quite different. The cities in California are still looking, fifteen years into the epidemic, at close to 90 percent of their cases among men who had sex with men, whereas now in New York one-half of the cases are related to injection drug use; also, a far greater proportion of the cases in New York are among people from African American and Latino populations.

2. In more than one conversation, Matt Mutchler (University of California, Santa Barbara) pointed out the necessity of these components in the successful development of AIDS prevention education for young gay men.

3. These cases were not updated, leaving us with a rather abrupt end to each of the narratives. Considerable work would be necessary to follow the trajectory of each city through the 1990s, particularly in the wake of the changing cultural and political climate in the country generally and with regard to AIDS.

4. I am familiar with more of the Santa Barbara story, only some of which can be told here. The Resource Center expanded to set up AIDSCAP offices in what is called "North County," the more conservative part of the county, focusing even further staff time and resources on AIDS. The Pride Mission, a project by and for young gay men to generate community and foster safe sex, was motivated by researchers from the University of California, San Francisco. This removed much of the burden of AIDS education for the gay community from the Center. And two group houses for people with HIV/AIDS without homes opened, taking donations that might have been given to AIDSCAP. After a brief flurry of gay-related activity, the Center has returned to providing only counseling for lesbians and gays and a hot line. By 1995, all the major projects in the city—the film festival, National Coming Out Day, the Pride events—were organized by people who at one time were involved with the Center but who were now working independently.

Though the board does not say as much, the Center staff and time are almost wholly devoted to AIDS. Once again, the name of the parent organization has been changed (to the Pacific Pride Foundation), and the Center is now a project of the larger organization.

References

Adam, Barry. (1992). "Sex and Caring among Men: Impacts of AIDS on Gay People." In K. Plummer (Ed.), *Modern Homosexualities* (pp. 175–183). New York: Routledge.

Adam, Barry. (1995). *The Rise of a Gay and Lesbian Movement.* (Revised Edition). Boston: G. K. Hall.

Altman, Dennis. (1994). *Power and Community: Organizational and Cultural Responses to AIDS.* London: Taylor and Francis.

Altman, Dennis. (1987). *AIDS in the Mind of America.* Garden City, NY: Anchor.

Arno, P. S. (1986). "The Nonprofit Sector's Response to the AIDS Epidemic: Community-Based Services in San Francisco." *American Journal of Public Health,* 76, 1325–1330.

Being Alive. (1992). "Being Alive Expands to the Valley." *Being Alive: People with HIV/ AIDS Action Coalition Newsletter,* August/September.

Berube, Allan. (1988). "Caught in the Storm: AIDS and the Meaning of Natural Disaster." *Out/Look,* 1, 3, 8–19.

Bull, Chris. (1992). "The Outing of a Family-Values Congressman." *Advocate,* 612, 38–45.

Cain, Roy. (1994). "AIDS Service Organizations and the Canadian State." Paper presented at the Annual Meetings of the Society for the Study of Social Problems, Los Angeles, August.

Callen, Michael. (1990). *Surviving AIDS.* New York: Harper Perennial.

Cruikshank, Margaret. (1992). *The Gay and Lesbian Liberation Movement.* New York: Routledge.

Davis, Kristine, & Stapleton, Jack. (1991). "Migration to Rural Areas by HIV Patients: Impact on HIV-Related Healthcare Use." *Infection Control and Hospital Epidemiology,* 12, 540–543.

Fernandez, Elizabeth. (1991). "A City Responds." In MacKenzie, N. F. (Ed.), *The AIDS Reader: Social Political and Ethical Issues* (pp. 577–585). New York: Meridian.

Foster, Jim. (1988). "Impact of the AIDS Epidemic on the Gay Political Agenda." In Corless, I. B. & Pittman-Lindeman, M. (Eds.), *AIDS: Principles, Practices, Politics* (pp. 209–219). Washington, DC: Hemisphere Publishing.

Gould, Peter. (1991). "Modeling the Geographic Spread of AIDS for Educational Intervention." In Ulack, R. & Skinner, W. F. (Eds.), *AIDS and the Social Sciences: Common Threads* (pp. 30–44). Lexington, KY: University Press of Kentucky.

Hackney, Edwin. (1991). "Low-Incidence Community Response to AIDS." In Ulack, R. & Skinner, W. F. (Eds.), *AIDS and the Social Sciences: Common Threads* (pp. 64–81). Lexington, KY: University Press of Kentucky.

Hays, Robert B., & Peterson, J. L. (1994). "HIV Prevention for Gay and Bisexual Men in Metropolitan Cities." In DiClemente, R. J. & Peterson, J. L. (Eds.), *Preventing AIDS: Theories and Methods of Behavioral Interventions* (pp. 267–296). New York: Plenum.

Herek, Gregory M., & Glunt, Eric K. (1995). "Identity and Community among Gay and Bisexual Men in the AIDS Era: Preliminary Findings from the Sacramento Men's Health Study." In Herek, G. M. & Greene, B. (Eds.), *AIDS, Identity and Community: The HIV Epidemic and Lesbian and Gay Men* (pp. 55–77). Thousand Oaks, CA: Sage.

Katoff, Lewis, Ince, Susan, & the staff of the GMHC Clinic Services Department.

(1991). "Supporting People with AIDS: the GMHC Model." In MacKenzie, N. F. (Ed.), *The AIDS Reader: Social, Political, and Ethical Issues* (pp. 543–576). New York: Meridian.

Kayal, Philip. (1993). *Bearing Witness: Gay Men's Health Crisis and the Politics of AIDS.* Boulder, CO: Westview.

King, Edward. (1993). *Safety in Numbers: Safer Sex and Gay Men.* New York: Routledge.

Kirp, David L. (1989). *Learning by Heart: AIDS and Schoolchildren in America's Communities.* New Brunswick, NJ: Rutgers University Press.

Kobasa, Suzanne C. Ouellette. (1991). "AIDS Volunteering." In *A Disease of Society: Cultural and Institutional Responses to AIDS,* edited by D. Nelkin, D. P. Willis, and S. V. Parris. New York: Cambridge University Press.

Kramer, Larry. (1989). *Reports from the Holocaust: The Making of an AIDS Activist.* New York: St. Martin's.

Levine, Martin P. (1992). "The Life and Death of Gay Clones." In Herdt, Gilbert (Ed.), *Gay Culture in America: Essays from the Field* (pp. 68–86). Boston: Beacon Press.

Lynch, Frederick. (1992). "Nonghetto Gays: An Ethnography of Suburban Homosexuals." In Herdt, Gilbert (Ed.), *Gay Culture in America: Essays from the Field* (pp. 165–201). Boston: Beacon Press.

Marks, Robert. (1988). "Coming Out in the Age of AIDS: The Next Generation." *Out/Look,* Spring, 66–74.

Miller, Neil. (1989). *In Search of Gay America: Women and Men in a Time of Change.* New York: Harper and Row.

Moerkerk, Hans, with Aggleton, Peter. (1990). "AIDS Prevention Strategies in Europe: A Comparison and Critical Analysis." In Aggleton, P., Davies, P., & Hart, G. (Eds.), *AIDS: Individual, Cultural and Political Dimensions* (pp. 181–190). London: Falmer Press.

Navarro, Mireya. (1993). "Healthy, Gay, Guilt-Stricken: AIDS Toll on the Virus-Free." *New York Times,* 11 January, A1.

Odets, Walt. (1995). *In the Shadow of the Epidemic: Being HIV Negative in the Age of AIDS.* Durham, NC: Duke University Press.

Omoto, Allen M., & Crain, A. Lauren. (1995). "AIDS Volunteerism: Lesbian and Gay Community-Based Response to HIV." In Herek, G. M. & Greene, B. (Eds.), *AIDS, Identity, and Community: The HIV Epidemic and Lesbians and Gay Men* (pp. 187–209). Thousand Oaks, CA: Sage.

Patton, Cindy. (1996). *Fatal Advice: How Safe-Sex Education Went Wrong.* Durham, NC: Duke University Press.

———. (1990). *Inventing AIDS.* New York: Routledge.

Petrow, Steven, with Frank, Pat, & Wolfred, Timothy. (1990). *Ending the HIV Epidemic: Community Strategies in Disease Prevention and Health Promotion.* Santa Cruz, CA: Network Publications.

Poole, William. (1992). "Bringing It Back Home." *Out/Look,* 4, 4, 36–44.

Preston, John. (1991). *Hometowns: Gay Men Write about Where They Belong.* New York: Dutton.

Rist, Darrell Yates. (1989a). "Darrell Yates Rist Replies." *The Nation,* 19 June, 834.

———. (1989b). "AIDS as Apocalypse: The Deadly Costs of an Obsession." *The Nation,* 13 February.

Rofes, Eric. (1990). "Gay Lib vs. AIDS: Averting Civil War in the 1990s." *Out/Look,* Spring, 8–17.

Rounds, K. (1988). "AIDS in Rural Areas: Challenges to Providing Care." *Social Work,* May–June, 257–261.

"Rural New York and HIV: Issues Faced by the Heartland." (1992). *Focus on AIDS: A Newsletter of the New York State Department of Health AIDS Institute.* Albany, NY.

Schmidt, William. (1987). "North Dakota Girds to Keep AIDS at Bay." *New York Times,* 22 December.

Schneider, Beth E. (1992). "Lesbian Politics and AIDS Work." In Plummer, K. (Ed.). *Modern Homosexualities* (pp. 160–174). New York: Routledge.

Spiro, Ellen, & Lane, Michael. (1992). "Homespun Homos." *Advocate,* 25 February, 34–40.

Vaid, Urvashi. (1995). *Virtual Equality: The Mainstreaming of Gay and Lesbian Liberation.* New York: Anchor.

Verghese, Abraham. (1994). *My Own Country: A Doctor's Story of a Town and Its People in the Age of AIDS.* New York: Simon and Schuster.

Watney, Simon. (1994). *Practices of Freedom: Selected Writings on HIV/AIDS.* Durham, NC: Duke University Press.

SEVEN

From Feminism to
Polymorphous Activism:
Lesbians in AIDS
Organizations

NANCY E. STOLLER

Understanding lesbian involvement
in the AIDS epidemic requires analysis beyond questions of either sexual identity or ethical choice. Participation in any social movement,
including the response to AIDS, is highly determined both by internal
movement factors such as recruitment and mobilization techniques,[1]
and by external factors such as potential recruits' shared values, sympathy for political goals, and existing organizational memberships.
Thus the values, social location, and occupation of a lesbian significantly affect the possibilities of her involvement in AIDS work. In addition, during the decade of the epidemic's presence in North America,
the culture (including values and sexual identity) of the lesbian population has itself changed. These changes have configured the positions
of lesbians in the social world of AIDS. Although cultural and other
progressive feminisms dominated the practice of early lesbian AIDS
activists, a more radical and increasingly queer politics emerged in the
work and culture of women who came to the movement in the late
eighties and early nineties. To understand the history of the complex
relationship of lesbian activists to AIDS, we first need to know the
dominant networks, cultures, and institutions of North American lesbians when AIDS was first identified in the United States.

Feminism

During the 1970s, the combination of the second wave of feminism
with the emergence of the gay liberation movement led to a complex

This chapter was published in a slightly different form under the title "Lesbian
Involvement in the AIDS Epidemic: Changing Roles and Generational Differences," in
Beth E. Schneider & Nancy E. Stoller (Eds.), *Women Resisting AIDS: Feminist Strategies
of Empowerment* (Philadelphia: Temple University Press, 1995).

flowering of culture and social organization by women. Many of the leadership roles in the women's movement were filled by lesbians (part time, occasional, emerging, temporary, long term, and otherwise). This was a mutual love affair by lesbians for feminism (the idea that women matter) and of feminism for the essence of the lesbian vision (women are first in time, emotional interest, and political commitment). The slogan that "feminism is the theory and lesbianism the practice" may not be perfectly true, but its emotional validity brought the two movements together. In addition, most feminist organizations during this period attempted to include both heterosexuals and lesbians. On the subject of the body, the motto of feminism was "Our Bodies, Our Selves," which was not just a health slogan, but also a call for self-determination, expressed in forms ranging from self-examination to sexual experimentation. Not surprisingly, "political lesbianism" was born in this milieu.

In a concrete sense, what combined aspects of the two movements—and especially linked lesbians to feminism—was precisely what had drawn lesbians to work with women and girls throughout the nineteenth and twentieth centuries in the United States: feminism, and particularly feminist institution-building, represented the opportunity to express a lesbian's love of women both at work and in politics, even though the work and politics said "women" and not the sub-category, "lesbians." This sort of work for women and girls provided the opportunity for a (universalistic) sublimated love that could exist in a universe parallel to one's private life and (particularistic) love. With this match, lesbians became the leaders in many of the feminist institutions formed in the seventies: the women's health movement, with its self-examination and self-help movements, its collectives and health centers; the feminist press; bookstores; restaurants; music. It is through the work of such women that these feminist institutions have survived into the eighties and nineties.

In many cases, the language of the movement itself conflated women and lesbians. For example, during the mid-seventies, as lesbian culture went public, it was labeled "women's culture" by its promoters, *viz.* "women's music," which was really lesbian music, and music for a predominantly White and college-educated audience at that. That this conflation still exists is shown by the fact that Olivia Records, the primary vector for lesbian/women's music, now sells "women's cruises" (no pun acknowledged), which are designed for lesbians, not for women or even feminists in general.[2]

The feminist movement and the lesbian movement were parallel and interconnecting; they were linked to other movements and had considerable diversity within them, which is often lost in more superficial reporting.[3] For example, there is a widespread notion that the "women's movement" was White and middle class,[4] but as I experienced the radical political movements of the seventies, they were intentionally cross-class and multiracial. Feminists and lesbians in all segments of the population were active in prison reform and organizing, especially the segment that worked with women; battered women's shelters; anti-racist organizing; ethnic liberation struggles; school board fights; and reproductive rights that addressed sterilization abuse.[5]

Despite some invisibility in the eyes of the left and many White gay men, it was during the seventies that both lesbians and women (at least the feminists in the name of women) "went public."[6] Gaining experience in their "own" movements, as well as other struggles, they began to create new sets of institutions for women. As a result, for lesbians, alternate and additional institutions beyond women's bars and the sports clubs associated with them emerged. Separatist settings and services for women (health clinics, therapy services, restaurants, book stores, retreats, land groups, classes, caucuses) were suddenly everywhere. Women's studies courses and programs were invented. Gay and straight women mingled. Lesbianism was presented as a legitimate option for women; many lesbian-inclined women chose it, and did so openly, in ways that their older sisters could not have done so easily.

Feminism helped make this development of women's "spaces" and lesbian lifestyle and culture possible, because it brought the energies of women of all sexual persuasions together in the name of "women," therefore making available many more resources than either straight women or lesbians could generate by themselves. Each group had access to different types of resources. In a certain way, the reason why lesbians have led the women's movement and its institutions is that lesbians have more labor, more focused attention, and less distraction to offer: they are not so torn by the need to return to men. On the other hand, the connections of straight women to men brought a different set of resources, especially financial aid. Since women's salaries ranged from 59 to 63 percent of men's during this period, a woman with a man was almost inevitably in a wealthier household than a woman with a woman. (Regardless of what we think of fish and bicycles.)

Gay Liberation

The movement for gay liberation, which emerged as a powerful force in 1969 and spread internationally within a few years, further affected lesbian visibility, politics, economics, and culture. Although men dom-

inated the movement, women were assertive in many of its political organizations and other institutions. The movement's effects on
lesbian-gay solidarity varied by location: in larger urban areas, men
dominated the economy and the institutions of the gay community;
socializing by men and women was predominantly segregated and reflected different sexual, political, and social values. Lesbian culture, in
both its older and its new institutions, such as the bars, was characterized by a more socially critical stance—beyond lesbian/gay assertion.
Because women had fewer institutions to call their own, their gather-
ing places continued to be more mixed racially and in terms of class
than were male institutions, which as they multiplied replicated the
class and racial character of the larger society more thoroughly than
did women's institutions. Lesbians were also just plain worse off economically than gay men, consequently their interests, alliances, and
culture reflected this difference.

Gay male culture, except for that segment affected by groups such
as the Radical Fairies, the Gay Liberation Front, and a few other
groups, was more a celebration of male and gay culture without the
radicalizing addition of feminism.[7] A major distinction between lesbians and gay men, as articulated in publications and politics of the seventies, was in their notions of what sexual freedom meant. In fact, to
understand lesbians and the AIDS epidemic, it is important to spend
some time looking at these different meanings.

Lesbians and Gay Men: Sexual Difference in the Seventies

Despite some more radical critiques, the models of sexuality for lesbians that dominated the seventies came from women's socialization and
feminism. Recent theorists have argued that female development
moves in the direction of a relational orientation in contrast to male
developmental emphasis on individuation and separation.[8] Gilligan,
for example, argued that within Western culture, male moral development has emphasized an ethic of justice, although that of women has
greater emphasis on caring. Even though some feminist theorists
emphasize the role of oppression in developing this orientation in
women,[9] it is still true that regardless of the structural sources, almost
all women, including lesbians, have been strongly affected by a pattern
of socialization that emphasizes the importance of relationships and
networks, as well as care-giving and nurturance. Although lesbians
may resist certain aspects of female socialization (males as sexual ob-
ject choices, for example), they are not immune from these cultural
pressures.

Common wisdom in lesbian culture of the late seventies and early eighties asserted that lesbians form couples and model their coupleship on romantic love and enduring relationships. This popular notion was complemented, and perhaps strengthened, by research on "fusion" in lesbian relationships, which emphasizes the tendency to blur boundaries between self and other and identifies female socialization as a source for this tendency.[10] A second pervasive aspect of female socialization has been the historical and contemporary emphasis on monogamy, tied partly to patriarchal possessiveness but also to the risk of pregnancy and the need for legitimate fathership.

In contrast to these two aspects of female socialization (relatedness and monogamy as values and life orientations), male socialization has emphasized individuation and non-monogamy. Although gay men, like lesbians, challenge traditional sex roles, they are, similarly and simultaneously, drawn to them. Gay male sexuality in the seventies was historically marked by less emphasis on the creation of "family" or on sexual monogamy. The impact of gay liberation movements on gay male sexuality has recently been discussed in many venues, primarily because of the belief that patterns of sexuality among gay men have been responsible for the rapid spread of the epidemic.[11] Although a detailed look at this topic is outside the scope of this chapter, gay male and lesbian sexualities and the value systems associated with them were important sources of separation between men and women within the social and cultural landscape of gay life.

For women who emerged as lesbians in the seventies, feminism had several primary sexual messages: communication, equality, androgyny, and nonviolence. Beyond the burst of radical energy associated with the first few years of early seventies feminism, radical sexual experimentation was not prominent among the explicit messages of feminism.[12] Nor did monogamy suffer a sustained critique. Although gay liberation provided the opportunity for lesbians to be more out, female socialization seemed to insure that they would move primarily in the directions that were already expected of women: to seek long-term close relationships. The critique of male-female sexual relationships led to an emphasis in feminism on equality and, for some women (both lesbian and straight), a fear of repeating the same oppressive forms found between men and women in traditional nonfeminist couples. Struggles against sexism, sexual abuse, and oppression were pitted against the right to have one's own sex life and to be creative without being censored.[13] Lesbians who were out before the seventies reacted variously to these messages and conflicts depending on their interest, class, ethnicity, education, and commitment to previous patterns.[14]

Differences within lesbian and feminist communities concerning sexual expression created major divisions that lingered into the nineties. One strand of feminists gravitated toward a severe critique of power; some became involved in the antipornography movement that supported censorship and regulation.[15] Other feminists rallied to protect free speech and self-expression as cornerstones of women's rights to determine their own sexuality. The conflicts escalated in the late seventies and early eighties, especially among the more political and academic segments of the feminist world. Lesbians were actively engaged in this debate. In addition, lesbians involved in femme-butch and the growing S&M community felt attacked by those who emphasized androgyny and equality as the only proper expressions of female sexuality.[16]

The message of gay liberation for men, however, was more one of self-expression of male socialization within the arena of gay sex. This meant multiple partners, self-assertion, and "individuation" (i.e., experimentation). Gay male sexuality had involved multiple sex partners before gay liberation; the gay movement, which basically legitimized gay life "as it was," focused on gaining full rights (again a "male" theme of justice) for gay men to live their lives—and discover them—as they wished. In the early seventies, gay male liberation provided a critique of traditional male sexuality. This critique included the presentation of the possibility that gay men might form their own families, whether of the communal type or more "nuclear" versions. By the end of the decade, more gay men had created families (in some cases linked to lesbians), which included children. As the gay movement became institutionalized, however, it lost much of its radical critique of sexism. There was no movement comparable to feminism to effectively challenge male socialization—although some segments of the gay male community adopted the critique of domination and oppression; they applied this critique to gay male social relations as well as to those between gay men and lesbians.

The seventies marked a rapid increase in public gay male culture, political influence (including Harvey Milk's successful supervisorial campaign in San Francisco), and institutions. Within these new institutions, struggles over the appropriate nature of gay male life—What was the meaning and appropriateness of camp? Of "super-masculine" behavior? Of clone culture?—appeared. Writers began to speak of gay identity and community replacing homosexual behavior and populations. Although gay men were in some cases able to claim physical and geographic locations—the Castro, the Village—for their community culture, lesbians existed more as a relationship or fictional community, often on the geographical fringe of gay men's areas, but usually spread more widely and less distinctly as a community.

Although lesbians were ideologically connected to many feminist goals, many gay men accepted the semipermanent dominance of heterosexual society and patriarchy in its more traditional forms, including its "use" of women as nurturers and "helpmates." Possibly the lack of challenge by gay men to sexism made it easy for them to appreciate the nurturing they received from lesbians and straight women when the epidemic hit, but harder to acknowledge women as intellectual equals.

Thus when the seventies ended and the AIDS epidemic exploded, most lesbians and gay men were living essentially parallel lives, organized primarily around the separate themes of female values and feminism for the women and masculinity and justice for the men.

The AIDS Epidemic

Although AIDS has struck men in higher numbers than women, women have been among the ill since the beginning. They have also been involved as caretakers, educators, physicians, public health officials, and community activists. As a diverse social group linked by gender in an epidemic in which gender and sexuality are key, women, and lesbians in particular, have played powerful symbolic, sexual, and social roles.

From the start, lesbians were involved not only in their occupational functions—nurses, activists, social workers, etc.—but also as "women" and "lesbians," two potential master statuses. Simultaneously active and self-conscious, lesbians were often seen as representing "the" feminist stance. Their social-psychological backgrounds, the nature of the lesbian/gay community, and the broader social and political context of the early eighties affected the roles that lesbians could, and did, play in the epidemic. These roles have changed substantially over the first decade of AIDS activism.

The basic arenas of AIDS activity might usefully be sorted into five institutional foci: medical (including research), public health, educational, caring services, and political. As the eighties began, women in the United States (including lesbians) were occupationally placed in large numbers where they would be likely to encounter men with HIV. In medical settings they comprised most of nurses, as well as a significant proportion of nurse aides, home health workers, medical clerical staff, and an increasing number of physicians. Women also dominated the front-line workforce in social work and therapy. They were well represented in public health, especially in health education. Within the lesbian and gay community, most of the service organizations that were cosexual had numerous female staff (primarily because women outnumber men in the helping professions).

The above-noted professional roles, whether in straight or gay institutions, draw on traditional nurturing and service models for female activity. Although some of the lesbians in these roles may have been completely traditional in their attitudes toward their work, it is likely that most had been influenced both by the enormous changes in lesbian culture and institutions caused by the gay liberation movement and by the impact of seventies feminism on medicine and other health care work.

Within the primary arenas for AIDS work, and especially among activist segments in the political arena, we can delineate four dominant lesbian perspectives in the eighties on whether and how to make AIDS a social priority:

1. Women/lesbians make a distinctive contribution;
2. Equal rights for women (or lesbians) within the AIDS world;
3. Lesbians and gay men must form coalitions;
4. Lesbians need separatism.

These phrases summarize four approaches, which are best understood as ideal types. I have constructed this typology inductively on the basis of my field research and participation in AIDS work over the past ten years. The typology is complemented and supplemented by the findings of other researchers, although they may not use my language.[17] These perspectives have developed somewhat chronologically during the course of the epidemic as women have participated in various institutional and social movement responses.[18]

In addition to these four primarily feminist approaches to AIDS, there are the nonfeminist and anti-feminist conservative approaches to AIDS, some of which have specific positions on women and AIDS. Conservative approaches argue, for example, that certain infected adults (such as gay men, prostitutes, drug users, and "the promiscuous") deserve their infection and death. The holder of such a view may argue for quarantine of the "guilty" infected; in California, for example, prostitutes who test positive for HIV become felons instead of the misdemeanants they would be were they uninfected. These conservative positions are less common among lesbians who are involved in public responses to AIDS and are therefore not explored in depth in this chapter.

In addition, there are some lesbian AIDS activists who have been labeled "nonfeminists" because they were too "femme," or too "into roles" or "power," or "soft" on pornography. In fact, most of these women did identify themselves as feminists and were critical of those whom they call "lesbian feminists." The sex radicals (as members of this group occasionally called themselves) felt rejected by lesbian separatist and lesbian feminist organizations, many of which were dominated by the philosophy of androgyny and equality. They are the political descendants of the radical feminists of the early seventies. Their early eighties interest in AIDS politics and the organizational milieu of AIDS work was fueled by a belief that AIDS organizations would be groups that were more open about sexual diversity. Some were drawn to these (gay) organizations rather than to "mainstream" lesbian organizations in which they felt invisible or criticized. Their activity is included in the following discussion of feminist rationales for AIDS work.

1. The Distinctive Contribution of Women

This approach characterized the first few years of the epidemic. It was (and continues to be) most commonly expressed by women working in the medical and caring services. Shorthand versions of this approach are "AIDS needs women" and "To get the best man for the job, call a woman." Believers in women's distinctive contribution argue that women have special skills to bring to the AIDS response, which should be brought and taught or shared with "the guys," our gay brothers.

In this model, what do women bring? Compassion; women's health movement experience; health skills; nurturing skills; experience with illness; ability to express emotions; relational abilities; an understanding of organizational growth and change. Many lesbians did bring these skills and styles with them to their work in AIDS. The AIDS organizations for the first half of the decade (1981–86) were focused on medical care, social and mental health services, and education. Initially, most of the clients were men. Within the organizations, lesbians played a variety of nurturing and relational roles. In some cases, women acted as leaders; however, their contribution was generally underreported and underrated.

The Women's AIDS Network, located in the San Francisco Bay Area, was founded by a mixed group of lesbians and straight women in 1982 at an early national AIDS conference. Members of this organization, led primarily by lesbians, were overwhelmingly highly educated AIDS professionals:[19] nurses, doctors, therapists, health educators. Similar to the women in Melissa McNeill's study of nineteen prominent lesbian AIDS activists,[20] almost all WAN members arrived with experience in feminism, health organizing, and/or lesbian and gay civil rights work.

They began by giving all they could from what they knew. Such an approach, giving all you've got, is compatible with conservative feminism, and with the "neoconservative" or "post-modern" feminism, which seeks full rights for women but views radical activism with ironic detachment. In fact, some of the lesbians who worked at the San Francisco AIDS Foundation, as either staff or volunteers, are most appropriately described as nonfeminists and in some cases hostile to feminists. Their political commitment was more as "homosexuals" who were part of gay/lesbian culture and less connected to feminist culture. They saw feminism itself as periodically hostile to gay men (because feminism criticized the men for camp and/or sexual promiscuousness) or as opposed to their own individual (economic) success. Their involvement was more often a result of connection to the gay male community, and less a result of a political analysis. These women were sometimes unsympathetic to their more feminist coworkers, especially when those women presented feminist agendas concerning services for women. The "homosexual" women interpreted such behavior as uncaring of men.[21]

Most of the lesbians who got involved in AIDS research, service, and policy work in the early years, however, were both feminists and nurturers who saw themselves connected politically and ethically to the various populations at risk for AIDS.

The idea that women have special nurturant skills has frequently been expressed and appreciated in AIDS organizations, including those dominated by men. But the special skills associated with women's organizational experience was less acknowledged. This finding held true in McNeill's study as well as in my own research in San Francisco.

2. Equal Rights for Women/Lesbians in the AIDS World

Soon after women became engaged in the work of the epidemic, a second perspective began to be expressed: that women, as AIDS workers and as people at risk for AIDS, were the victims of sexism and secondary status.

This perspective holds that we need to examine every AIDS response strategy to make certain that women's unique needs are met and that potential oppression and/or exploitation are prevented. Reproductive rights; civil liberties issues; the role of motherhood, HIV and maternal transmission; the scapegoating of prostitutes; equal access of women— and children—to AIDS education, treatment, social services, food banks, and so forth: These are all issues that lesbians and straight women addressed in the epidemic. They saw the equal rights approach as necessary because most AIDS policy was being determined by and for men, whether it was being set within community-based organizations (CBOs) or by governmental organizations.

One example of such sexism played out in the San Francisco AIDS Foundation in 1985-'86. At that time, I was the coordinator of the women's program and the supervisor of educational materials development and distribution. I had supervised the development of most of the brochures for the foundation, which were being distributed nationally: the first HIV test brochures (English and Spanish versions); a multiracial heterosexual brochure (also English and Spanish); "Sex, drugs, and AIDS"; a women and AIDS brochure (drafted by the Women's AIDS Network); and other materials for people with AIDS. The Women's AIDS Network had just agreed to work with the foundation to produce what would be the first brochure specifically for lesbians. But when I went to my supervisor, a gay man who was director of the Education Department, to show him the text and get formal permission for printing, for the first time in my work at the foundation, I was told that my brochure would not be approved for printing because unlike the other groups "lesbians are not at risk for AIDS." I was shocked by his response. I called members of the Women's AIDS Network. Within a week, WAN was using its contacts within and without the organization to reverse the decision and eventually (but only after three months of lobbying), the brochure was published. One rationalization that the director held onto was "well, lesbians aren't really at risk, but since they are working so hard in AIDS services, they deserve a brochure." Thousands of copies were distributed or sold within the first year. The brochure was reprinted and widely distributed for six years. The conflict indicated how invisible lesbians were as women at risk, as activists, and as experts, even within a gay—and lesbian—organization.

In North American AIDS work, championing the equal rights focus for women often means emphasizing class and race issues because most women with HIV are poor and of either African American or

Latino descent. Lesbians, who were often the primary advocates for straight women as well as themselves, walked a fine line when they spoke about their needs for visibility. What did it mean to speak for "women" if one were also lesbian? Lesbian networking (through organizations like WAN), as well as direct service by lesbians to women of all sorts, has resulted in a situation in which straight women have increasingly championed lesbian needs as well as their own in terms of HIV/AIDS advocacy. As the international demographic and epidemiological facts have hit home (although slowly) in the United States, heterosexual women received consistently more attention. Lesbians, though, continue to lag far behind. In 1992, the Centers for Disease Control still excluded any woman from its "lesbian" category if she had sex even once with a man since 1977.

The last two major stances held by lesbians in regard to the epidemic emerged most strongly during the second half of the decade, although, as will be seen, they (like the equal rights approach) have their roots in feminist activist movements that flourished in the seventies.

3. Lesbians and Gay Men Must Form Coalitions

By the middle of the first decade of AIDS, many AIDS organizations had begun to feel the stress of inadequate funding. Additionally, the dream of quick medical solutions and rapid research advances had faded. As a result, direct action tactics became more popular. ACT-UP and its clones were born and spread rapidly throughout the United States and Europe.

Coalition lesbians argue that lesbians (and for that matter, everyone) should work on improving AIDS policies (even if a specific policy change will benefit men primarily) because the public repressive response to the epidemic is a response to communities and populations that include lesbians as well as gay men. Therefore it is in the interests of women, as well as the more often affected men, to have better AIDS policies.

Such women often see AIDS as a "homosexual" issue. They argue that many recent civil rights restrictions are based on homophobia and justified because of AIDS. Furthermore, the concomitant rise in antigay violence, the loss of community leaders, friends, and family through illness and death: all affect lesbians as well as gay men. An additional argument is that focusing on AIDS discrimination is the best strategy for ending discrimination against gay people because the two discriminations (AIDS discrimination and homophobia), as well as the prejudice, stigma, and marginalization associated with both, are completely entangled, and there is funding and some political interest in dealing with AIDS discrimination. So one can reverse antigay discrimination and prejudice by working on AIDS.[22]

Many AIDS activist women who share the coalition perspective also view the AIDS epidemic as an opportunity to move toward broader social agendas: national health care, local housing and shelters, effective and humane drug policy. They see these changes as key to improving the role of women and gay people in society.

The coalition approach to AIDS work is often associated with an activist position. McNeill found that of the half of her sample who were primarily involved in ACT-UP and OUT! (the Washington, D.C. version of ACT-UP), a major appeal was the activism. Many stated positions that indicated that they saw AIDS work as a way of approaching the broader society and making changes in it. In my own interviews with lesbian members of ACT-UP in New York, all stated that they saw their work as part of coalition politics. All were feminists and aligned with the sexual radical side of feminism.

Divisions with the ACT-UP organizations of several cities indicate that the definition of coalition politics varies: although some women support the narrow definition of lesbians, gay men, and others working together around AIDS (the initial perspective of ACT-UP New York), others are more attuned to the broader critique of society. They are more likely to be found in the descendants of ACT-UP that have taken on the wider health and/or political issues beyond AIDS.

It is out of the bonds between lesbian and gay male activists, symbolized in organizations such as ACT-UP, that Queer Nation, gay antiviolence patrols, and queer culture have been formed. This new culture, in which women fill many leadership roles and which is explicitly multicultural, speaks primarily with the voice of the second generation since Stonewall. It is led by women and men who have come of age during the eighties. But the legacies of racism and sexism (so alive in the seventies) have not been overcome in these newer organizations; they continue to break apart over challenges to the maintenance of white male systems of power.

While these political developments emerged, a previously traveled route was being explored by the "older generation" of lesbians: withdrawal and separatism.

4. Separatist Approach

The final perspective has strong roots in lesbian and feminist separatism. Separatist lesbians holding this perspective argue that feminist and lesbian health priorities should not be focused on AIDS, but on worse problems affecting women. For example, breast cancer strikes and kills many more women than does AIDS.[23] And our poverty and powerlessness are more serious health problems than HIV disease. Violence against women is endemic. This is the perspective presented in Jackie Winnow's speech at the 1988 Lesbians and AIDS conference in San Francisco, which was reprinted in *Out/Look* magazine.[24] Although her comments were directed primarily at lesbians, she argued that all women suffered from the current AIDS funding and organizing focus, due to loss of funds for and diminished attention to women's health issues.

Additionally, some lesbians argue that even if they themselves see AIDS as a major threat to their communities, this is not the way the average person feels in communities which are not primarily gay-identified (e.g., African Americans, Latinos, the homeless, poor Whites). Therefore AIDS-focused organizing is not an effective way to move toward organizing these communities, including their lesbian members, for survival.

Although some lesbians may have stayed "out of AIDS" from the beginning because they were unconnected to gay men, did not see themselves at risk, or just wanted to avoid the whole thing, others who were engaged have left full-time work, some to work in other areas and some to do part-time volunteer activity. Of McNeill's subjects, despite their leadership roles, 25 percent (five) were turning their attention elsewhere. By 1991, fifteen had reprioritized their AIDS work to focus on women and were involved in other health issues affecting women and lesbians.[25]

No matter what size or type of AIDS response organization one examines, these four perspectives appear. In the more radical activist organizations (e.g., the ACT-UP chapters), one is more likely to find the coalitionists. Nevertheless, in three months of field work with New York ACT-UP in 1989, I found that the "distinctive contribution" idea was one of the strongest motivators for highly political women. Their distinctive contribution happened to be their organizing experiences gained in other direct action and civil disobedience movements. Consistently contributions were identified feminist "inventions," such as consciousness-raising and affinity groups, as well as various techniques to assure participatory democracy.

There was—and is—no one lesbian perspective on AIDS. Even within fairly cohesive AIDS organizations with explicit values and priorities concerning the epidemic and women, there has been considerable variation.

The priorities of women who have been active in AIDS response organizations have been undergoing considerable change as the organizations themselves grow—and shrink—and as the nature of the epidemic
and the federal, state, and local responses to it, have changed. We
should expect these transformations in priorities to continue.

Generational Differences

Of lesbians who got involved in the AIDS epidemic in the first five
years, some have stayed within the field, even if they have moved to
other organizations (as many gay men have done). They have become
career AIDS professionals. A second group has moved into allied fields
(health education, public health, systems management), in some cases
with a focus on women. A third group has left AIDS and health alto-
gether, an option that, as far as I can tell, is being pursued primarily
by those women who were more tangentially or "accidentally" engaged, either because of a single friendship or a coincidence of employment (a lesbian takes a job in a food bank in an AIDS agency, but
really wants to be a graphic designer and eventually succeeds at this).

Although some have become simultaneous AIDS professionals and
direct action activists, this does not seem to be common. McNeill
found considerable hostility between the professionals and the activists
in her sample. The professionals referred to the activists as irresponsible and ill-informed, and some of the activists thought that the professional women were co-opted. I would argue that although there may
have been predictable hostility between members of the AIDS activist
movement and the institutionalized service sector, there is also a generational split, reflecting major societal transformations that have
changed the politics and culture of lesbian life during the past twenty
years.

The differences between the older lesbians and the younger generation are deep, widespread, and in many cases quite antagonistic. They
affect how and why lesbians do—or don't do—AIDS work. They also
help to explain how lesbians not involved with AIDS organizations
view the epidemic, sex, including safe sex, and those lesbians who are
"connected" to HIV and AIDS issues. Although the epidemic itself has
helped to shape these differences, other social, economic, and cultural
factors have also been at work. To explain this, I will compare the two
generations as they have emerged in this study of women engaged in
AIDS activity.

The first group of lesbians (predominantly in their late thirties and
forties) grew up in the sixties, when they were influenced both by more

traditional female socialization and by the radical activism of the civil rights movement, antiwar demonstrations, and nascent feminism. In the seventies, when many came of age and came out, feminism was strong and the opportunity to be out relatively easily as a lesbian was new. For many of these women, simply "being" a lesbian and being public about it was a revolutionary sexual step.

The second generation, on the other hand, has come of age—and come out—in the eighties, a decade marked by explicit sexuality debates, much greater openness about what would have been called deviant behavior ten years ago, broad female access to education, a deepening economic recession, and a growing radicalism both among gay men (as the epidemic remains "uncured" and the failed health economy slams into their lives) and other segments of the population. These lesbians have less faith in education or government, less of a sense of individual futures; their sexual radicalness goes beyond being a lesbian. Being able to be a lesbian is more of a given than it was ten years ago, and for many lesbians of the current generation, it is a very limiting identity.

During the eighties, gay men explored "safe sex" and brought fisting, dildos, rimming, nipple rings, golden showers, and S&M scenes into public discussion, especially within the gay community—which by now had a shared press read by both men and women. Increasingly lesbians, especially the younger ones, have sought access to this world of experimentation. Sexual activities that go far beyond the feminist notions of equality and nonviolence have become exciting options to the new generation. By the early nineties, while some older feminist lesbians looked on in disappointment, younger women (and a few of their older friends) attended clubs with names such as Faster Pussycat, the G-Spot, and the Ecstasy Lounge, where cruising, S&M, public sex, and such skills as the safe use of dildos were being (re)introduced to a new generation.

The new generation of AIDS activist lesbians carries a different psychology, culture, politics, and sexuality from those who came to the movement in the early eighties. These activists are connected to the older women by the term "lesbian" and by some similarities of sexual practice. Many, however, see their elders as sexually repressed, conservative, and somewhat anti-male. In addition, they see themselves as moving beyond categories of gender, sexual orientation, and racial division to a new multicultural and queer life. If there is any political movement that characterizes this culture, it is anarchism.

The two groups of lesbians may be separated by certain predictable sources of cross-generational conflict (the inevitable activist mellowing that comes with age and the fact that the older women can be—and in some cases are—the parents of the younger women). But it is the social changes of the eighties that have provided a different sexual and political framework and have led to the new sexuality and its political expression, both of which include an ever more pointed critique of sexual identities and practices that are anything less than polymorphous. It is this changed context of greater poverty and social service constriction, together with a greater openness to radical sexuality, that increasingly informs younger lesbian perspectives and gives shape to their involvement in the epidemic.

Lesbians with AIDS career longevity continue to work as educators, therapists, social workers, doctors, nurses, administrators, and policy advocates. Meanwhile the younger women activists provide the energy and focus that help insure the funding and policy decisions that create the services and fight the expansion of the epidemic. The lesson of the first decade of lesbian activism in AIDS work is that the two strategies of service and direct action are complementary, dialectical, and mutually productive.

Notes

1. Doug McAdam, John McCarthy, & Meyer Zald, "Social Movements."

2. In 1987 I went on a one-week women's kayak trip, attended by a nonfeminist, recently divorced, fifty-three-year-old straight woman who was horrified that everyone but her and the tour guide were lesbians. "What did she expect?" one dyke kayaker asked.

3. See especially Alice Echols, *Daring to be Bad: Radical Feminism in America, 1967–1975* (1989), for an excellent analysis of the radical side of seventies feminism.

4. This approach, which obscures the activity of those who do not command major amounts of resources and media, is repeated in the histories of many movements, in which the roles of the poor, the oppressed, and the companions of the powerful are repeatedly denigrated or made invisible because they have produced fewer material records of their role (fewer books, films, newspapers, paintings) that are easily accessible to historians and journalists of dominant classes and races. The nonwriters are then proclaimed nonexistent as activists and creators.

5. See B. Epstein, "Lesbians Lead the Movement," 1988, pp. 27–32.

6. It is interesting that when straight White men write the history of the 1970s, again and again they record the death of "the movement." What movement do they mean? Perhaps it is "their" movement (the antiwar movement built on the civil rights movement) that was moribund. Of the active movements of the 1970s, which they did not lead, they seem to see little, perhaps because they were not in their center. Feminism, gay rights, movements in Latino and Native American communities, the rise of mass-based antinuclear activism, and environmentalism seem to have passed them by until they were labeled "identity politics" and somehow diffused into "culture" and no longer "real" politics. Defining these movements as being primarily about identity gives the incorrect impression that they are simply about the assertion of community, and not about structural issues at all.

7. John D'Emilio, "The Gay Community After Stonewall," 1992; Estelle Freedman & John D'Emilio, *Intimate Matters: A History of Sexuality in the United States* (1988).

8. Carol Gilligan, *In a Different Voice: Psychological Theory and Women's Development* (1982).

9. See S. Hoagland, *Lesbian Ethics* (1988).

10. See Beverly Burch, "Psychological Merger," 1982, pp. 201–277; J. Krestan & C. Bepko, "The Problem of Fusion," 1980, pp. 277–289; and S. Smalley, "Dependency Issues," 1987, pp. 125–136.

11. Cf. Randy Shilts, *And The Band Played On* (1987); Larry Kramer, *Faggots* (1978); Larry Kramer, *Reports from the Holocaust* (1989).

12. See Echols for an excellent review of this period and of the beginning of the demise of radical feminism as a major force in feminist politics.

13. See especially Snitow, Stansell, & Thompson, eds., *Powers of Desire: The Politics of Sexuality,* and Carole S. Vance, ed., *Pleasure and Danger: Exploring Female Sexuality,* to get a sense of the nature of these debates.

14. See for example, the conflicts described by Lillian Faderman in *Odd Girls and Twilight Lovers* (1991) and the critiques of "politically correct" lesbian feminism by butches and femmes writing in Joan Nestle, ed., *The Persistent Desire: A Femme-Butch Reader* (1992).

15. See works by Andrea Dworkin (e.g., *Pornography: Men Possessing Women*) and Catharine MacKinnon for the detailed expression of this perspective.

16. The best accounts of this conflict and the confusion experienced by femmes and butches of the seventies and eighties are found in Nestle's excellent anthology, *The Persistent Desire.*

17. Cf. Melissa A. McNeill, *Who Are "We"?* (1991).

18. The alert reader will note the parallelism between my typology and recurrent value constructs concerning appropriate women's roles: traditionalism, liberal feminism, socialist feminism (coalition-building), and radical/separatist/lesbian feminism. Such constructs are widespread and associated with various (sub)cultures and social systems for those who adhere to them.

19. By this term I mean people who received their primary income from AIDS activities and who meet the sociological definition of a professional, someone whose primary value is in his or her education and receives honorific payment.

20. McNeill, p. 50.

21. In 1992, the notion that lesbians have little risk from AIDS and are suffering from "virus envy" resurfaced in England, where it was evident in posters from the Terrence Higgins Trust that proclaimed "Oral sex is very low risk, so throw away those dental dams." Lesbian inventors of the posters claimed that safe-sex emphasis for lesbians was part of a combined negative attitude toward sex and a desire by some to be a greater part of the epidemic.

22. Katy Taylor interview, 1989.

23. "About 142,000 American women develop [breast cancer] each year and 43,000 die of it. Only lung cancer causes more cancer deaths among American women." *New York Times,* November 9, 1989, referring to an article in the *New England Journal of Medicine* for November 9, 1989.

24. Jackie Winnow, "Lesbians Working on AIDS," 1989, pp. 10–18.

25. McNeill, p. 55.

References

Burch, Beverly. (1982). "Psychological Merger in Lesbian Couples: A Joint Ego Psychological and Systems Approach." *Family Therapy, 9* (3), 201–277.

D'Emilio, John. (1992). "After Stonewall." In D'Emilio (Ed.), *Making Trouble* (pp. 234–274). New York: Routledge.

Dworkin, Andrea. (1981). *Pornography: Men Possessing Women.* New York: Perigee.

Echols, Alice. (1989). *Daring to be Bad: Radical Feminism in America, 1967–1975.* Minneapolis: University of Minnesota Press.

Epstein, Barbara. (1988). "Lesbians Lead the Movement." *Out/Look, 1* (2), pp. 27–32.

Faderman, Lillian. (1991). *Odd Girls and Twilight Lovers.* New York: Penguin.

Freedman, Estelle, & D'Emilio, John. (1988). *Intimate Matters: A History of Sexuality in the United States.* New York: Harper & Row.

Gilligan, Carol. (1982). *In a Different Voice: Psychological Theory and Women's Development.* Cambridge, MA: Harvard University Press.

Hoagland, Sarah. (1988). *Lesbian Ethics.* Palo Alto, CA: Institute of Lesbian Studies.

Kramer, Larry. (1978). *Faggots.* New York: Random House.

———. (1989). *Reports from the Holocaust.* New York: St. Martin's Press.

Krestan, Jo Ann, & Bepko, Claudia. (1980). "The Problem of Fusion in the Lesbian Relationship." *Family Process, 19* (3), 277–289.

McAdam, Doug, McCarthy, John & Zald, Meyer. (1988). "Social Movements." In Neil J. Smelser (Ed.), *Handbook of Sociology,* pp. 695–739. New York: Sage.

McNeill, Melissa A. (1991). *Who Are "We"? Exploring Lesbian Involvement in AIDS Work.* Master's thesis, School of Social Work, Smith College.

Nestle, Joan (Ed.). (1992). *The Persistent Desire: A Femme-Butch Reader.* Boston: Alyson Publishers.

Shilts, Randy. (1987). *And the Band Played On.* New York: St. Martin's Press.

Smalley, Sondra. (1987). "Dependency Issues in Lesbian Relationships." *Journal of Homosexuality, 14* (1/2), 125–136.

Snitow, Ann, Stansell, Christine, & Thompson, Sharon (Eds.). (1983). *Powers of Desire: The Politics of Sexuality.* New York: Monthly Review Press.

Taylor, Katy, New York Human Rights Commission. (Personal interview). (1989).

Vance, Carole S. (Ed.). (1984). *Pleasure and Danger: Exploring Female Sexuality.* Boston: Routledge and Kegan Paul.

Winnow, Jackie. (1989). "Lesbians Working on AIDS: Assessing the Impact on Health Care for Women." *Out/Look, 5,* 10–18.

EIGHT

The HIV Epidemic and Public Attitudes Toward Lesbians and Gay Men

Gregory M. Herek

Most of the chapters in this book describe the lesbian and gay community's encounters with HIV—how the community has been affected by the AIDS epidemic and has responded to it. This chapter, in contrast, focuses on heterosexuals. I consider how heterosexuals' attitudes toward lesbians and gay men have been affected by the epidemic, and how they have shaped societal response (and, in many cases, nonresponse) to AIDS. These attitudes and the behaviors, laws, and policies related to them are important components of the context in which gay people have experienced and responded to AIDS in the United States.

Much as perceptions of the nineteenth-century American cholera epidemics were influenced by majority attitudes toward Catholics, Blacks, and other minorities that were both disliked and disproportionately affected by the disease (Rosenberg, 1987), so have public attitudes toward homosexuality shaped cultural constructions of AIDS in the United States (Blendon & Donelan, 1988; Herek, 1990; Herek & Glunt, 1988; Sontag, 1989). Hostility toward gay men and lesbians has influenced institutional responses. During the epidemic's first decade, for example, the Reagan administration refused to request funds for AIDS and, when Congress appropriated funds anyway, delayed their expenditure (Panem, 1987; Shilts, 1987). During the same period, a majority of the Senate supported amendments by Jesse Helms (R-NC) that prohibited federal funding for AIDS education materials that "promote or encourage, directly or indirectly, homosexual activities" ("Limit Voted on AIDS Funds," 1987).

The original empirical data reported in this chapter were collected for a project supported by a grant to the author from the National Institute of Mental Health (R01 MH43253), and by additional resources provided by the late Harold Proshansky, president of the Graduate Center of the City University of New York. I thank John Capitanio for his assistance with data analysis.

Attitudes toward homosexuality have also been reflected in individual heterosexuals' AIDS-related attitudes and behaviors. Members of the U.S. public who express negative attitudes toward gay people repeatedly have been found to be more poorly informed about AIDS than are others and more likely to stigmatize people with AIDS (D'Augelli, 1989; Goodwin & Roscoe, 1988; Herek & Glunt, 1991, 1993; Herek & Capitanio, forthcoming; Price & Hsu, 1992; Pryor, Reeder, Vinacco, & Kott 1989; Stipp & Kerr, 1989). Furthermore, gay men with AIDS are more likely to be negatively evaluated than are heterosexuals with AIDS (Anderson, 1992; Crandall, 1991; Fish & Rye, 1991; St. Lawrence et al., 1990; Triplet & Sugarman, 1987). When public awareness about AIDS increased during the mid-1980s, antigay harassment and victimization began to include verbal references to AIDS. Of the 7,031 incidents of antigay harassment and victimization reported to the National Gay and Lesbian Task Force (NGLTF) in 1989, 15 percent were AIDS-related; the proportion was 17 percent in 1988, 15 percent in 1987, 14 percent in 1986, and 8 percent in 1985 (Berrill, 1992). Because the NGLTF subsequently changed its data collection procedures, more recent reports are not directly comparable to earlier findings. Nonetheless, AIDS-related stigma continues to figure in antigay crimes. In both 1992 and 1993, AIDS bias was documented in 8 percent of the incidents recorded by NGLTF in eight metropolitan areas (NGLTF Policy Institute, 1994).

AIDS-related stigma clearly is linked to antigay prejudice. But has AIDS affected heterosexuals' attitudes toward gay people? Before considering this question, it is important to recall the situation of gay men and lesbians in the United States when the epidemic began.

The gay community entered the 1980s with a mixture of optimism and pessimism, following a decade of significant social and personal change. Throughout the 1970s, gay visibility had increased as never before. Lesbians and gay men came out in the professions, academia, churches, and the military in unprecedented numbers. Gay organizations, associations, and self-help groups proliferated. During the decade, more than half of the states had repealed their sodomy laws, and many municipalities passed legislation prohibiting discrimination on the basis of sexual orientation. In 1973, the American Psychiatric Association declared that homosexuality per se is not a mental illness; this action was strongly endorsed by the American Psychological Association (Bayer, 1987).

Meanwhile, businesses and social organizations catering to a gay clientele blossomed. The number of such institutions listed in *Bob*

Damron's Address Book increased nearly threefold between 1970 and 1980, from 1,500 to almost 5,000 (Darrow, et al. 1986; D'Emilio, 1983). "Gay ghettoes" thrived in New York, San Francisco, and Los Angeles and began to develop in Boston and Chicago (Levine, 1979). These communities and institutions were largely White and middle to upper class. They were also predominantly male, although lesbians began to define new physical spaces for themselves as well (Faderman, 1991). Reflecting the radical questioning of earlier sexual norms and rules that characterized the 1960s, the culture of the gay male communities that developed during the 1970s emphasized the importance of sexual expression and exploration as a form of personal liberation.

Despite their gains, gay people remained at the margins of American society. By the late 1970s, under attack from increasingly powerful political conservatives and religious fundamentalists, many of the community's recent victories appeared to be unraveling (Adam, 1987). Anita Bryant led a successful, nationally visible campaign in 1977 to overturn a gay rights ordinance in Dade County, Florida. Soon after, similar laws were overturned or defeated in St. Paul, Minnesota; Wichita, Kansas; Eugene, Oregon; Davis, California; and Santa Clara County, California. The gay community enjoyed some political success in staving off organized attacks. For example, the 1978 Briggs Initiative, which would have barred gay teachers from California schools, was soundly defeated at the polls (Adam, 1987; Shilts, 1982).

Within weeks of the Briggs vote, however, openly gay San Francisco Supervisor Harvey Milk and gay-sympathetic Mayor George Moscone were murdered by antigay Supervisor Dan White. With Dianne Feinstein newly installed in the mayor's office and the liberal establishment in disarray, the city that had become a major cultural and political center for lesbians and gay men shifted to more conservative policies. The country as a whole followed suit. By 1981, Ronald Reagan was president of the United States, having been elected with strong support from antigay fundamentalist Christians. Thus by the beginning of the 1980s, gay men and lesbians were achieving unprecedented visibility in American society, many heterosexuals were first developing or articulating their personal attitudes toward gay people, and the religious right was emerging as an increasingly powerful adversary of the gay community.

It was in this context that scattered reports began to appear of a new, deadly disease that initially seemed to single out gay men. As the medical and social implications of AIDS became apparent, gay men and lesbians wondered whether they would all soon be targeted for greater hostility, discrimination, and violence. Many feared that AIDS would be used by the political right to destroy the gay community or drive it underground, perhaps by reinstating sodomy statutes and enacting quarantine laws. They saw mandatory testing as a possible step toward developing government lists of gay people for subsequent enforced isolation or discrimination.

Their concerns were not unfounded. Despite persistent educational efforts by public health officials, a significant minority of the American public consistently endorsed repressive measures, such as general quarantine of HIV-infected persons, universal mandatory testing, and even tattooing of infected individuals (e.g., Blendon & Donelan, 1988; Price & Hsu, 1992; Schneider, 1987; Singer & Rogers, 1986; Singer, Rogers, & Corcoran, 1987; Stipp & Kerr, 1989).

Today, well into the epidemic's second decade, it is clear that the gay community's worst fears never materialized. The use of quarantine and other coercive measures proved to be the exception rather than the norm, implemented by public health officials only in individual cases as a last resort (National Research Council, 1993). Repressive quarantine and mandatory testing laws were proposed, but in most cases, gay men and lesbians formed coalitions with public health advocates and civil libertarians to prevent their enactment. In California in the 1980s, for example, such coalitions effected the statewide defeat of Propositions 64, 69, and 102—each of which would have restricted the civil liberties of people infected with HIV and each of which was sponsored by individuals and organizations widely perceived to be antigay (see Herek & Glunt, 1993; Krieger & Lashof, 1988).[1] Although the United States Supreme Court's 1986 decision upholding the constitutionality of state sodomy laws had serious consequences for gay rights litigation in general (Rubenstein, 1993), it was not followed by wholesale reinstatement of sodomy statutes.

What, then, has been the impact of AIDS on heterosexuals' attitudes toward gay men and lesbians? Did the epidemic create a backlash of prejudice and hostility? Or did it simply provide a focus for prejudice, a convenient hook upon which some people could hang their preexisting hostility toward homosexuality?

Ideally, empirical data to answer these questions would have been collected beginning in the 1970s, before the onset of the AIDS epidemic. Interviews would have been conducted at regular intervals with representative samples of heterosexual Americans. Multiple facets of attitudes would have been measured (e.g., affective reactions, opinions about civil liberties, beliefs in stereotypes). Attitudes toward both lesbians and toward gay men would have been assessed. And the interviews would have included questions about a wide range of other variables (e.g., religiosity, political ideology, attitudes about gender) to permit evaluation of how factors apart from AIDS have influenced heterosexuals' attitudes.

Unfortunately, no empirical research was ever conducted that even approximates these criteria. In this chapter, therefore, I examine existing data—recognizing their limitations—to assess the effect of AIDS stigma on antigay prejudice. I present data from three sources: (1) trend data from national surveys conducted throughout the AIDS era; (2) cross-sectional data from a 1988 national telephone survey that I conducted at the Graduate Center of the City University of New York (Herek & Glunt, 1991, 1993); and (3) panel data from a two-wave study that I conducted through the Survey Research Center at the University of California, Berkeley, in 1990 and 1991 (Herek & Capitanio, 1993, 1994, 1995, 1996, forthcoming).

Longitudinal Trends in Attitudes toward Homosexuality

To begin, let us consider the direction and intensity of attitudes toward homosexuality before the AIDS epidemic became part of the public consciousness, using data from the Roper Center archives. Although the Roper database contains hundreds of items about homosexuality from national telephone surveys during the past twenty years, only a few of these items have been included in multiple surveys and thus permit assessment of time trends.

Table 8.1 lists eight such items. Four are taken from the General Social Survey (GSS) conducted by the National Opinion Research Center (NORC) at the University of Chicago (Wood, 1990). The remaining four are taken from the Gallup poll ("Backlash against gays," 1987; Colasanto, 1989; Hugick, 1992; "Majority say opinion of gays unchanged," 1986; "Sharp decline found," 1986).[2] In all cases, these were national surveys with large samples (usually at least one thousand respondents) drawn from the forty-eight contiguous states. The Gallup poll was conducted by telephone, whereas the GSS involved face-to-face interviews. Response data for these items are summarized in Figures 8.1 through 8.6 and Tables 8.2 and 8.3.

Rights of free expression. The GSS includes three items concerning respondents' willingness to grant basic free-speech rights to "a man who admits that he is a homosexual." Respondents are questioned about whether they would allow such a man to "make a speech in your

Table 8.1. Attitudes toward homosexuality: National survey items

GSS series

1. There are always some people whose ideas are considered bad or dangerous by other people. What about a man who admits that he is a homosexual? Suppose this admitted homosexual wanted to make a speech in your community. Should he be allowed to speak, or not? (see Figure 8.1)
2. Should such a person be allowed to teach in a college or university, or not? (see Figure 8.2)
3. If some people in your community suggested that a book he wrote in favor of homosexuality should be taken out of the public library, would you favor removing this book, or not? (see Figure 8.3)
4. What about sexual relations between two adults of the same sex? Do you think it is always wrong, almost always wrong, wrong only sometimes, or not wrong at all? (see Figure 8.4)

Gallup series

5. Do you feel that homosexuality should be considered an acceptable alternative lifestyle, or not? (see Figure 8.5)
6. As you know, there has been considerable discussion in the news lately regarding the rights of homosexual men and women. In general, do you think homosexuals should or should not have equal rights in terms of job opportunities (see Figure 8.6)
7. Do you think homosexuals should or should not be hired for each of the following occupations: Salesperson? Armed Forces? Doctors? Clergy? Elementary school teachers? (see Table 8.2)
8. Do you think homosexual relations between consenting adults should or should not be legal? (see Figure 8.7)

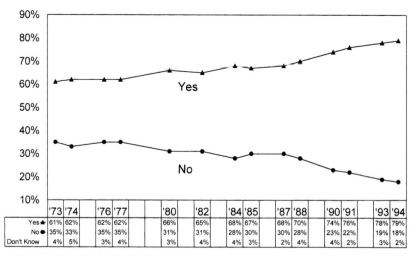

Fig. 8.1. Should an admitted homosexual be allowed to make a speech?
Source: National Opinion Research Center data.

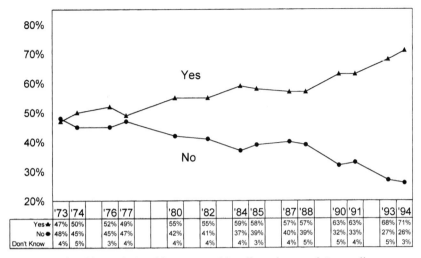

Fig. 8.2. Should an admitted homosexual be allowed to teach in a college or university? *Source:* National Opinion Research Center data.

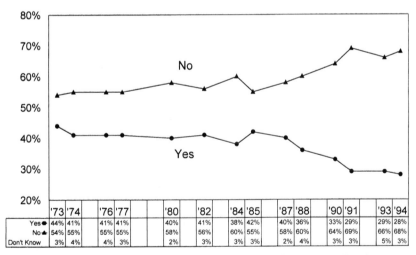

Fig. 8.3. Would you favor removing a book in favor of homosexuality from the public library? *Source:* National Opinion Research Center data.

community" or "teach in a college or university," and whether they would favor removing "a book he wrote in favor of homosexuality" from the public library. Responses to these items for selected years since 1973 are depicted in Figures 8.1 through 8.3.

In the responses prior to 1983—that is, before the time when AIDS emerged as a topic of national interest (Albert, 1986; Baker, 1986)—

it is noteworthy that support for First Amendment rights in connection with homosexuality was relatively strong even in 1973. In that year, 61 percent would have allowed a homosexual man to speak, 47 percent would have allowed him to teach in a college, and 54 percent would have opposed censoring a book that he wrote in favor of homosexuality.

The trend between 1973 and 1983 indicates a slight increase in public support for civil rights. By 1982, the proportion that would have allowed a homosexual man to speak had increased by 4 percent, the proportion that would have allowed him to teach in a college was up by 8 percent, and the proportion that would have opposed censoring a book that he wrote in favor of homosexuality was up by 2 percent.

This same trend continued throughout the 1980s and into the 1990s. By 1994, the proportions endorsing First Amendment rights regarding homosexuality had grown to 79 percent for speech, 71 percent for teaching, and 68 percent against censorship. These were increases from 1973 of 18 percent, 24 percent, and 14 percent, respectively. The percentage of respondents opposing rights for a male homosexual showed a corresponding decrease.

Judgments of wrong and right. Figure 8.4 shows the trend in responses to a GSS question concerning whether sexual relations between two adults of the same sex are "always wrong, almost always wrong, wrong only sometimes, or not wrong at all." To simplify the graphic depiction of the trend, the "wrong only sometimes" and "not wrong at all" responses are combined in Figure 8.4.

Perhaps the most remarkable feature of these data is their consistency over time. Between 1973 and 1982, the proportion responding "always wrong" ranged between 70 and 73 percent (median = 72.5 percent). The proportion responding "never" or "only sometimes" wrong varied between 19 and 24 percent (median = 21.5 percent). Throughout the remainder of the 1980s, the proportions remained fairly steady except for a slight increase in "always wrong" responses between 1985 and 1988. Data from 1993 and 1994 indicate that public condemnation of adult homosexual relations diminished in those years, but a solid majority still regards homosexual behavior as wrong.

Any interpretation of responses to this item must acknowledge the response bias invited by its wording: the question's phrasing strongly suggests that homosexual relations are wrong to at least some extent. Data from other surveys with differently worded items assessing the morality of homosexual behavior, however, are consistent with responses to the GSS item (Herek, 1994).[3]

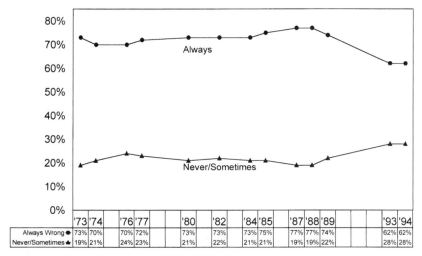

Always Wrong ●	'73	'74		'76	'77			'80		'82		'84	'85		'87	'88	'89				'93	'94
Always Wrong ●	73%	70%		70%	72%			73%		73%		73%	75%		77%	77%	74%				62%	62%
Never/Sometimes ▲	19%	21%		24%	23%			21%		22%		21%	21%		19%	19%	22%				28%	28%

Fig. 8.4. Are sexual relations between two adults of the same sex wrong?
Source: National Opinion Research Center data.

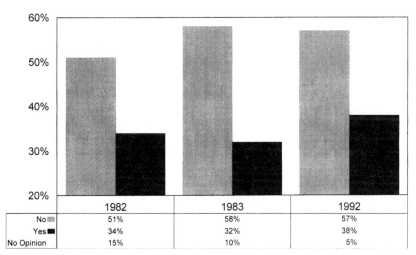

	1982	1983	1992
No ▨	51%	58%	57%
Yes ■	34%	32%	38%
No Opinion	15%	10%	5%

Fig. 8.5. Should homosexuality be considered an acceptable alternative life-style? *Source:* Gallop Poll data.

Acceptable lifestyle. Turning to items included in the Gallup poll, let us begin by considering respondents' opinions about whether homosexuality should be considered an acceptable alternative lifestyle. As with the GSS question on whether homosexual relations are wrong, responses to this item have been fairly consistent over time (see Figure 8.5). By a margin of 17 points (51 percent to 34 percent), respondents did not consider homosexuality an acceptable lifestyle in 1982. In 1992, the margin was 19 points (57 percent to 38 percent), with roughly equal numbers of undecided respondents having shifted to a positive or negative response.

Employment rights. The Gallup poll also assessed attitudes toward equal employment opportunities. The majority of respondents expressing general support for employment rights grew slightly from 56 percent in 1977 to 59 percent in 1982. The proportion opposing employment rights was initially a minority (33 percent in 1977), and decreased to 28 percent in 1982. Support for equal rights in job opportunities increased dramatically throughout the first decade of the AIDS epidemic. By 1992, 74 percent supported such rights and only 18 percent opposed them (see Figure 8.6).

The public's support for employment equality was less enthusiastic when questions were asked about specific occupations (see Table 8.2). Nevertheless, the trend still has been toward steadily increasing support, both before and after the start of the epidemic. Increases in support for employment rights range from six percentage points (for the military)[4] to 14 points (for salespeople and elementary school teachers). One of the most remarkable changes has been in the proportion of Americans who feel homosexuals should be hired as elementary school teachers: it has grown from 27 percent in 1977 (when 65 percent were

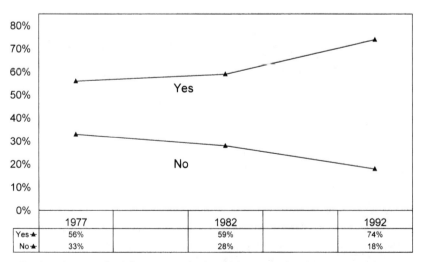

Fig. 8.6. Do you think homosexuals should have equal rights in terms of job opportunities? *Source:* Gallop Poll data.

Table 8.2. Support for job rights in specific occupations by year (Gallup Poll data)

Occupation	Year				Change (1977–92)
	1977	1982	1987	1992	
Sales	68%	70%	72%	82%	+14%
Military	51%	52%	55%	57%	+6%
Doctors	44%	50%	49%	53%	+9%
Clergy	36%	38%	42%	43%	+7%
Teachers	27%	27%	33%	41%	+14%

Source: Gallup Poll

opposed and 8 percent undecided) to 41 percent in 1992 (when 54 percent were opposed and 2 percent undecided).

Sodomy laws. The Gallup poll asked whether homosexual relations between consenting adults should be legal. This issue displays greater volatility than any of those considered above (see Figure 8.7). In 1977, respondents were evenly split, with 43 percent favoring legalization and 43 percent opposing it. By 1982, a plurality favored legalization (45 percent to 39 percent opposed). By 1987—well into the epidemic—legalization was strongly opposed (55 percent to 33 percent). The trend appeared to reverse again in 1992, however, with a plurality favoring legalization (48 percent to 44 percent).[5]

Trends in undecided respondents. Another possible indicator of

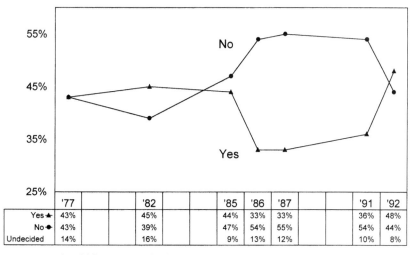

Fig. 8.7. Should homosexual relations between consenting adults be legal? *Source:* Gallop Poll data.

Table 8.3. Proportion undecided about job rights in specific occupations by year (Gallup Poll data)

Occupation	Year				Change (1977–92)
	1977	1982	1987	1992	
Sales	10%	12%	8%	2%	−8%
Military	11%	12%	8%	4%	−7%
Doctors	12%	12%	7%	9%	−3%
Clergy	10%	11%	7%	5%	−5%
Teachers	8%	9%	4%	2%	−6%

Source: Gallup Poll

changes in attitudes over time is the proportion of respondents who are undecided about their attitudes. It is possible, for example, that Americans became increasingly polarized in their opinions concerning homosexuality after the beginning of the AIDS epidemic, which would be indicated by progressively smaller proportions of respondents in the "undecided" or "unsure" category.

Such a trend was not apparent in the GSS data. For the items summarized in Figures 8.1 through 8.3, the proportion of "don't know" responses remained consistently between 2 and 5 percent. For the morality item, the proportion of "other" responses was reported as 0 for most years. In the Gallup data, however, we see a possible trend toward fewer undecideds, as shown in Figures 8.5, 8.6, and 8.7. Table 8.3 displays the proportion of undecided respondents for each of the five occupational questions. With the exception of attitudes toward allowing gay people to be doctors, the proportion of undecideds declined by at least 5 points between 1977 and 1992. That 9 percent of respondents remained undecided about the "doctors" item in 1992 may well be related to public concerns about HIV infection through medical and dental procedures, which received considerable media attention around that time.

Discussion

The patterns in responses to these few survey items suggest some tentative conclusions about public opinion trends during the AIDS epidemic. First, most attitudes appeared to be unaffected by the AIDS epidemic. Public support for First Amendment rights and employment rights for gay people increased steadily, whereas moral condemnation of homosexuality remained consistently high through the 1980s. It is impossible to know, of course, how these patterns might have been different in the absence of AIDS. But with the exception of a small increase in moral disapproval in 1987, no discontinuities are obvious in the data after AIDS became a major focus of popular discourse in the early 1980s.

Second, public attitudes toward the legalization of homosexual behavior have fluctuated dramatically. During the late 1970s and early 1980s, opposition to legalization began to decrease while the proportion supporting legalization remained around 45 percent. By the mid-1980s, opposition to legalization surged. By 1992, this trend had reversed and the distribution of responses resembled what it had been in 1977.

The shift toward greater opposition to legalization in 1985 may well have reflected public concern about the AIDS epidemic. In the 1985 Gallup poll, 37 percent of respondents said that the epidemic had changed their opinion about homosexuals for the worse; only 2 percent said it had changed their attitudes for the better ("Majority Say Opinion of Gays Unchanged," 1986). *The Gallup Report* noted that the 1985 poll "found no decrease since 1982 in the proportion who feel homosexual relations between consenting adults should be legal, and only a minor increase in those who disagree" and that "the survey found no increase since 1982 in [support for] job discrimination against homosexuals" ("Majority Say," 1986:2). When public support for legalizing homosexual relations declined sharply to 33 percent in the next Gallup poll, the drop was attributed to "growing public antipathy toward the gay community" ("Sharp Decline Found in Support," 1986:24).[6]

However, opposition to legalizing homosexual behavior in the mid-1980s may have reflected fear of HIV contagion more than a desire to persecute gay people. Schneider (1987) made this argument, noting that an overall increase in antigay prejudice would have been evidenced in public opinion about issues unrelated to sexual conduct, such as employment discrimination. As already noted, however, support for employment rights increased during this period. Other factors probably were also influential. Most notably, the Supreme Court decision upholding the Georgia sodomy law in *Bowers v. Hardwick* (1986) was released in June, less than one month before the Gallup poll was conducted. (In that July survey, 51 percent of Americans said that they approved of the ruling, compared to 41 percent who disapproved and 8 percent who were undecided.)

In summary, Gallup and GSS surveys suggest that the AIDS epidemic principally affected national attitudes concerning legalization of homosexual behavior, which may also have been influenced by other events not directly related to AIDS. This is not to minimize the significance of antigay attitudes during the 1980s. Apart from legalization of same-gender sexual activity, however, the data suggest that AIDS probably served primarily as a vehicle for expressing preexisting hostility toward gay people rather than as a cause of negative attitudes.

A Cross-Sectional National Survey

I turn now to data from a second source, a national telephone survey that I conducted between July 5 and August 10, 1988 (see Herek & Glunt, 1991). In that study, telephone interviews were conducted by the staff of the New York City Study at the City University of New York Center for Social Research with a random sample of 1,078 English-speaking American adults (see Herek & Glunt, 1991, for a detailed description of the methodology and sample selection). The response rate was only 47 percent, which dictates that the data be interpreted cautiously. A total of 960 interviews contained sufficiently complete data for the analyses relevant to the present paper.[7]

The survey included a five-item AIDS Stigma scale. Items on this scale ascertained respondents' agreement or disagreement that people with AIDS should be quarantined, that their names should be made public, that they are getting what they deserve, that they are a serious risk to the rest of society, and that they have only themselves to blame. Responses were summed to form a Likert-type scale (*alpha* = .70), with higher scores indicating greater stigmatization of people with AIDS.

Respondents were also asked whether they agreed, disagreed, or were "in the middle" for the five items constituting the short form of the Attitudes Toward Gay Men (ATG) scale (Herek, 1988, 1994). The five-item ATG scale displayed an acceptable level of internal consistency in this, its first telephone administration to a national sample (*alpha* = .85).

The results of greatest relevance to this chapter were obtained in regression analyses designed to assess the relationship between attitudes toward gay men and AIDS-related stigma. Antigay attitudes were second only to overestimates of the risks of casual contact in predicting AIDS stigma. Moreover, the latter variable was itself predicted by antigay attitudes. Thus antigay attitudes appeared to exert a direct effect on AIDS stigma as well as an indirect effect, the latter through their influence on beliefs about casual contagion.

These results indicated a strong relationship between AIDS-related stigma and antigay prejudice. Because the data were cross-sectional, I could not determine directly whether respondents' attitudes toward gay men had developed before or after their attitudes concerning AIDS, or whether both sets of attitudes evolved concurrently. Before discussing these results further, I describe results from another survey study.

A Panel Study

Between 1990 and 1992, I conducted a two-stage panel study of public reaction to AIDS. The Wave 1 sample ($n = 538$) was drawn from the population of all English-speaking adults (at least eighteen years of age) residing in households with telephones within the forty-eight contiguous states. Interviews were conducted by the staff of the Survey Research Center at the University of California, Berkeley between September 12, 1990, and February 13, 1991, using their computer-assisted telephone interviewing (CATI) system (for a detailed description of sampling and data collection procedures, see Herek & Capitanio, 1993, 1994, 1995, 1996, forthcoming).[8]

The Wave 2 data were collected approximately one year later using the same sample. Wave 2 interviews were successfully completed with 382 (69 percent) of the Wave 1 respondents. Analysis of demographic variables revealed that the respondents who could not be successfully interviewed in Wave 2 had reported significantly lower educational levels than other respondents in Wave 1. Otherwise, the Wave 2 respondents did not systematically differ from those who were lost to attrition. Of the 382 Wave 2 respondents, 361 identified themselves as heterosexual and provided complete responses for the variables analyzed below.

Equation of Homosexuality and AIDS

Two items were included in the Wave 1 survey to assess the extent to which respondents equated homosexuality with AIDS. Each item was based on the following scenario: "Think of two healthy homosexual men—neither of whom is infected with the AIDS virus. Now suppose they have sexual intercourse." The first item then asked: "If they use condoms, would you say that at least one of them is (a) *almost sure to become infected,* (b) *has a fairly strong chance,* (c) *very little chance,* or (d) *no chance of becoming infected?*" The second item was: "Now suppose the same two healthy men have sexual intercourse but this time they do not use condoms. Would you say at least one of them is *almost sure to get infected*," etc.

Because both men were explicitly described as not infected with HIV, neither of them could be infected by their sexual encounter. Nevertheless, 19.1 percent of the respondents believed that at least one of the men was almost sure to get infected or had a fairly strong chance of doing so—even if they used condoms. If condoms were not used, 47.5 percent of the respondents believed infection was likely.[9]

These results were sufficiently surprising that I revised the wording of the items at Wave 2 to eliminate any possible confusion about the hypothetical couple's HIV status. The Wave 2 wording for the first scenario was: "First, think of two healthy homosexual men—neither of whom is infected with the AIDS virus. Now suppose they have sexual intercourse with each other *only one time*. If they use a condom, would you say that at least one of them is (a) *almost sure to become infected from having intercourse that one time*, (b) *has a fairly strong chance*, (c) *very little chance*, or (d) *no chance of becoming infected from having intercourse that one time?*" The second item was revised to "Think of two *different* healthy homosexual men—neither of whom is infected with the AIDS virus. Suppose they have sexual intercourse with each other *only one time* but they do not use a condom. Would you say that at least one of them is (a) *almost sure to get infected from having intercourse that one time*," etc. With these more explicitly worded items, 9 percent of the respondents still believed that—even if the men used condoms—at least one of them was almost sure to get infected or had a fairly strong chance of getting infected. If condoms were not used, 26.2 percent of the respondents believed infection was likely.

I added a new item in Wave 2: "Now think of two healthy homosexual women—neither of whom is infected with the AIDS virus. Suppose they have sex with each other only one time. Would you say that at least one of them is (a) *almost sure to get infected from having intercourse that one time*," etc. Of the respondents, 12.3 percent gave the incorrect response to this item, slightly more than had done so for the first scenario (i.e., unprotected sex between uninfected men).

Some respondents' Wave 2 answers may reflect simply an inability to understand the question, despite the revised wording. Yet even if we assume this to have been the case for all Wave 2 respondents who stated that infection was likely to occur when condoms were used by the uninfected men (9 percent), still another 17.2 percent believed AIDS could result from a single sexual act between two uninfected men if they do not use condoms. This response pattern suggests that a small but significant minority of the public does not clearly understand that AIDS results from transmission of a virus rather than from homosexual activity per se. If this interpretation is valid, it has disturbing implications. It suggests that many Americans equate homosexuality (even female homosexuality) with AIDS, and that many Americans do not believe that homosexual sex can ever be safe. Such a belief is likely to affect the public's willingness to support AIDS prevention programs targeting men who have sex with men.[10]

Affective Responses to People with AIDS

In Wave 1, respondents were asked about the extent to which they felt sympathetic toward PWAs (people with AIDS), disgusted by them, and afraid of them. Four response alternatives were provided (e.g., *very sympathetic, somewhat, a little, not at all sympathetic*). Eighty-one percent felt very or somewhat sympathetic (only 5.5 percent felt not at all sympathetic); 28.2 percent felt very/somewhat disgusted (52.8 percent felt not at all disgusted); and 34.2 percent felt very/somewhat afraid of PWAs (40 percent felt not at all afraid).[11]

In the Wave 2 survey, respondents were asked about the same three feelings toward persons with AIDS, but separate questions were posed about feelings toward people who got AIDS through two different routes: "through homosexual behavior" and "from a blood transfusion." Respondents expressed considerably more negative feelings toward a person who got AIDS through homosexual behavior. Whereas 98 percent felt sympathy for a blood transfusion recipient (and fewer than 1 percent felt no sympathy at all), only 58.3 percent felt sympathy for someone who had engaged in homosexual behavior (22.8 percent felt not at all sympathetic).[12] Comparable results were obtained for disgust (7.3 percent for blood transfusion vs. 40.4 percent for homosexual behavior). For fear, however, the difference between transmission routes was fairly small (23.4 percent for blood transfusion vs. 27.6 percent for homosexual behavior).

These data indicate that the notion of "innocent victims" is alive and well. Clearly, many Americans who are inclined to feel positively toward a generic person with AIDS are affected by learning that the person contracted HIV through homosexual behavior.

Attitudes toward Gay Men and Lesbians and AIDS-Related Stigma

The interviews for both Waves 1 and 2 included three items from the Attitudes Toward Gay Men (ATG) scale. Respondents were provided four alternatives for each item: *agree strongly, agree somewhat, dis-*

agree somewhat, and *disagree strongly.* The responses were summed to yield a scale score (*alpha* = .76), with higher scores indicating higher levels of antigay feelings.

Attitudes toward lesbians were not assessed in Wave 1. In Wave 2, however, a three-item short form of the Attitudes Toward Lesbians (ATL) scale (*alpha* = .76) was included. It consisted of three ATG items reworded to apply to lesbians. The ATL and ATG items are: (1) "Sex between two women [men] is just plain wrong;" (2) "I think lesbians [male homosexuals] are disgusting;" and (3) "Female [male] homosexuality is a natural expression of sexuality in women [men]" (for a general discussion of the ATL and ATG scales, see Herek, 1994).

In addition, three items from the AIDS Stigma scale (described above for the 1988 study) were included in the survey. Respondents were asked how much they agreed or disagreed that: (1) "People with AIDS should be legally separated from others to protect the public health" (QUARANTINE); (2) "The names of people with AIDS should be made public so others can avoid them" (NAMES); and (3) "People who got AIDS through sex or drug use have gotten what they deserve" (BLAME). Four response alternatives were provided (*agree strongly, agree somewhat, disagree somewhat, disagree strongly*).

Results. Attitudes toward gay men did not change substantially between Wave 1 and Wave 2. At Wave 1, 69.2 percent of the heterosexual respondents felt that male homosexuality is wrong (compared to 68.3 percent at Wave 2), 53.5 percent that it is disgusting (compared to 59.9 percent at Wave 2), and 75.6 percent that it is not natural (compared to 75.4 percent at Wave 2). Attitudes toward lesbians were very similar to attitudes toward gay men; the percentages were 64.3 percent (wrong), 59.9 percent (disgusting), and 73.2 percent (not natural).

A significant minority of the sample in both waves manifested AIDS-related stigma. At Wave 1, roughly one-third of the sample agreed that people with AIDS should be quarantined (35.5 percent) and that their names should be made public (29.1 percent). One-fifth (20.1 percent) agreed that PWAs deserved their illness. Willingness to enact coercive policies decreased somewhat at Wave 2, to 25.3 percent supporting quarantine and 22.4 percent wanting to make PWAs' names public. Blame for people with AIDS did not change.[13]

The influence of AIDS attitudes on attitudes toward gay people was assessed in three sets of regression equations.[14] The first set replicated the regression analyses for the 1988 study (described above), with the three indicators of AIDS stigma (quarantine, names public, blame) as dependent variables, and ATG scores—along with a variety of other demographic and attitudinal variables—as independent variables. Attitudes toward gay men emerged as the primary predictor for BLAME and as one of the principal predictors for QUARANTINE and NAMES.[15]

In the second set of equations, we assessed the extent to which attitudes toward homosexuality explained changes over time in attitudes concerning AIDS. Using the Wave 2 QUARANTINE, NAMES, and BLAME items as dependent variables, we constructed three hierarchical regression equations. On the first step, we entered the Wave 1 item corresponding to the dependent variable (e.g., for the equation with Wave 2 QUARANTINE as the dependent variable, we entered the Wave 1 QUARANTINE response as the independent variable). This procedure controls for the variance in Wave 2 attitudes that can be explained by preexisting attitudes. In other words, any statistical significance associated with the remaining independent variables can be interpreted as reflecting the importance of that variable in explaining changes in AIDS attitudes between Waves 1 and 2. On the second step, we entered Wave 1 ATG scores along with relevant Wave 1 demographic variables (gender, age, education, race, income, number of children, attendance at religious services, political ideology).

The results did not indicate a strong role for ATG scores in predicting changes in AIDS stigma. As expected, Wave 1 responses strongly predicted Wave 2 responses, accounting for 42.4 percent of the variance in the QUARANTINE, 28 percent of the variance in the NAMES item, and 21.1 percent of the variance in the BLAME item. Controlling thus for Wave 1 responses, attitudes toward gay men accounted for less than 1 percent of the variance in Wave 2 agreement with QUARANTINE, NAMES, or BLAME.[16]

In the third set of regression equations, we reversed the analysis and assessed the extent to which AIDS-related attitudes and beliefs accounted for change in attitudes toward gay men and lesbians over time. We constructed hierarchical regression equations with Wave 2 ATG and ATL scores as the dependent variables. On the first step of each equation, we entered Wave 1 ATG scores to control for the variance in Wave 2 attitudes that can be explained by preexisting attitudes.[17] On subsequent steps, we entered AIDS-related (i.e., QUARANTINE, NAMES, BLAME, feelings toward PWAs, beliefs about casual contact) and demographic variables.

The results did not indicate a significant effect for the AIDS variables. As expected, Wave 1 ATG scores explained most of the variance in Wave 2 ATG (49.2 percent) and ATL (40 percent). None of the independent variables explained at least 1 percent of the variance in changes in ATG scores. In contrast, three variables explained more than 1 percent of the variance in ATL scores after controlling for Wave 1 ATG scores: religious attendance (1.5 percent), political ideology (1.2 percent), and education (1 percent). Respondents were more likely to express increasingly negative attitudes toward lesbians to the extent that they attended religious services frequently, were politically conservative, and had a lower educational level.[18]

Discussion

The regression results suggest that although AIDS-related attitudes are strongly correlated with attitudes toward gay men and lesbians, one type of attitude cannot be characterized as "causing" the other. AIDS-related attitudes did not predict subsequent changes in attitudes toward gay men or lesbians. Similarly, attitudes toward gay men strongly predicted contemporaneous willingness to blame, quarantine, and publicly identify people with AIDS, but did not predict changes in such stigma one year later.

It is important to recognize the limitations inherent in these data due to the relatively small sample size and the brief interval (one year) between surveys. In addition, the timing of the data collection may have affected the outcome. A similar survey conducted in the early years of the epidemic when public opinion was newly forming might have revealed significant attitudinal shifts, even over a one-year period. By the early 1990s, however, Americans' attitudes concerning AIDS probably were much more stable than had been the case only five years before.

Obviously, the data described here are not definitive in the way that the findings might be if they were derived from an ideal study, such as the one sketched earlier in this chapter. Nevertheless, three tentative conclusions can be offered. First, AIDS-related attitudes were strongly correlated with attitudes toward homosexuality throughout the epidemic's first decade. Second, by the 1990s, short-term changes in heterosexuals' AIDS attitudes could not be explained by their prior attitudes toward gay people, and short-term changes in attitudes toward gay people could not be explained by prior attitudes concerning AIDS.

Third, with one possible exception, the AIDS epidemic has not had an obvious direct impact on longitudinal trends in public attitudes toward homosexuality. The exception is in the area of public support for the repeal of sodomy laws in the late 1980s; fear of AIDS may have (temporarily) reversed a trend toward support for repeal. AIDS appears to have had little effect on moral judgments about homosexuality, which continue to be strongly negative. And it appears to have had little impact on support for civil liberties in employment and speech, which have consistently increased. Public opinion in these areas might be different today had the AIDS epidemic never occurred, of course, but no dramatic discontinuities are evident in data collected since the early 1970s.

AIDS may have had minimal impact on the direction and intensity of heterosexuals' attitudes toward lesbians and gay men, but the epidemic clearly has affected the nature, content, and rhetoric of those attitudes. Early in its history, AIDS was defined principally in terms of homosexuality. Before adopting the AIDS acronym, the Centers for Disease Control initially called the new disease Gay-Related Immune Deficiency, or GRID (Shilts, 1987). In early AIDS discourse, the phrase "the general public" was frequently used as a counterpart to "risk groups," clearly conveying the distinction between dominant in-group and stigmatized out-group. Furthermore, people with AIDS were dichotomized into the guilty and the innocent. A *Newsweek* caption early in the epidemic, for example, described a teenage hemophiliac and an infant with AIDS as "the most blameless victims" ("Social Fallout From an Epidemic," 1985). In contrast, those whose HIV infection occurred as a result of stigmatized behavior—gay men, injection drug users, and their sexual partners—were considered neither blameless nor part of the general public.

As the data reported in this chapter show, homosexuality and AIDS continue to be equated in the minds of many Americans. A minority of the public believes that sex between two people of the same gender is sufficient for transmitting AIDS, even when neither person has HIV. Gay men with AIDS continue to evoke less sympathy and more disgust than other PWAs. To regard AIDS stigma as synonymous with antigay prejudice, however, is an oversimplification. Some individuals do indeed manifest stigma toward persons with AIDS as a way of symbolically expressing prejudice against social groups linked to AIDS—the latter including not only gay people, but also drug users, the poor, people of color, and foreigners (e.g., Herek & Glunt, 1993; Jelen & Wilcox, 1992; Pryor et al., 1989). Others, however, do so out of a genuine fear of contracting HIV (e.g., Bishop, Alva, Cantu, & Rittiman, 1991), perhaps based on their distrust of scientists and public health officials (Herek & Capitanio, 1994).

To the extent that AIDS stigma serves as a vehicle for expressing preexisting antigay prejudice, it is a consequence of hostility toward gay men and lesbians rather than a cause of it. Thus the AIDS epidemic's effect on heterosexuals' attitudes toward gay men and lesbians may be primarily in the new forms of expression it has provided for prejudice. For example, AIDS provided Patrick Buchanan, a conservative columnist and 1996 candidate for the Republican presidential nomination, with an opportunity to decry "the willful refusal of homosexuals to cease indulging in the immoral, unnatural, unsanitary, unhealthy, and suicidal practice of anal intercourse" (Buchanan, 1987:23; see also Schwartz, 1992). Even without AIDS, however, Buchanan and others sharing his ideology probably would have found ways to express their hostility toward the gay community.

It would be inaccurate to assume that AIDS has had only negative effects on heterosexuals' attitudes. AIDS may also have created a cultural context in which many heterosexuals developed more favorable attitudes toward lesbians and gay men. The epidemic probably has motivated many lesbians and gay men to come out to their loved ones, with the likely consequence that many of the latter have adopted more positive feelings toward gay men and lesbians in general (Herek & Capitanio, 1996; Herek & Glunt, 1993). Furthermore, by creating new visibility for gay people, their relationships, and communities, the epidemic may have hastened the emergence of new public identities and roles for gay men and lesbians. Media coverage, for example, has documented the rich and varied lives led by people with AIDS. It has also reported on the devoted care that many people with AIDS have received from their lovers and their extended gay and lesbian families, often while biological relatives rejected them because of their homosexuality. As a consequence of this coverage, new images of gay people—as contributors to society, as partners in relationships, and as members of a community—are widely available. These images may help to create new social identities for gay people, supplanting earlier identities that were defined almost exclusively in terms of sexual behavior (Herek, 1992, 1996). The consequence may be that heterosexuals humanize and individuate gay people to a greater extent, psychological processes that are associated generally with the reduction of prejudice toward minority groups (Brewer & Miller, 1984).

AIDS could have created a major backlash of prejudice and hostility against gay men and lesbians, but it did not. If anything, AIDS appears to have provided yet one more arena in which the political right could attack the gay community. The reasons why, despite AIDS, public opinion continued to move toward greater support for civil liberties and remained stable concerning moral judgments are undoubtedly complex. Part of the explanation must lie in the actions taken by the gay and lesbian community from the beginning of the epidemic. The community recognized early on that AIDS could be used to eradicate the hard-won victories of the 1970s, and it organized quickly to prevent such an outcome. Gay people were supported in this effort by largely sympathetic public health and medical establishments that incorporated civil rights safeguards into their traditional responses to communicable disease (National Research Council, 1993). Any explanation of why the worst fears of the gay community failed to materialize must also take account of the American public's apparent reluctance to deprive even an unpopular group of its civil liberties without good reason. Although members of the political right attempted repeatedly to use AIDS as a justification for repressive measures, they failed because the public became convinced that such measures were unnecessary and ineffective (e.g., Krieger & Lashof, 1988).

The proliferation of AIDS among heterosexuals in the United States probably signals an impending respite for the gay community on this battlefront. As public perceptions of AIDS increasingly associate the disease with nongay populations and communities, the likelihood diminishes that AIDS will exert a significant negative impact on public reactions to homosexuality. This prediction is offered cautiously, with recognition that future changes in the course of the epidemic could revitalize the prospects for AIDS-based repressive measures against the gay community. For example, a calamitous new wave of AIDS cases among young gay men might arouse sufficient public alarm to revive calls for quarantine or mandatory testing. Even without such events, the gay community will continue to be confronted by antigay rhetoric that includes images of disease and blame. Such rhetoric will affect public debate, especially in cities and towns where AIDS is only now being recognized as an important public health problem.

In short, AIDS will continue to figure in public discourse surrounding homosexuality. But the principal impact of AIDS on heterosexuals' attitudes toward gay men and lesbians has probably already been felt and has been surprisingly small.

Notes

1. A fourth ballot measure—Proposition 96, which required HIV testing of anyone who was both charged with a crime and accused of having interfered with the official duties of a police officer, firefighter, or emergency medical worker—passed in 1988 by a margin of 62 percent to 38 percent (see Herek & Glunt, 1993).

2. In addition to the GSS and Gallup polls, data from several other national surveys

are cited throughout this chapter. Recognizing that many readers will not have access to the Roper archives, I have tried whenever possible to include additional bibliographic references for these data. Data without an accompanying citation are taken from the Roper Center archives. I thank Professor Bliss Siman of Baruch College of the City University of New York for her assistance in obtaining the Roper Center data.

3. In a 1978 Gallup poll, 62 percent of the respondents felt that "homosexual relations between consenting adults is wrong." A 1978 poll by Yankelovich, Skelly & White found that 53 percent of respondents felt that such relationships were wrong, compared to 38 percent who felt that they are "not a moral issue." In a 1980 poll by Research and Forecasts, 72 percent felt that homosexuality is morally wrong, whereas 28 percent felt it was not a moral issue. In a 1986 ABC News/Washington Post poll, 66 percent felt that "homosexuality is morally wrong." A 1987 ABC poll with the same item found that 63 percent agreed, but this proportion was reduced to 43 percent when respondents were asked about the morality of homosexuality if "the individual voluntarily agrees to abstain from sexual activity."

4. Public opinion about military service by gay men and lesbians has been volatile since late 1992 (Herek, 1993; Herek, Jobe, & Carney, 1996; National Defense Research Institute, 1993).

5. I exclude the 1989 Gallup survey data from the figures and from my discussion because they are so inconsistent with other trends in the Gallup series that I suspect they reflect sampling bias, methodological artifact, or a temporary fluctuation in attitudes for that year. Pro-gay responses increased substantially in the 1989 survey, but then dropped back to their previous levels in 1991. In 1989, legalization of homosexual relations was favored by a margin of 47 percent to 36 percent (17 percent no opinion); respondents strongly approved of general employment rights (71 percent to 18 percent opposed) and of employment in sales (79 percent to 13 percent), the military (60 percent to 29 percent), and medicine (56 percent to 32 percent); smaller proportions favored having homosexuals as clergy (44 percent to 43 percent) or elementary school teachers (42 percent to 48 percent).

6. Other survey data indicate that AIDS-related antigay sentiment may have been at its height around this time. Between 1985 and 1987, for example, approximately one-fourth of the respondents to *Los Angeles Times* national polls agreed that "AIDS is a punishment God has given homosexuals for the way they live" (28 percent on December 5, 1985; 24 percent on July 9, 1986; and 27 percent on July 24, 1987). And approximately 12 percent of Americans indicated that they were avoiding homosexuals as a way of protecting themselves from getting AIDS (12 percent in a 1987 *ABC News/Washington Post* poll, 12 percent in a 1987 Gallup poll, and 11 percent in a 1988 Gallup poll). In a 1990 *ABC News/Washington Post* poll, only 5 percent said they were avoiding such contact.

Many Americans believed a shift was occurring in popular attitudes. In a 1987 *Los Angeles Times* survey, 54 percent agreed that "AIDS has set off a wave of antigay sentiment in the general public," with another 5 percent believing that AIDS had led both to increased bigotry and increased sympathy for homosexuals.

7. Using the United States Census Bureau's Current Population Survey for March 1988, the data were post-stratified by sex, race, and age. The post-stratified data are used for the analyses described in this paper.

8. The cases were post-stratified by gender and racial category (White, Black, other), using 1990 Census Bureau data.

9. For purposes of comparison between Waves 1 and 2, the proportions reported in the text refer only to the respondents who completed both years of the survey. If data from all of the Wave 1 respondents (including those lost to attrition at Wave 2) are considered, the proportions believing transmission was likely were 15.5 percent when condoms were used and 41.9 percent when condoms were not used.

10. These data are consistent with the results from other surveys conducted in 1991. In a Gallup poll sponsored by Gay Men's Health Crisis, 34 percent of the respondents felt that "gay men will always be at higher risk for AIDS, regardless of what they do" (60 percent felt that "safer sex for gay men would reduce their risk of AIDS"). In a separate 1991 Gallup poll, 58 percent believed that "homosexual males who practice 'safe sex' with many male sex partners" were at high risk (compared to 31 percent who felt such activity carried moderate risk and 8 percent who felt it carried little or no risk).

11. As with the transmission scenarios, these proportions are based only on heterosexual respondents who completed both interviews. When respondents who did not complete the Wave 2 interview are included, the proportions are: 78.8 percent very/somewhat sympathetic; 27.7 percent very/somewhat disgusted; 35.7 percent very/somewhat afraid.

12. A few years earlier, in a 1988 *CBS/New York Times* poll, the proportion of respondents with "a lot" of sympathy for people with AIDS was 46 percent; asked specifically about sympathy for "people who get AIDS from homosexual activity," however, the proportion dropped to 17 percent. The proportion of respondents who replied "not much" or who volunteered that they felt no sympathy at all for people who get AIDS from homosexual activity was 60 percent, in contrast to 20 percent when homosexuality was not mentioned in the question. In a 1991 poll by the same organizations, 51 percent felt "a lot" of sympathy for "people who have AIDS," but only 19 percent felt similarly for people who get AIDS from homosexual activity. As in 1988, 60 percent replied "not much" or volunteered that they felt no sympathy at all for people who get AIDS from homosexual activity, in contrast to 11 percent when homosexuality was not mentioned in the question.

13. The Wave 1 proportions are not substantially altered if we include the respondents who were lost to attrition at Wave 2. With all Wave 1 respondents (including those who did not complete the Wave 2 survey) included, the Wave 1 results were as follows: for the Attitudes Toward Gay Men items, 69.8 percent agreed that male homosexuality is just plain wrong, 54.1 percent agreed that it is disgusting, and 74.4 percent felt that it is not natural. For the AIDS Stigma items, 33.7 percent agreed that people with AIDS should be quarantined, 28.8 percent agreed that their names should be made public, and 20 percent agreed that PWAs deserved their illness.

14. For all of the regression analyses described below, $n = 361$. These were the heterosexual respondents who completed both Wave 1 and Wave 2 interviews and provided complete responses for all of the items used in the regression analyses.

15. For QUARANTINE, the independent variables explained 33.3 percent (adjusted R^2) of the variance, with 9.7 percent accounted for by casual contact beliefs, 6.5 percent by ATG scores, and 3 percent by educational level. For NAMES, the independent variables explained 13.3 percent of the variance, with 3.9 percent accounted for by casual contact beliefs, 2.2 percent by education, and 1.6 percent by ATG scores. For BLAME, the independent variables explained 21.2 percent of the variance, with 9.4 percent accounted for by ATG scores, 2.9 percent by religious attendance, and 3.7 percent by race (Blacks were less likely than others to blame PWAs).

16. For QUARANTINE, none of the independent variables explained at least 1 percent of the variance after controlling for Wave 1 attitudes. For NAMES, age explained 2.1 percent of the variance and educational level explained 1.9 percent. Respondents were likely to decrease their support for publicly identifying PWAs to the extent that they were younger and better educated. For BLAME, race was an important predictor, with the dummy variable for WHITE accounting for 2.2 percent of the variance, and the dummy variable BLACK explaining 1.6 percent after controlling for Wave 1 attitudes. Religious attendance explained an additional 1.9 percent of the variance and education explained an additional 1.2 percent. Examination of the regression coefficients revealed that respondents were more likely to increase their blame for PWAs if they were neither

White nor Black (i.e., if they were in the "Other Race" category, which included Latino, Asian, and Native Americans; these groups were combined for the analysis because of their small numbers in the sample) and to the extent that they attended religious services frequently and were not highly educated.

17. Because attitudes toward lesbians were not measured at Wave 1, we used ATG scores as a proxy variable. This decision is justified by the high correlation between ATG and ATL scores.

18. We also computed the regression equations with only the four AIDS variables (casual contact beliefs, BLAME, QUARANTINE, NAMES, and negative feelings toward PWAs) as independent variables. Those analyses indicated that changes in attitudes toward gay men were predicted to a slight extent (0.92 percent of variance explained) by respondents' support for coercive policies (QUARANTINE and NAMES): greater support for such policies in Wave 1 predicted an increase in hostile attitudes toward gay men in Wave 2. For both ATL and ATG scores, however, none of the AIDS variables accounted for 1 percent of the variance.

References

Adam, Barry D. (1987). *The Rise of a Lesbian and Gay Movement.* Boston: Twayne.

Albert, Edward. (1986). "Illness and Deviance: The Response of the Press to AIDS." In Douglas A. Feldman & Thomas M. Johnson (Eds.), *The Social Dimensions of AIDS: Method and Theory* (pp. 163–178). New York: Praeger.

"Backlash against Gays Appears to Be Leveling Off." (1987). *Gallup Report,* March (258), 12–18.

Baker, Andrea J. (1986). "The Portrayal of AIDS in the Media: An Analysis of Articles in the *New York Times.*" In Douglas A. Feldman & Thomas M. Johnson (Eds.), *The Social Dimensions of AIDS: Method and Theory* (pp. 179–194). New York: Praeger.

Bayer, Ronald. (1987). *Homosexuality and American Psychiatry: The Politics of Diagnosis* (2nd Ed.). Princeton, NJ: Princeton University Press.

Berrill, Kevin T. (1992). "Anti-Gay Violence and Victimization in the United States: An Overview." In Gregory M. Herek & Kevin T. Berrill (Eds.), *Hate Crimes: Confronting Violence Against Lesbians and Gay Men* (pp. 19–45). Newbury Park, CA: Sage.

Bishop, George D., Alva, Albert L., Cantu, Lionel, & Rittiman, Telecia K. (1991). "Responses to Persons With AIDS: Fear of Contagion or Stigma?" *Journal of Applied Social Psychology, 21,* 1877–1888.

Blendon, R. J. & Donelan, K. (1988). "Discrimination against People with AIDS: The Public's Perspective." *New England Journal of Medicine, 319,* 1022–1026.

Bowers v. Hardwick. (1986). 106 S. Ct. 2841.

Brewer, Marilynn B. & Miller, Norman. (1984). "Beyond the Contact Hypothesis: Theoretical Perspectives on Desegregation." In Norman Miller & Marilynn B. Brewer (Eds.), *Groups in Contact: The Psychology of Desegregation* (pp. 281–302). Orlando, FL: Academic Press.

Buchanan, Patrick J. (1987). "AIDS and Moral Bankruptcy." *New York Post,* December 2, p. 23.

Colasanto, D. (1989). "Tolerance of Homosexuality Is on the Rise among the Public." *The Gallup Report,* October (289), 11–15.

Darrow, William W., Gorman, E. M. & Glick, Brad P. (1986). "The Social Origins of AIDS: Social Change, Sexual Behavior, and Disease Trends." In Douglas A. Feldman & Thomas M. Johnson (Eds.), *The Social Dimensions of AIDS: Method and Theory* (pp. 95–107). New York: Praeger.

D'Augelli, Anthony R. (1989). "AIDS Fears and Homophobia among Rural Nursing Personnel." *AIDS Education and Prevention, 1,* 277–284.

D'Emilio, John. (1983). *Sexual Politics, Sexual Communities: The Making of a Homo-*

sexual Minority in the United States, 1940–1970. Chicago: University of Chicago Press.

Faderman, Lillian. (1991). *Odd Girls and Twilight Lovers: A History of Lesbian Life in Twentieth-Century America.* New York: Columbia University Press.

Fish, Thomas A. & Barbara J. Rye. (1991). "Attitudes toward a Homosexual or Heterosexual Person with AIDS." *Journal of Applied Social Psychology, 21,* 651–667.

Goodwin, M. P. & B. Roscoe. (1988). "AIDS: Students' Knowledge and Attitudes at a Midwestern University." *Journal of American College Health, 36,* 214–222.

Herek, Gregory M. (1988). "Heterosexuals' Attitudes toward Lesbian and Gay Men: Correlates and Gender Differences." *The Journal of Sex Research, 25,* 451–477.

———. (1990). "Illness, Stigma, and AIDS." In Paul T. Costa Jr. & Gary R. Vanden Bos (Eds.), *Psychological Aspects of Serious Illness: Chronic Conditions, Fatal Diseases, and Clinical Care* (pp. 103–150). Washington, DC: American Psychological Association.

———. (1992). "The Social Context of Hate Crimes: Notes on Cultural Heterosexism." In Gregory M. Herek & Kevin T. Berrill (Eds.), *Hate Crimes: Confronting Violence against Lesbians and Gay Men* (pp. 89–104). Thousand Oaks, CA: Sage.

———. (1993). "Sexual Orientation and Military Service: A Social Science Perspective." *American Psychologist, 48,* 538–549.

———. (1994). "Assessing Attitudes toward Lesbians and Gay Men: A Review of Empirical Research with the ATLG Scale." In Beverly Greene & Gregory M. Herek (Eds.), *Lesbian and Gay Psychology: Theory, Research, and Clinical Applications* (pp. 206–228). Thousand Oaks, CA: Sage.

———. (1996). "Why Tell If You're Not Asked? Self-Disclosure, Intergroup Contact, and Heterosexuals' Attitudes toward Lesbians and Gay Men." In Gregory M. Herek, Jared Jobe, & Ralph Carney (Eds.), *Out in Force: Sexual Orientation and the Military* (pp. 197–225). Chicago: University of Chicago Press.

Herek, Gregory M. & Capitanio, John P. (1993). "Public Reactions to AIDS in the United States: A Second Decade of Stigma." *American Journal of Public Health, 83,* 574–577.

———. (1994). "Conspiracies, Contagion, and Compassion: Trust and Public Reactions to AIDS." *AIDS Education and Prevention, 6,* 365–375.

———. (1995). "Black Heterosexuals' Attitudes toward Lesbians and Gay Men in the United States." *The Journal of Sex Research, 32,* 95–105.

———. (1996). " 'Some of My Best Friends': Intergroup Contact, Concealable Stigma, and Heterosexuals' Attitudes toward Gay Men and Lesbians." *Personality and Social Psychology Bulletin, 22,* 412–424.

———. (Forthcoming). "AIDS Stigma and Contact with Persons with AIDS: The Effects of Personal and Vicarious Contact." *Journal of Applied Social Psychology.*

Herek, Gregory M. & Glunt, Eric K. (1988). "An Epidemic of Stigma: Public Reactions to AIDS." *American Psychologist, 43,* 886–891.

———. (1991). "AIDS-Related Attitudes in the United States: A Preliminary Conceptualization." *The Journal of Sex Research, 28,* 99–123.

———. (1993). "Public Attitudes toward AIDS-Related Issues in the United States." In John B. Pryor & Glenn D. Reeder (Eds.), *The Social Psychology of HIV Infection* (pp. 229–261). Hillsdale, NJ: Lawrence Erlbaum Associates.

Herek, Gregory M., Jobe, Jared & Carney, Ralph (Eds.). (1996). *Out in Force: Sexual Orientation and the Military.* Chicago: University of Chicago Press.

Hugick, Larry. (1992). "Public Opinion Divided on Gay Rights." *The Gallup Poll Monthly,* June, pp. 2–6.

Jelen, Ted G. & Wilcox, Clyde. (1992). "Symbolic and Instrumental Values as Predictors of AIDS Policy Attitudes." *Social Science Quarterly, 73,* 736–749.

Krieger, Nancy & Lashof, Joyce C. (1988). "AIDS, Policy Analysis, and the Electorate:

The Role of Schools of Public Health." *American Journal of Public Health,* 78, 411–415.

Levine, Martin P. (1979). "Gay Ghetto." *Journal of Homosexuality,* 4(4), 363–377.

"Limit Voted on AIDS Funds." (1987). *New York Times,* October 15, p. B12.

"Majority Say Opinion of Gays Unchanged by AIDS Epidemic." (1986). *Gallup Report,* January (244–245), 2–9.

National Defense Research Institute. (1993). *Sexual Orientation and Military Personnel Policy: Options and Assessment.* Santa Monica, CA: RAND.

National Gay and Lesbian Task Force Policy Institute. (1994). *Anti-Gay/Lesbian Violence, Victimization, & Defamation in 1993.* Washington, DC: Author.

National Research Council. (1993). *The Social Impact of AIDS in the United States.* Washington, DC: National Academy Press.

Panem, Sandra. (1987). *The AIDS Bureaucracy.* Cambridge, MA: Harvard University Press.

Price, Vincent & Hsu, Mei-Ling. (1992). "Public Opinion about AIDS Policies: The Role of Misinformation and Attitudes toward Homosexuals." *Public Opinion Quarterly,* 56, 29–52.

Pryor, John B., Reeder, Glenn D., Vinacco, R. Jr., & Kott, T. L. (1989). "The Instrumental and Symbolic Functions of Attitudes toward Persons with AIDS." *Journal of Applied Social Psychology,* 19, 377–404.

Rosenberg, Charles E. (1987). *The Cholera Years: The United States in 1832, 1849, and 1866* (2nd ed.). Chicago: University of Chicago Press.

Rubenstein, William B. (Ed.). (1993). *Lesbians, Gay Men, and the Law.* New York: New Press.

Schneider, William. (1987). "Homosexuals: Is AIDS Changing Attitudes?" *Public Opinion,* 10(2): 6, 7, 59.

Schwartz, J. (1992). "Buchanan Calls AIDS 'Nature's Retribution.'" *San Francisco Examiner,* February 28, p. A18.

"Sharp Decline Found in Support for Legalizing Gay Relations." (1986). *Gallup Report,* November (254), 24–26.

Shilts, Randy. (1982). *The Mayor of Castro Street: The Life and Times of Harvey Milk.* New York: St. Martin's.

———. (1987). *And the Band Played On: Politics, People, and the AIDS Epidemic.* New York: St. Martin's.

Singer, Eleanor & Rogers, Theresa F. (1986). "Public Opinion and AIDS." *AIDS and Public Policy Journal,* 1, 1–13.

Singer, Eleanor, Rogers, Theresa F. & Corcoran, Mary. (1987). "The Polls: AIDS." *Public Opinion Quarterly,* 51, 580–595.

"Social Fallout from an Epidemic." (1985). *Newsweek,* August 12, pp. 28–29.

Sontag, Susan. (1989). *AIDS and Its Metaphors.* New York: Farrar, Straus and Giroux.

Stipp, Horst & Kerr, Dennis. (1989). "Determinants of Public Opinion about AIDS." *Public Opinion Quarterly,* 53, 98–106.

Triplet, R. G. & Sugarman, D. B. (1987). "Reactions to AIDS Victims: Ambiguity Breeds Contempt." *Personality and Social Psychology Bulletin,* 13, 265–274.

Wood, F. W. (Ed.). (1990). *An American Profile: Opinions and Behavior, 1972–1989.* Detroit: Gale Research.

PART THREE

IDENTITIES

NINE   Latino Gay Men and Psycho-
                              Cultural Barriers to AIDS
                              Prevention

                    RAFAEL MIGUEL DIAZ

                                     As overlapping members of two
"high-risk" groups—Latinos and men who have sex with men—Latino gay/bisexual men in the United States have been highly and disproportionately affected by the AIDS epidemic. During 1990, the death
rate (per 100,000) from HIV-related causes was 22.2 for Latinos compared to 8.7 for Whites (National Commission on AIDS, 1992). By
June 1994, 17 percent of all diagnosed AIDS cases in the country were
Latino, an ethnic group that constitutes only about 9 percent of the
population (CDC, 1994). Similarly, since the very beginning of the
HIV epidemic, men who have sex with men (MSM) have carried
the largest and most disproportionate share of AIDS cases in the nation; as of June 1994, 65 percent of all male diagnosed AIDS cases in
the United States have been among MSM.
    Little is known about Latino gay/bisexual men in the United States,
but we now have a number of studies that report both quantitative and
qualitative (ethnographic and clinical) data on knowledge, behavior,
and attitudes of Latino gay men in relation to the AIDS epidemic (see

    I want to thank, first of all, the Latino gay men who participated in the individual
and group interviews; thank you for sharing in truth and generosity your life histories
and courageous struggles in the midst of a devastating epidemic. I am indebted to Victor
Gaitan of Latino AIDS Services (Instituto Familiar de la Raza) for facilitating access to
individuals and friendship networks, especially *Vestidas,* in San Francisco's Mission district. *Mil gracias por tu ayuda, Victor!*
    The project was made possible through a National Institute of Mental Health post-
doctoral traineeship at the Center for AIDS Prevention Studies (CAPS), University of
California, San Francisco. I am deeply grateful to the faculty, fellows and staff at CAPS
for providing a highly stimulating and friendly work environment. Special thanks go
to Dr. Barbara V. Marin for her sponsorship, guidance, editorial work and deeply felt
enthusiasm for all aspects of this project. I also want to thank Dr. Alex Carballo-
Dieguez, Dr. Joseph Carrier, Dr. Cynthia Gomez, Dr. Eduardo Morales, Dr. Reinaldo
Ortiz-Colon, and Dr. Ron Stall for their careful reading and insightful comments on
the manuscript.

Diaz, 1995 for a review). Even though the number of studies is admittedly small, and the information quite limited, there is a need to review critically and integrate the available findings. Thus, a first goal of the present chapter is to review briefly the existing literature and integrate the findings into a coherent picture of Latino gay men as they face the challenges posed by the AIDS epidemic.

A second goal of the chapter is to present the findings from focus group and individual interviews the author conducted with Latino gay/bisexual men in the San Francisco Bay Area. This qualitative study assessed barriers to the practice of safer sex in the context of cultural guidelines, values, and beliefs about homosexuality in Latino communities. These qualitative data bring out the voices of Latino gay/bisexual men, giving meaning and understanding to the troublesome numbers and statistics reported in quantitative studies. A major theme that emerges from the qualitative analysis is that sexual risk behavior in Latino gay/bisexual men is not a matter of "deficits" in knowledge, motivation or skills; it is behavior that has meaning and logic from a given sociocultural context.

A Review of the Quantitative Literature

The available quantitative literature has yielded three reliable findings:

1) As we move through the second decade of the epidemic, there is still a worrisome increase in the number of AIDS cases and HIV seroconversion among Latino gay men;

2) Consistent with the first finding, Latino gay men report alarming rates of unprotected anal intercourse;

3) High-risk practices occur in the presence of a relatively high degree of knowledge regarding the modes of HIV transmission and means of effective prevention.

Before we review the findings with some detail, it is important to clarify the use of the terms men who have sex with men (MSM) and gay/bisexual men throughout the chapter.

In Latino communities, as well as in many other communities, there are men whose same-sex behavior has no impact on their heterosexual identity. And it is for this reason, and for the fact that HIV is transmitted through behavior and not identities, that the label MSM is widely, and sometimes appropriately, used. But the overwhelming majority of participants in the studies reviewed below, including those in my qualitative study, *do* self-identify as gay or bisexual, and the findings do not apply to the more generic, over-inclusive MSM category. Through most of the chapter, I will use the term Latino gay/bisexual men or gay men, rather than men who have sex with men (MSM). On the other hand, because of current government practices in HIV surveillance, I will have to use the label MSM when reporting government-collected statistics on AIDS cases and HIV seroprevalence.

AIDS Prevalence

According to a recent report of the Centers for Disease Control and Prevention, (CDC) by June 1994, a total of 29,432 AIDS cases had been diagnosed among Latino men who have sex with men; Latino MSM thus constitute 52 percent of all reported Latino male AIDS cases in the nation (CDC, 1994). Percentages of Latino AIDS cases accounted for by MSM vary substantially across the major ethnic subgroups. In 1992, for example, 70 percent of Cubans, 59 percent of Mexican, and 18 percent of Puerto Rican AIDS cases were among MSM (CDC, 1993). The relatively low percentage of MSM among Puerto Rican AIDS cases reflects the higher incidence of HIV transmission through injection drug use in this Latino subgroup.

The numbers are even more striking when they are examined for cities with a high concentration of Latinos and homosexuals. In San Francisco, for example, the number of Latino AIDS cases diagnosed during a given year continued to rise from 168 cases diagnosed in 1989 to 334 cases diagnosed in 1992; approximately 80 percent of these cases are Latino gay and bisexual men. This unfortunate increase in AIDS cases among Latino gay and bisexual men stands in contrast to the slower, though also unfortunate, increase of cases for non-Latino Whites in the city during the same time period (an increase from 1,533 cases diagnosed in 1989 to 2,239 cases diagnosed in 1992; of these cases, 87 percent are gay/bisexual males). In other words, the number of yearly reported AIDS cases in the city increased 99 percent for Latinos, but only 46 percent for non-Latino Whites within the same four-year period. Based on numerous epidemiological studies in the region, the AIDS Office of the San Francisco Department of Health (SFDH) has recently estimated the HIV seroprevalence among Latino gay/bisexual men at 43 percent (SFDH, 1933).

It is important to note that the above statistics are most likely conservative estimates for two important reasons. First, Lindan et al. (1990) have shown that in California about 20 percent of Latino AIDS cases were incorrectly reported and recorded as non-Latino Whites. Second, as recently recognized by the National Commission on AIDS (1992), different definitions of homosexuality and gay identity among Latinos, a central problem to be addressed in greater detail below, "may skew statistics dealing with homosexual/bisexual infection rates since there are Hispanic/Latino men who fit these categories but do not identify themselves accordingly" (p. 40).

Rates of Unprotected Anal Intercourse

Five studies that have measured rates of unprotected anal intercourse in Latino gay/bisexual men (Doll, et al., 1991; Fairbank, Bregman & Maullin, 1991; Lemp et al., 1993; National Task Force on AIDS Prevention, 1993; Richwald et al., 1991) agree that these men have had enormous difficulties adjusting to condom use and adopting less risky forms of sexual behavior. In all five studies, Latinos had the highest rates of unprotected anal intercourse, when compared to samples of non-Latino Whites, African Americans, or men from other minority groups.

For example, in a survey of knowledge, attitudes, and behavior conducted in the summer of 1990 in San Francisco's American Indian, Filipino and Latino gay/bisexual male communities, Latinos reported the highest rates of unprotected anal intercourse (35 percent) during the last thirty days as compared to 25 percent of Filipinos and 12 percent of American Indians (Fairbank, Bregman, & Maullin, 1991). Unfortunately, this situation has not changed much for Latinos in San Francisco during the last few years, even though AIDS education/prevention programs in the city are well established and represent state-of-the-art programs. In Lemp et al.'s (1993) recent study of young gay men in San Francisco, 40 percent of Latinos reported engaging in unprotected anal intercourse during the last six months, as compared to 38.5 percent of African Americans and 28.1 percent of non-Latino Whites.

A similar situation is found in southern cities, not considered AIDS epicenters, as evidenced in a recent study of gay men of color sponsored by the National Task Force on AIDS Prevention (NTFAP, 1993). Sampled in eight urban centers, in five states ranging from Texas to Florida, Latinos reported the highest rates of both insertive and receptive anal intercourse without condoms. For insertive anal intercourse, 37.6 percent of Latinos reported engaging in this activity without condoms during the past month, as compared to 32.4 percent of African American and 28.7 percent of non-Latino Whites. Differences were even more striking for receptive anal intercourse: 37.2 percent of

Latinos, 21.2 percent of African American and 24.9 percent of non-Latino Whites reported engaging in this activity without condoms during the last month.

Studies of special groups of gay men, such as bathhouse patrons or sexually transmitted disease (STD) patients, have replicated the findings regarding the HIV vulnerability of Latino gay/bisexual men. In a study of patrons exiting gay bathhouses in Los Angeles, Richwald et al. (1988) found that, of all ethnic groups interviewed, Latinos accounted for the greatest proportion of men practicing anal sex without condoms. In fact, approximately 25 percent (20 of 81) of Latinos interviewed reported engaging in unprotected anal intercourse during the bathhouse visit, as compared to 10 percent (10 of 99) of African American, and 9 percent (50 of 576) of White men. Finally, when predicting anal sex without condoms in predominantly Hispanic and Black clients of urban STD clinics, Doll et al. (1991) found three major predictors: number of drugs each month, sex within a steady relationship, and being of Latino ethnicity.

Inconsistency between AIDS Knowledge and Risk Behavior

The most consistent finding in the available data about Latino gay/bisexual men is the occurrence of high-risk behavior in the presence of substantial knowledge about the modes of HIV transmission and means of prevention. For example, in a study of one hundred Latino gay men in San Francisco, Sabogal et al. (1991) reported the following knowledge-behavior incongruences: 89 percent agreed with the statement that "Condoms are the best protection for HIV," but only 45 percent said that they used condoms consistently and 47 percent reported they had unprotected anal intercourse, at least once, with a male partner during the last twelve months; 89 percent agreed that "Not being promiscuous/having only one sex partner is the best protection from HIV," but the mean number of sexual partners was 2.46 for the past month and 13.71 for the past year; 70 percent responded "A great deal" to the question "How much would you say you know about AIDS?", but, based on analyses of sexual behavior during the past year, 71 percent of the sample was classified as either "definitely at risk" (50 percent) or "possibly at risk" (21 percent).

Similar knowledge-behavior incongruences have been reported in the study of 137 Latino gay/bisexual men in eight southern cities. The men responded quite accurately to items assessing the effectiveness of latex versus lambskin (78 percent correct) condoms and the protection utility of non-oxynol 9 (83 percent correct). They were also accurate in indicating that unprotected intercourse with withdrawal before ejaculation does not prevent transmission (82 percent correct), that the inserter or "top" partner in unprotected intercourse is also at risk (83 percent correct), and that it is not possible to tell by appearances alone whether a sex partner has AIDS (85 percent correct). Nonetheless, 38 percent of the sample reported unprotected insertive anal intercourse and 32 percent unprotected receptive anal intercourse in the last thirty days (NTFAP, 1993). Thus, the available data suggest that the overwhelming majority of Latino gay men have a rather sophisticated, specific and practical knowledge about HIV/AIDS, even though they live in cities other than major AIDS epicenters. For a large number of men, however, such knowledge does not serve as a protective factor against the spread of AIDS.

Barriers to Safer Sex: A Qualitative Analysis

Accurate knowledge about what constitutes right action, although necessary, is not sufficient to explain human activity. In fact, psychologists have been aware for a long time that cognitive factors such as knowledge and attitudes tend to be poor predictors of human behavior (Mischel, 1973). Furthermore, the literature on self-regulation and action control (Bandura, 1976; Kuhl & Beckmann, 1985), as well as common sense and personal experience, has long recognized that a multitude of personal and contextual/environmental variables can influence or undermine the enactment of even quite strong behavioral intentions. In the study of behavior change for protection against HIV transmission, the AIDS Risk-Reduction Model (ARRM) (Catania et al., 1990) has included the "enactment" of intentions as a distinctive and crucial phase of risk reduction. The model recognizes that safe-sex intentions, formulated on the basis of individuals' perceived risk and accurate knowledge about risk-reduction strategies, still must be enacted in the face of competing sources of difficulty such as the presence of strong internal impulses or peer pressure.

   A second goal of the chapter is to explore the apparent inconsistency between AIDS knowledge and risk behavior in Latino self-identified gay men, based on observations I recently collected in the context of focus groups and individual open-ended interviews in San Francisco. It is important to note that even though an inconsistent relationship between knowledge and behavior is by no means unique to the Latino gay population (see e.g., Kelley, et al., 1991), the reasons for this par-

ticular inconsistency are most likely different and perhaps unique to
the sociocultural situation of Latino gay men in the United States.
There are major differences in sexual practices, gay identity formation,
and social organization between Latino and White gay men (Almaguer, 1991); findings from one group cannot be simplistically generalized to the other. Thus, the task at hand is to define the sources of
disconnection between knowledge and behavior for this particular
group of men, as well as to document their attempts to act congruently
to protect themselves against the threat of HIV infection.

The quantitative data on Latino gay men raise an important set of
questions. What are the sources of incongruency between knowledge
and behavior for this population? What are the personal and contextual influences that compete against their desire and intention to protect themselves against HIV infection? What are the cultural barriers
against the consistent use of condoms and the practice of safer sex?

To begin answering these questions, the author interviewed sixty-
two Latino gay men from November 1992 through June 1993; fifty-
three men were interviewed in the context of ten focus groups; nine
men were interviewed in the context of individual in-depth interviews.
The men were recruited through establishments, organizations, agencies and friendship networks, ensuring that both Spanish-speaking,
nonacculturated men and English-speaking, acculturated men were included; accordingly, focus groups and interviews were conducted in
either Spanish or English. Approximately half of the sample was Mexican or of Mexican descent; the rest of the sample included eight different nationalities from the Caribbean, Central and South America. One
focus group was done with five *Vestidas* ("the ones who dress up"),
which is the collective name for transvestite/transgender men within
the nonacculturated Latino gay/bisexual community. Another focus
group included five men who had worked for some time with other
gay/bisexual men as health educators and outreach workers within
Latino-identified AIDS education/prevention programs in the city.

Focus group and interview questions were formulated to elicit the
subjective experiences of Latino men regarding their developmental
and social histories as self-identified gay/bisexual men in Latino communities; their past and current sexual behavior; their perceptions of
risk for AIDS infection; their level of commitment to practice safer
sex; the perceived difficulties and barriers to safe-sex practices; and the
major sources of social support, including the relationships to their
own families and friends, to the Latino community, and to the mainstream gay community in San Francisco. (A copy of the interview pro-

tocols, for both focus group and in-depth individual interviews, can be obtained from the author.)

Psycho-cultural Barriers to AIDS Prevention

Even though the qualitative data collection and analyses are still under way, based on my observations to date, I would like to propose as preliminary findings that four major psycho-cultural factors (described in detail below) constitute important sources of incongruence between knowledge and behavior in Latino gay men. The label *psycho-cultural* underscores the fact that cultural values and social structures become internalized in human development, giving shape to individuals' construction of their sense of self and their relation to the social world. I am constructing a psychometric questionnaire that will assess quantitatively individual variability in the internalization of the four psycho-cultural factors. It is my intention to test for their prevalence among Latino gay men, as well as for their ability to predict unprotected anal intercourse in this population. In the meantime, the four factors and my reflective statements about them should be considered as hypotheses that must be confirmed with further quantitative observations and analyses.

Machismo's Double Bind

Beginning early in their socialization process, through multiple channels and on repeated occasions, Latino males are given two important and powerful messages. The first message is that to be a male is a major and highly regarded advantage. Indeed, the male gender and its essence, "masculinity," are associated by the culture with positive characteristics and virtues such as strength, courage, dependability, assertiveness, and power. To be born male, so the message goes, is to begin life with a number of quite distinctive advantages and privileges. Latino parents are not shy in expressing great pride and delight in their sons and in their expression of attributes associated with masculinity.

Closely connected to this first message of affirmation and delight in boys' genetic endowment, a second message as powerful as the first is conveyed: "You are not a man until you prove it!" This disempowering and, at times, devastating message completes what I call the "double bind" of Latino machismo. The combined message stating "It's great to be a man, but you are not one until you prove it" constitutes a powerful predictor and explains much of the behavior, psychological

characteristics, and emotional wounds attributed to Latino males, homosexuals not excepted.

In fact, because of the culture's definition of homosexuality in terms
of gender identification rather than sexual orientation (Almaguer,
1991), boys who experience same-sex desires tend to be tortured with
doubt about their masculinity. The machismo double bind message is,
therefore, perceived as particularly relevant and accusatory by homosexual boys, leading to a more pronounced need to prove their masculinity. Some boys, especially those with more effeminate characteristics, may give up early in their attempts to prove manhood, and
construct a feminine identification. Others, less extreme, grow up believing that they are not truly *hombres hombres* (men men) or "real
men" like their heterosexual counterparts, constructing the idea that
their masculinity is in reality a show or facade that hides more or less
successfully the *loca* (crazy woman, queen) within. Thus, even though
it may appear somewhat counterintuitive, my working hypothesis is
that gay-identified men who grow up in Latino cultures are more vulnerable to the machismo double bind and therefore would be more
concerned and compelled to prove their masculinity than their hetero-
sexual- or feminine-identified peers.

The culture not only poses the challenge to prove maleness, but also
provides specific means and avenues for doing so. The culture's definition of what constitutes manly or masculine behavior is acquired with
particular poignancy by young Latino boys in the world of elementary
school. Thus a great deal of time and effort in the lives of Latino youths
is devoted to proving or showing off their masculinity through excel-
lence in sports, through fights that establish hierarchies of power,
through stories of defiant risk-taking activities and, above all, through
boasting of sexual prowess.

Boys' stories about their sexual activity take on a particularly important role in establishing that they are indeed masculine macho men.
It is not unusual for Latino youths to boast their sexual prowess
through stories of sexual intercourse with older women who seduced
them, stories of penetrating homosexual/effeminate boys who "let
them do it" or older men who may "pay them to do it," and, in rural
areas, even stories of penetrating animals. Stories abound about fathers
taking their sons early in their teenage years to be with prostitutes "so
that they can finally become men." Needless to say, in this world of
Latino male culture, sexual penetration becomes, to paraphrase Freud,
the royal road to "machohood."

The strong connection between masculinity and penetration leads to a construction of sexuality as the favored locus to prove masculinity, an optimal place to restore the often-wounded male ego. I believe that this construction is also present in men who enjoy passive intercourse. For them, the macho characteristics of the insertive partner and the potential strong/rough qualities of anal intercourse between two men play a major role in what is defined as pleasurable and erotic. The preoccupation of the insertive partner to maintain a long and strong erect penis for penetration, and the preoccupation of the receptive partner to be penetrated, hard and heavy, by a "real man," constitute two sides of the same coin: a sexuality designed to create, mend, and restore masculinity and macho ideal that are always under threat by the machismo double bind.

It is no surprise, then, that for many men in my sample, sex was defined narrowly and exclusively as penetration practices. Other sexual activity, such as deep kissing, caressing, and mutual masturbation were seen simply as preludes to the "real thing," penetration. Some men spoke about their sexual encounters as if orgasm and ejaculation were possible only in the context of penetration. Many feared that unless penetration occurred, their partners would be disappointed, that is, partners would perceive the encounter as bad sex or as having no sex at all. In fact, sexual activity without penetration was described often as "nothing really happened."

Consequently, the men whom I interviewed expressed a great deal of concern about the negative effects of condoms on the sexual act. The main concern is that condoms, and their implicit connection to illness and death, would make them lose their erection. This is perceived as a source of great embarrassment by the insertive partner— yet another failure at masculinity. The loss of an erection is apparently equated with the collapse of the macho facade that reveals the true *loca pasiva* inside, giving precisely the wrong message to the demanding, now disappointed, receptive partner.

It is clear that the construction of sexuality as a place to create and prove masculinity poses some major challenges and obstacles for the enactment of safe sex intentions. The machismo double bind given by the culture does not allow much space for the kind of caring and nurturing that is needed for the negotiation of safer sex between sexual partners. The concern with maintaining erections at all cost does not allow the time needed for the gradual familiarization with and erotization of condoms. The exclusive focus on penetration does not allow Latino gay men to explore and develop a repertoire of nonpenetrative safer-sex practices that can be enjoyed as true expressions of sexual desire. Thus, the machismo double bind, unless confronted and dealt with, leads men to increasing risk-taking with an increasing number of partners because ultimately how could anyone—or any one act—successfully prove manhood?

Passion and Control

A consistent theme throughout the interviews I conducted was the perception that Latino men have little control of their sexuality. The belief is that Latino men are supposed to experience intense feelings, urges, and sensations that cannot or should not be controlled. For example, the men I interviewed often used the notion of being "passionate" as a justification for unprotected intercourse. "Passionate," however, refers not only to the intensity of the feelings and sensations experienced, but also to the surrender of inhibitions, self-control, and regulation in the presence of intense sexual feelings. In other words, "passionate" meant that intense "hot" feelings took precedence over and were not mediated by "cold" decision-making or thinking processes that could temper the intensity of the experience. I should add that this self-perception of intense, passionate, and personal surrender to the dictates of sexual arousal is often reinforced when projected on Latino gay men by members of the mainstream gay culture in a stereotypical fashion.

The perception of low sexual control is, I believe, also strongly connected to the machismo values of the Latino culture. The idea is that men's sexual urges are delightfully but painfully strong and thus require immediate release; men's sexual urges cannot be ignored, postponed, or ultimately controlled. Accordingly, males are expected to have multiple casual partners and their sexual activity is expected to occur more often as a response to strong biologically based impulses, rather than as an expression of love and affection in the context of interpersonal relationships. Females, in contrast, are expected to control, and not even feel, their sexual desires; if their sexual desires or behavior do not occur in the context of relationships, then they are considered immoral, depraved, or prostitutes.

In support of a self-perception of low sexual control, the men interviewed shared the belief that regulatory control of sexual behavior is not possible at times of high sexual arousal; the higher the arousal, the less control possible. This perception was epitomized by the well-known phrase "*cuando la de abajo se calienta, la de arriba no piensa*," literally translated as "when the one on the bottom gets hot, the one on the top can't think." The "one" refers to "head," of which males have two: the head of the penis (on the bottom), and the head that contains the thinking brain (on the top). The belief is that sexual arousal interferes with or inhibits thinking processes, as if sexual arousal and rational decision-making processes cannot happen simultaneously within the person. It is not surprising that many men used this perception or colorful phrase as a way to justify instances of unprotected sex in what they believed was a socially accepted pattern of male behavior.

Quite consistent with the self-perception of low sexual control, there is a complementary belief that any attempt at regulatory control of their sexuality would lead to a decline of sexual arousal or loss of erection. When describing the difficulties he had with condoms, one of the men described how the mere act of thinking he had to use a condom interrupted the flow of events during a sexual encounter:

> Here we are, in the foreplay, getting hotter and hotter in preparation for penetration and then all of a sudden I say, "Oh condoms! Where are they? Where did you put them? And by the time I think where they are and look for them, I lose interest, I lose my erection, and tell my partner, "Can we do this tomorrow?"

Thus the perception of low sexual control also involves a belief in the incompatibility between thinking processes and sexual arousal. This incompatibility was reflected in one man's distinction between "participants" and "spectators" in a sexual encounter. "When you think about the need to use condoms, you become a spectator, and you can't participate. You can't be both; you are either a participant or a spectator." The distinction between spectator and participant roles for people who are actual participants in a sexual act is a troublesome one, especially when it equates regulatory awareness or control with the spectator role. The underlying mental representation is that any attempt at controlling or regulating the sexual encounter will lead to a psychological distancing from the situation and a consequent loss of physical sexual arousal. Needless to say, when taken to its ultimate consequences, this perception or belief constitutes a major psychological barrier to the practice of safer sex among self-identified as "passionate" Latino gay men.

La Familia

It is a well-known and documented fact that Latinos have an enormous regard for, and place a very high value, on family life and the interpersonal relations among family members. This central value of Latino culture has been termed *familismo* by researchers in the field. According to Marin and Marin (1991), *familismo* is "a cultural value that involves individuals' strong identification with and attachment to their nuclear and extended families, and strong feelings of loyalty, reciprocity, and solidarity among members of the same family" (p. 13). The importance of family relations and the actual close involvement of families in the lives and affairs of the individual members is not considered a temporary situation of youth, but a lifelong commitment that connects individuals, even after marriage, to a relatively large and supportive social network of caring and concerned human beings.

Latinos are highly aware and proud of this shared cultural value. For example, when Latinos talk about themselves in comparison to the Anglo mainstream culture—as I have witnessed in many of my interviews—they often refer to the distance and coldness of relations among Anglo family members, and about their puzzlement at how Anglos "leave their families behind when they turn eighteen" or how "even some of them talk bad about their parents."

It is important to note that in Latin American culture, as explained by Carballo-Dieguez (1989), the concept of family

> encompasses more than the immediate family. Grandparents are considered an integral and important part of the family . . . Aunts, uncles, their children, and even more distant relatives are also considered part of what is known as the "extended family." Then there are the *compadres* and *comadres*, people very close to the family, because they are the godparents of a child, because they come from the same hometown, or simply because they are good old friends (p. 28).

Membership in such an extensive and resourceful social network provides individuals with a sense of security and social connectedness that protects them from both economic hardship and social isolation or loneliness. Marin and Marin (1991) note that *familismo* provides a natural support system that protects individuals from both physical and emotional stress. For Latinos in the United States, social support within the family system constitutes one of the most important protective factors against the health risks posed by poverty and minority status (Garcia-Coll, 1990).

For homosexuals, however, *familismo* values can represent something other than an asset, especially when families perceive their children's homosexuality as sinful and shameful. The strong ties within Latino families and the major role that families play in the care and support of Latino individuals can become (and usually are) major sources of conflict and tension for homosexuals (Ceballos-Capitaine, et al. 1990). Social support within homophobic families can be achieved only at the expense of self-expression and openness about the individual member's homosexuality; often, as will be discussed below, acceptance and social connectedness are achieved or maintained only at the price of silence. When talking to Latino gay men about their family conflicts, I often heard the statement, "I'm sure they know, but we can't talk about it."

Familismo values, strong in Latino homosexuals as in any other member of the Latino culture, prevent homosexuals from denouncing the family's homophobia and demanding acceptance. Instead, for the sake of psychological connectedness and identification with the family, homophobia tends to become internalized in a self-punitive way. I believe that is why my interviews seldom complained about their parents' and family members' rejection. Instead, taking the point of view of the family, they talked about how difficult it is to live with the fact that their homosexuality hurts their parents. "My parents have worked very hard, they have lived a very hard life, sacrificing themselves for their children, and now they have to deal with this shame . . . it is a very serious blow to them," one said. In this way, the majority of men interviewed spoke with great sadness about the pain that their homosexuality has caused their family. In contrast, they seldom expressed anger at the families for the pain that they themselves have experienced due to their families' homophobic rejection.

In my view, there are three major consequences of having such a strong bond to homophobic families. First, personal and social identification as homosexual, that is, coming out to oneself and to others, becomes extremely difficult. Because coming out to the family involves the risk of hurting or losing them, it often happens only partially, only with selected people and in selected places that have no direct connection or contact with the family. For example, a substantial number of immigrant men I talked to came to the United States to come out and live more open and relaxed lives. Many of these men were not able to deal with society's and their families' homophobia and chose the difficulties of exile and immigration as a better or less painful alternative.

Since closeted and hidden lives do not allow individuals to deal effectively with and recover from their own internalized homophobia, issues of low self-esteem and personal shame about homosexual desire are abundant among Latino gay men. Homosexual feelings are experi-

enced with some resentment because these feelings are recognized as
the source of disruption and estrangement from the highly valued and
potentially protective family support system.

For those individuals who remain in close connection with their
families, identification with and participation in family life requires
that their sexual lives, their sexual partners or lovers, and their gay
friends be excluded from the social/affective network of family membership. Thus a second consequence of relating to homophobic families is a forced separation between individuals' sexuality and their so-
cial/affective life. It is no surprise that for Latino gay men who try to
keep a strong and active connection to family life, sex and relationships
become progressively disconnected, that is, sexual behavior is pushed
towards the context of anonymous, hidden encounters and out of the
affective/social domain. Many of these men participate in family re-
unions, family dinners, family holiday events, at times bringing "girlfriends" to those events to please (or not hurt) their parents and cover
up their homosexuality. Frequently, right after the family events, right
after taking their girlfriends home and kissing them goodnight, these
men go to parks, truck stops, or public rest rooms to have sex with
other men, typically with strangers and in strange hidden places. Sexuality is thus constructed as the domain of the secret and the forbidden,
mentally and functionally disconnected from affective and social relationships.

Some homosexual men, well aware of their strong homosexual desires and orientation, get married to participate more fully and more
comfortably in the social life of their extended family. Through marriage they can partake of the immense protective benefits and social
support of family life. These men's sexual release and fulfillment can
happen only "on the side," either by having secret lovers whom they
meet for quick sexual encounters or by having anonymous sex. It
seems clear that the high frequency of bisexual behavior found among
Latinos is due not only to the fact that heterosexual men are allowed
to find sexual release with other men, but also to the large number
of truly (but secretly) homosexually identified men who have chosen
married life as a way to solve the homophobic family dilemma. The
perceived loss of family life as one of the consequences of accepting
and living one's homosexuality is so strong that even gay-identified
Latino men who live openly within the gay community often talk about
their frustrated dreams of getting married and having children not only
to create their own families, but also to reconnect with their own extended families.

A third consequence of *familismo* is that the building of gay community among Latino men can become a difficult endeavor. As shown by Sabogal et al. (1987), *familismo* includes three types of value orientations: "a) perceived obligations to provide material and emotional support to the members of the extended family; b) reliance on relatives for help and support; and c) the perception of relatives as behavioral and attitudinal referents" (cited in Marin & Marin, 1991, p. 14). In other words, among Latinos, the family is seen as *the* main source of social support and is considered *the* social referent group. Thus the notion that a group or community other than the family group could become the main source of support or referent group is somewhat alien to the Latino culture.

For many homosexual men in the Western industrialized world, support for their gay selves and social identification has been found within the context of a strongly constituted gay community, in some cases coupled with the visible presence of gay neighborhoods, gay establishments, and gay organizations. Help with coming out issues, as well as support for working through the personal shame due to internalized homophobia, has been given in the context of membership in the gay community. Such membership, however, requires a shift of referent group from the family to the peer group, a reworking of social support systems and personal loyalties away from the family of origin.

I believe that the strong values of *familismo* could present major obstacles to the sense of participation in gay community and the benefits that Latino gay men could derive from it. The shift away from support of family groups toward support from gay peer groups would require a deep revision of the *familismo* value these men so deeply share. Latino gay men are often puzzled by the fact that Latino organizations and community-building efforts are difficult and plagued with a great deal of interpersonal conflict and tension. It is plausible (though admittedly speculative at this time), that *familismo* and the construction of the role of family as the ultimate referent group are two of the major obstacles to gay community-building.

It may seem puzzling that I have discussed the family as a source of risk when, for Latinos as a whole, the family constitutes a substantive protective factor against the stresses of poverty and minority status. But when one considers the implications of *familismo* for Latino homosexuals, namely, internalized homophobia, a sense of personal shame, the separation of sexuality and affective life, and the lack of a gay peer referent group, then it becomes clear how such cultural values might be strongly related to difficulties in the practice of safe sex. Research has shown that issues of self-esteem, difficulties in coming out, and a lack of social support are predictors of high-risk practices (Catania et al., 1991; Coates et al., 1988). The time has come to examine how some of these predictors may be closely tied to the shared beliefs and values about the importance of family life, when defined in heterosexual terms.

It is important to end this section by noting that not all Latino families are homophobic, and that great variability thus exists in the Latino community regarding family acceptance of their children's homosexuality. Similarly, there is great variability in how many and how much Latino gay men have been able to integrate their sexual and affective lives by dealing with internalized homophobia, participating in gay culture, and creating gay families. The gay liberation movement has indeed developed, though with many difficulties, in Latin America (see e.g., Carrier, 1989; Lumsden, 1991) and in the U.S. Latino community. With it, Latino gay organizations have begun to emerge in major urban cities, promoting and supporting their members' coming out and its consequences for family life.

Nonetheless, from the interviews I have conducted so far, it is my impression that Latino gay men still feel pretty isolated, do not feel part of a community, and have difficulties participating in gay events and other community-building activities. More important, the relationship to family is still highly problematic for most of them, and the consequences of family conflict mentioned above are still highly prevalent among this group. Invariably, men who spoke with pride about their homosexuality and seemed well connected to the gay community were men who had spoken openly to their families and either experienced acceptance or consciously walked away from the familia with a sense of personal dignity. It was clear to me that for many Latino gay men, the homophobic conflict with *la familia* was very much at the root of high-risk sexual practices.

Sexual Silence

I was struck and somewhat puzzled, especially during the focus group interviews, by the difficulties men experienced when talking openly about sex. More often than not, men spoke about their sexual experiences without explicit reference to specific sexual activities, that is, they either became silent or strongly hesitated when they needed to use sex words. An example of this difficulty can be seen in the moving story of one focus group participant, who told the group about his sexual initiation around the age of seven with an older man, a friend of the family. After explaining the different contextual elements of the story, the sexual act was described with the following phrase: *y cuando paso lo que tenia que pasar* . . . ("and when what needed to happen, happened . . ."). Similarly, especially among men of Mexican origin, the word *relaciones* ("relations") was often used to describe sex: *tuvimos relaciones* ("we had relations"), meaning "we had sex." During the interviews, men often paused, apologized, or giggled with embarrassment at explicit words that describe sexual practices.

In line with the behavior observed during the interviews, men often expressed difficulties in talking about sex with casual partners. Men discussed how frequently, even though it was very much on their minds, the topics of condoms and/or limitations on sexual practices were difficult to discuss or not discussed openly with their potential sexual partners. When I inquired about the use of condoms in casual sex, a man described a pickup at a Latino gay bar that ended in an unprotected sexual encounter, saying: *y de eso, ni se hablo* . . . ("and of that, we didn't even talk . . .") referring to condom use.

It seems that outside the domain of jokes or boasting about conquests, serious discussions about sexuality are extremely difficult and rare among Latino gay men. These observations are consistent with recent survey findings regarding high rates of "sexual discomfort" among Latinos, and findings regarding the silence about sexuality found within Latino families (Baumeister, Flores, & Marin, 1993; CDC, 1991; Padilla, 1987). Sexual silence, especially about homosexuality, is not surprising in light of the observations about homophobia within Latino families. As discussed in the previous section, acceptance of homosexuality within Latino families can be achieved only if it remains underground, not talked about, "under the carpet"; silence about sexuality is no doubt a most efficient way to keep shameful behavior under the carpet of public discourse and removed as much as possible from the world of conscious reality.

Sexual silence can be understood also in light of a well-recognized Latino value known as *simpatia*, which expresses the importance of smooth, conflict-free, and non-confrontational interpersonal relations. In the words of Marin and Marin (1991):

> *Simpatia* emphasizes the need for behaviors that promote smooth and pleasant social relationships. As a script, *simpatia* moves the individual to show a certain level of conformity and empathy for the feelings of other people. In addition, a person with *simpatia* ("*simpatico*") behaves with dignity and respect to-

wards others and strives to achieve harmony in interpersonal relations. Researchers have operationally defined *simpatia* as a general tendency toward avoiding interpersonal conflict, emphasizing
positive behaviors in agreeable situations, and de-emphasizing
negative behaviors in conflictive circumstances. (p. 12)

Because conversations about sexuality can bring to the surface potentially embarrassing, sensitive or private matters of individuals, the
Latino *simpatia* script promotes silence rather than open and frank
discussion about sexuality. I believe *simpatia* is directly relevant to understand the lack of discussion about safe-sex practices, especially between casual sex partners. Many men in the interviews mentioned that
asking their partners to use condoms felt very uncomfortable because
they were afraid that their partners would get offended. Apparently
these men were concerned that the request for condom use would be
interpreted by their partners as an accusation of being promiscuous,
infected or sick. In many cases, acting *simpatico* toward a desirable
potential sex partner, especially an unfamiliar person, and protecting
their partners from uncomfortable feelings seemed to take precedence
over protection from HIV infection.

I have often wondered why the sexual silence exists, that is, why
sexuality is such a difficult topic for open discussion among Latinos,
especially within the context of the family. I would like to state my
current thinking as hypotheses that need to be validated with further
systematic observations. There are at least three facts of our communities that are not particularly sources of cultural pride among Latinos:
a high frequency of homosexual/bisexual behavior among men who
identify as heterosexuals, a high incidence of sexual abuse or sexual
initiation of relatively young children by older relatives or family
friends, and a high incidence of marital infidelity with the justifications
that men need to find sexual release with multiple partners and that it
would be "unmanly" to resist any female advances. It is possible that
these three facts are considered "ugly" or "dirty laundry" by the culture, and need to be kept outside the realm of public discourse and
awareness, especially in light of the *simpatia* script. It would be almost
impossible for the culture to initiate an open dialogue about sexuality
without confronting these three major facts, which for so long have
been kept "under the carpet" in the name of *simpatia* among respectful
families and individuals.

It is precisely the denial of these three problems, sexual abuse, bisexuality, and marital infidelity, with which the AIDS epidemic has confronted our culture. I believe that little progress in AIDS prevention

within the Latino community will be made until we are willing to break the sexual silence and discuss openly, with dignity and compassion, the reality of our sexual lives and the factors that may prevent our further spreading the AIDS virus. In the meantime, Latino gay men are specially at risk to the extent that they participate in the culture and are willing to conspire with the silence. Needless to say, the by-now familiar phrase "silence = death" is especially relevant to the Latino community.

In Summary

In closing this section, I would like to propose that the four "psycho-cultural" experiences discussed above constitute major barriers that prevent Latino gay men from enacting their knowledge about AIDS prevention. I want to argue that the Latino values of machismo, *familismo*, homophobia, and *simpatia*, internalized by Latino gay men through their socialization experiences, are indeed major sources of difficulty in the practice of safer sex. I have tried to show how these internalized values *prevent* men from eroticizing condoms, from perceiving themselves as self-regulating agents within the domain of sexuality, from discussing sexual matters openly, and from finding or receiving support through participation in a gay community. Knowing that positive attitudes toward condoms, a sense of self-efficacy, communication about sex, and open identification with the gay community are major predictors of protected sexual practices (Coates, 1990), it should come as no surprise that a large number of Latino gay men are having enormous difficulties in protecting themselves against HIV infection.

A Note on Gaps and Limitations

Some important matters relevant to AIDS prevention and education have been omitted or only briefly mentioned in my discussion of the situation of Latino gay men in the United States. Of special concern is the experience of racism and objectification that many Latino gay men have experienced in the context of the mainstream White gay community. This topic deserves much more coverage and in-depth analysis. During my interviews, I heard not only how often Latino gay men have been rejected by mainstream gay men for their looks, accents, or different levels of education and class status, but also how many of them have been objectified in sexual encounters, having been treated as "exotic, dark and passionate" objects of pleasure. I was able to see, through the interviews, how the experience of overt and covert racism within the mainstream gay community has had three unfortunate consequences for Latino gay men: it has prevented active and meaningful participation within the gay community, it has promoted the "passionate" stereotype that leads to unsafe practices, and it has prevented Latinos from enjoying the benefits of AIDS education/prevention efforts and the gradual change in group norms that has helped the gay community adopt safer sex practices (Coates, 1990).

A second major omission is the chapter's lack of coverage regarding the situation of Latino gay men who are infected with HIV or living with AIDS. The reactions to the news of infection, the fear of further discrimination with self-disclosure of a positive serostatus; the reactions of families as they need to face openly, and all at once, their children's homosexuality and devastating illnesses; the countless stories of courage and compassion as gay men support one another through illness, death and dying—without this side of the story, and its impact on the active construction of Latino gay identity and community, I cannot claim to have given the reader a complete picture of Latino gay men, as we face, live, and struggle with the AIDS epidemic.

Suggestions for Empowerment AIDS Education

Any AIDS education and prevention program aimed at this population must start with the recognition of the sociocultural forces, values, and experiences that shape and constrain the expression of sexuality and homosexuality within the Latino culture. Above all, AIDS prevention/education programs must be based on the recognition that knowledge is not enough, especially for a group that faces enormous barriers, endures competing social pressures, and does not have the social power or cultural support to translate such knowledge into effective action.

A good definition of empowerment is that empowered individuals have the capacity, ability, and support to formulate and enact their own intentions; empowered people are self-directed people. It seems clear to me that within the domain of sexuality, Latino gay men do not enjoy such power and self-direction. I am convinced, however, that most Latino gay men do want to practice safe sex; we intend to be and remain healthy, but we face enormous barriers in protecting ourselves. Those barriers have to do less with personal variables such as impulsivity or poor negotiating skills than with the internalization of cultural values and social structures that regulate the expression of sexuality and homosexuality within the Latino culture. Therefore, AIDS prevention/education must be oriented to help Latino gay men deal not only with sexual communication and the erotization of condoms, but also with the confrontation of the cultural forces that function as barriers to self-esteem, sexual communication, and community membership. That, I would say, is *empowerment* AIDS education.

I suggest four strategies that might prove effective in the empowerment of Latino gay men for the adoption and maintenance of safer sex:

1. *Conversation:* We must actively promote the open and frank discussion of sexuality and homosexuality within the Latino community. We must create places, contexts and situations where Latino gay men can discuss their sexuality beyond the realm of jokes or boasting conquests.
2. *Self-awareness:* Through those conversations, we must promote awareness regarding the internalized values of machismo, homophobia, *familismo*, and *simpatia*, helping Latino gay men relate those internalized values to the sense of personal shame and self-destructive behavior that put them at risk.
3. *Organization:* We need to help Latino gay men connect with one another, organize, and create a sense of community, promoting the reconstruction and redefinition of family values along gay rather than heterosexual terms and circumstances.
4. *Activism:* We need to help Latino gay men become active agents of change in their own communities, to fight machismo, homophobia, racism, and any other kind of discrimination that constitutes a source of shame and disempowerment.

Finally, we should explore how activism and volunteerism in the fight against AIDS within the Latino community can become a most effective avenue to promote the needed conversation, self-awareness, and organization that will empower Latino gay men in connecting their AIDS knowledge and behavior.

References

Amaro, H., & Gormemann, I. (1992). *HIV/AIDS Related Knowledge, Attitudes, Beliefs, and Behaviors among Hispanics in the Northeast and Puerto Rico: Report of Findings and Recommendations.* Boston University School of Public Health.

Almaguer, T. (1991). "Chicano Men: A Cartography of Homosexual Identity and Behavior." *Differences: A Journal of Feminist Cultural Studies,* 3 (2), 75–100.

Bandura, A. (1976). *Social Foundations of Thought and Action: A Social Cognitive Theory.* Englewood Cliffs, NJ: Prentice Hall.

Baumeister, L., Flores, E., & Marin, B. V. (1995). "Sex Information Given to Latina Adolescents by Parents." *Health Education Research,* 10 (2), 233–239.

Carballo-Dieguez, A. (1989). "Hispanic Culture, Gay Male Culture, and AIDS: Counseling Implications." *Journal of Counseling & Development*, 68, 26–30.

Carrier, J. (1989). "Gay Liberation and Coming Out in Mexico." *Journal of Homosexuality*, 17, (3–4), 225–252.

Carrillo, H. (1993). "Another Crack in the Mirror: The Politics of AIDS Prevention in Mexico." Manuscript, University of California, Berkeley.

Catania, J. A., Kegeles, S. M., & Coates, T. J. (1990). "Towards an Understanding of Risk Behavior: An AIDS Risk Reduction Model (ARRM)." *Health Education Quarterly*, 17 (1), 53–72.

Catania, J. A., et al. (1991). "Changes in Condom Use among Homosexual Men in San Francisco." *Health Psychology*, 10 (3), 190–199.

Centers for Disease Control (CDC). (1991). "Characteristics of Parents Who Discuss AIDS with their Children—United States, 1989." *Morbidity and Mortality Weekly Report*, 22 (40), pp. 789–791.

———. (1993). *HIV/AIDS Surveillance Report, First Quarter Edition*, 5 (1).

———. (1994). *HIV/AIDS Surveillance Report*, 6 (1), 1–27.

Ceballos-Capitaine, A., Szapocznik, J., Blaney, N. T., Morgan, R. O., Millon, C., & Eisdorfer, C. (1990). "Ethnicity, Emotional Distress, Stress-related Disruption, and Coping among HIV Seropositive gay Males." *Hispanic Journal of Behavioral Sciences*, 12 (2), 135–152.

Coates, T. J. (1990). "Strategies for Modifying Sexual Behavior for Primary and Secondary Prevention of HIV Disease." *Journal of Consulting and Clinical Psychology*, 58, 57–69.

Coates, T. J., Stall, R. D., Catania, J. A., & Kegeles, S. (1988). "Behavioral Factors in HIV Infection." *AIDS 1988*, 2 (Suppl. 1), S239–S246.

Diaz, R. M. (1995). "HIV risk in Latino gay/bisexual men: A review of behavioral research." Center for AIDS Prevention Studies, University of California, San Francisco.

Doll, L. S., Byers, R. H., Bolan, G., Douglas, J. M., Moss, P. M., Weller, P. D., Joy, D., Bartholow, B. N., & Harrison, J. S. (1991). "Homosexual Men Who Engage in High Risk Behavior: A Multicenter Comparison." *Sexually Transmitted Disease*, 18(3), 170–175.

Fairbank, Bregman & Maullin Inc. (1991). *A Survey of AIDS Knowledge, Attitudes, and Behaviors in San Francisco's American Indian, Filipino, and Latino Gay and Bisexual Male Communities*. Report prepared for the San Francisco Department of Public Health, AIDS Office.

Garcia-Coll, C. (1990). "Developmental Outcome of Minority Infants: A Process-Oriented Look into Our Beginnings." *Child Development*, 61, 270–289.

Kingsley, L. A., et al. (1991). "Temporal Trends in Human Immunodeficiency Virus Type 1 Seroconversion 1984–1989: A Report from the Multicenter AIDS Cohort Study (MACS)." *American Journal of Epidemiology*, 134 (4), 331–339.

Kuhl, J., & Beckmann, J. (Eds.) (1985). *Action Control: From Cognition to Behavior*. New York: Springer Verlag.

LaFramboise, T., Coleman, H., & Gerton, J. (1993). "Psychological Impact of Biculturalism: Evidence and Theory." *Psychological Bulletin*, 114 (3), 395–412.

Lindan, C., Hearst, N., Singleton, J., Trachtenberg, A., Riordan, N., Tokagawa, D., & Chu, G. (1990). "Underreporting of Minority AIDS Deaths in the San Francisco Bay Area, 1985–1986." *Public Health Reports*, 4, 400–404.

Lumsden, I. (1991). *Homosexuality, Society and the State in Mexico*. Toronto: Canadian Gay Archives and Mexico, DF: Solediciones, Colectivo Sol.

Marin, G., & Marin, B. V. (1991). *Research with Hispanic Populations*. Applied Social Research Methods Series, Vol. 23. Newbury Park, CA: Sage.

Mischel, W. (1973). "Toward a Cognitive Social Learning Reconceptualization of Personality." *Psychological Review*, 8, 252–283.

Morales, E. (1990). "Ethnic Minority Families and Minority Gays and Lesbians." *Marriage and Family Review,* 14, 217–239.

National Commission on AIDS (NCA). (1992). *The Challenge of HIV/AIDS in Communities of Color.* Washington, DC: NCA.

National Task Force on AIDS Prevention (NTFAP). (1993). *The 1991 Southern States AIDS Education Survey.* San Francisco: NTFAP.

Padilla, A. M. (1980). *Acculturation: Theory, Models, and Some New Findings.* Boulder, CO: Westview Press.

Padilla, E. (1987). "Sexuality among Mexican Americans: A Case of Sexual Stereotyping." *Journal of Personality and Social Psychology,* 52, 5–10.

Richwald, G. A., Morisky, D. E., Kyle, G. R., Kristal, A. R., Gerber, M. M., & Friedland, J. M. (1988). "Sexual Activities in Bathhouses in Los Angeles County: Implications for AIDS Prevention Education." *The Journal of Sex Research,* 25 (2), 169–180.

Rotheram-Borus, M. J., & Koopman, C. (1991). "Sexual Risk Behavior, AIDS Knowledge, and Beliefs among Predominantly Minority Gay and Bisexual Male Adolescents." *AIDS Education and Prevention,* 3 (4), 305–312.

Sabogal, F. et al. (1987). "Hispanic Familism and Acculturation: What Changes and What Doesn't?" *Hispanic Journal of Behavioral Sciences,* 9, 397–412.

Sabogal, F., Sandlin, G., Reyes, R., Aguirre, V., Bregman, G., & Lemp, G. (1991). "San Francisco Latino Gay/Bisexual Males' HIV Knowledge, Attitudes, and Behaviors." Paper presented at the American Psychological Association annual convention, San Francisco.

———. (1992). "Hombres latinos Gay y Bisexuales: Una comunidad de alto riesgo del VIH/SIDA." *Revista Latinoamericana de Psicologia,* 24 (1–2), 57–69.

T E N   **Intergenerational Relations
and AIDS in the Formation
of Gay Culture in the
United States**

GILBERT HERDT

Introduction

The emergence of gay and lesbian culture in the United States has pre-
cipitated a flood of social change, and although AIDS may have accelerated this change or moved it in somewhat different directions, for
the most part these transformations were in progress before the epidemic came along. This represents the outsider's view. From the insid-
er's view, however, I will contend that in one area, AIDS has created
unprecedented possibilities for the development of new gay/lesbian
cultural practice: social intergenerational relations, especially between
older and younger males.

Today, it is still argued that gay-identified adults and adolescents
who love the same gender are divided by a political and social gulf,
issued by homophobia and sanctioned by the law (Herdt, 1989). AIDS
is creating change, but not uniformly. After some fifteen years, the epidemic continues to exact such a terrible toll on the community of survivors who support and remember—lovers and friends, family and
buddies—that it will take generations to calculate the psychosocial
costs. But it is precisely in the effort to halt the transmission of HIV
that gay men and lesbians have created a variety of social relations.
I suspect that these practices, especially teaching about HIV and sex

The encouragement to write this chapter came from my friend, the late Marty Levine,
to whom this is dedicated. The writing was made possible by a sabbatical from the
University of Chicago, and I am especially grateful to former provost Edward O. Laumann for support. Most of the Chicago project information on gay youth and culture
presented here was collected under the auspices of the study, "Sexual Orientation and
Cultural Competence: A Chicago Study," and I thank the Spencer Foundation for its
support. I am very grateful to my collaborator Andrew M. Boxer for his assistance in
the project and his insights related to this chapter. For reflections on this chapter, I am
especially indebted to Peter Nardi and Jeff Weiss.

education, reached their zenith about 1990, for reasons having to do with changes in the epidemic itself, particularly the declining number of gay men infected with the disease as a percentage of the total population (Binson et al., 1995; Herdt & Boxer, 1996; Paul, et al. 1995). On the other hand, the amelioration of stigma resulted from the efforts of the gay community to right antigay prejudice (Herek, 1996). That the epidemic has produced a new level of cultural consciousness and sapped the vitality of the very same population is remarkable and may be a human catastrophe without parallel in history, as argued below. What matters here is that the gay community's efforts have socialized gay and lesbian youth—not only into safer sexual practices (see Davies et al., 1993, especially chapter 3), but also into prosocial gay cultural activism. In short, the emergence of gay-defined cultural spaces for teaching about the epidemic have brought together gay adults and youth as never before.

Over the past decade, several critical factors having to do with HIV/AIDS have informed sociocultural study of homosexuality and the emergence of lesbian/gay culture (Abramson & Herdt, 1990; Bolton, 1992; Carrier & Bolton, 1991; Farmer, 1992; Herdt & Lindenbaum, 1992; Levine, 1992; Brummelhuis & Herdt, 1995; Murphy & Poirier, 1993). First among these is the idea that "culture" is the primary organizer of sexual conduct. Not only do cultural settings and institutions provide support for sexual behavior, even sex that goes against the norm, but a sexual culture can serve as "magnet" to attract gay men to urban cores (Herdt, in press; Murray, 1996). Second and of equal importance is the recognition that "sexual identity" and "sexual behavior" as constructs are not the same, though for a long time these were conflated, creating a variety of analytical problems. Third is the notion that culture creates discontinuities in personal development, with sexuality being chief among the elements of individualism that may divide the individual agent from his or her "natal" community, such as an ethnic group or neighborhood (Tremble et al., 1989). They may switch allegiance to their friends and network in the gay community. Fourth is the idea that gender roles predict some, yet not all, of sexual behavior, a point that grew out of feminist anthropology in the 1960s, but has subsequently been documented with respect to the link between typical gendered behavior and insertive sexual behavior. Fifth is the idea that AIDS has mobilized the gay community in such a way as to become a predictive life event, creating age-cohort differences of such magnitude that they parallel the shared experiences of prior generations surrounding World War II and the Great Depression. Finally, there is the idea that bar culture sexualized relations between gay men, as well as inter-generational relations. As gay and lesbian culture has emerged, new social (nonsexual) relationships have become possible as never before.

In the late 1980s my research team and I undertook a major study of these questions in Chicago (Herdt & Boxer, 1996). Based upon an intensive study for two years of the gay community and a social support agency in the city (Horizons Social Services, Inc.), we were able to interview 202 people aged 14 to 20 in detailed, face-to-face interviews, which focused upon the cultural and personal development of same-gender desires and relationships. A study of families and parental relations, set within the social and historical conditions of Chicago during this century, constituted the larger outlines of the study. Most of the insights and sources of information in this chapter draw upon this study.

Clearly a sea change has been building, over the past two decades, in the formerly tabooed area of intergenerational relationships. Most of this is positive, as I shall show, but there are also negative indications. As Jay Paul and colleagues (1995: 376) have suggested, "Young gay men today live in a very different world from the previous generation of gay men. Young men have expressed feelings ranging from envy to bewilderment to disgust in reconciling the differences between their experience and that of the earlier generation." Thus it is most strategic to examine the sociocultural effects of HIV/AIDS upon gay male identity development through the study of two synergistic sociocultural processes explored in this chapter: (1) coming out as an increasingly formed and expected sequence of life course change that structures individual identity formation within the gay culture; and (2) AIDS/HIV teaching and education/prevention activities that signify gay and lesbian culture-building.[1]

Coming out processes. Individual sexual orientation/identity development is concerned with how people who claim the cultural identity of being gay or queer declare this to significant others or the public. Typically their ambition is to live openly for the rest of their lives. "Identity" means the usual configuration of publicly fashioned cultural symbols of the social personhood that hinge upon a presumably prior same-sex desire. Teens face the problem of locating a space in which to internally and then publicly negotiate their sexuality, similar to that of younger heterosexual females who are unable to find a safe context in which to define their own needs and desires (Fine, 1992). As we have shown in our study, gay and lesbian youth grow up presumptively straight and must constantly resist the effort to pass as straight. Only when they are able to locate the safe space of a coming-out group are they able to understand and express their desires for the first time (Herdt & Boxer 1996). The early days following Stonewall were revolutionary in this identity change; and although many aspects of living openly gay have since altered, the flavor of rebellion still clings to the pronouncement of being gay in the United States. In renouncing the closet, gay-identified men stepped onto the stage of social activism. As Martin Levine (1992) showed, this step was difficult for many of them; coming from the White middle class or ethnic minorities, they had been taught to blend, to pass as straight. When AIDS came along, it became increasingly clear that this process of acculturation had failed to produce solutions to their individual suffering. Community was needed.

Culture-building processes. The formation of lesbian and gay cultural communities has taken on greater impetus since the 1960s. Gay culture means a system of shared symbols and social practices that express and confirm same-sex desire as an intentional social reality. The expression of this socially constructed reality is then objectified and indeed celebrated through such practices as the Gay and Lesbian Pride Day Parade (Herrell, 1992). It is true that individual desires are a critical source of identity formation; however, these are typically expressed through social practices and cultural contexts. For example, competing desires to love the same gender and have a heterosexual marriage to produce children forms the basis of a developmental dilemma for many young lesbians (Herdt & Boxer, 1996). Participation in lesbian social networks and culture-building eases the dilemma (Kennedy & Davis, 1993). Although many persons may have become involved in culture-building activities or activism as part and parcel of their own personal identity formation, there were other individuals who came out many years later (Newton, 1993). At least this was the case until the later 1970s and early 1980s, prior to the AIDS pandemic. In general, this cultural renaissance assisted the work of gay and lesbian community formation in many American urban centers and smaller cities.

In the United States we can thus trace the emergence and elaboration of two broad processes of lesbian and gay cultural identity formation that continue to operate across the generations. First, passing as heterosexual is a process involving the lone individual in largely hidden social networks and secret social spaces. This is an older process, haphazard and opportunistic, a hiding of the self that gradually inhibits and inhabits all areas of adult lives, often with unfortunate outcomes; this is distilled in the nineteenth-century folk notion of the closet homosexual as a shadow creature. In many towns and cities, especially unsophisticated and traditionally conservative areas of the country, the possibilities are only now emerging for explicit gay identification and community building. Second, coming out as gay, lesbian, queer, or bisexual is a group process characterized by life-crisis ritual and dramatic ceremonials, such as the Gay and Lesbian Pride Day Parade (Herrell, 1992). The process is a sequence of ritual passages that may begin in adolescence or young adulthood, and leads to self-identification as gay or lesbian. Commitment to these ritual steps is tantamount to enculturation into the gay and lesbian community. The process has been described elsewhere and shall be only sketched here (Herdt, 1992; Herdt & Boxer, 1996).

Today, the individual's identity development as gay, lesbian, queer, or bisexual is inextricably tied to the fortunes of gay and lesbian culture. Efforts by adult gays and lesbians to teach AIDS education to protect youngsters from HIV infection is pivotal to the larger project of lesbian and gay culture-building. When AIDS education work was situated within the gay and lesbian community in the 1980s, gays and lesbians became more sophisticated as a cultural minority with a distinctive social consciousness. For more than a decade, concepts such as identity, desire, and culture have been debated and problematized in AIDS education and prevention work and gay and lesbian studies more broadly (Fuss, 1992; Herek, 1990; Plummer, 1992; Vance, 1991). A new ethic of individual involvement through AIDS activism has promoted gay culture, suggesting that across the generations involvement in gay and lesbian community activities has reduced alienation and enhanced positive mental health (Weinberg & Williams, 1974; reviewed in Herdt & Boxer, 1996; Gonsiorek, 1993; Paul et al., 1995). AIDS-related activities thus promoted a new intergenerational discourse, the transmission of knowledge and collective experience that issued from a new, positive, "gay cultural tradition."

Culture, Historical Age-Cohorts, and Sexual Life-Course

Rooted in a long historical tradition of expressive individualism, the United States has seen the rise of cultural minorities as a contentious but integral product of liberal democracy formation (Bellah et al., 1985; Rhode, 1990; compare the policies of the United Kingdom in Berridge, 1996). Gay and lesbian culture is a critical new extension of this process of democratization and individual claims to human rights, most recently contested around issues of AIDS and stigma, gay visibility in the military, gay and lesbian marriage, and gay adoption of children. As social change has accelerated via media and electronic technology, so have these issues defined current developmental experience and the intentional worlds of people coming of age.

A generation ago it was typical to ignore chronological age in the study of same-sex desire expression. Not until the late 1960s did studies begin to identify the chronological age of the actor as significant in understanding sexual identity development and cultural community (reviewed in Herdt, 1989; Boxer & Cohler, 1989). Moreover, as age was often conflated with the stage of life and generation, it was widely assumed that to come out meant that one had achieved adulthood, having delayed the events of coming out until college or beyond (Deisher, 1989). Today the correlation between age and declaration of same-sex desires is highly variable but socially significant. It is no longer strange to hear of a 14-year-old boy or a 16-year-old girl coming out; nor are we surprised to learn of a 52-year-old divorced woman who tells her teenage children that she is a lesbian, or a 66-year-old celebrity who comes out on television. In these individuals the difference between historical cohort and chronological age was probably exaggerated in their developmental experience, due to the strong cultural taboo on the expression of same-sex desire that for decades inhibited persons from being out. While the individual continues to mature and change, the society continues to change (Laumann et al., 1994).

The complicated flux between individuals and cultural minorities in a mass society raises the question of how divergent identity pathways lead to common cultural outcomes. The answer lies in showing that cultural history creates shared experiences for the life course, thus constricting social relations throughout adulthood (Weeks, 1985). Age-related distinctions are helpful here (Boxer & Cohler, 1989). Indeed, age is especially salient, given the prominent role of age-stratification in same-sex relations that is found in the early modern period of Western culture and in many non-Western cultures around the world (Adam, 1986; Herdt, 1993; Herdt, 1994). The concept of "historical age cohorts" (following the work of Elder, 1974) is most useful to the task of analyzing large scale societies. Historical cohorts indicate demographic categories of persons who are analytically grouped not by absolute age, but by discernible patterns of identity development in collective periods of significant social change. Wars, depressions, and cultural revivals such as the emergence of the gay and lesbian movement in the 1960s tend to be totalizing experiences or, more precisely, a sequence of events that structures decisions and outcomes, such that an indelible stamp upon identity remains.

For the coming out experience, in particular, historical cohorts aggregate individuals into broad categories of identity necessary for understanding their relevant sexual histories of "coming of age." By "coming of age" I mean the general parameters of their sexual narratives as discursively folded into daily life. These narratives address such questions as: In what cultural community did the actor as a child grow up? How was the person influenced by the general fabric of sex/gender roles, norms, and religious beliefs? In what community and historical age did the person sexually mature, constrained or freed, as the case may be, in the expression of his or her intimate desires (Gagnon, 1989)? And lastly, in what milieu does the actor live (urban or suburban, heterosocial or gay-positive settings)? In general the answers help us to understand the match between the person and the normatively constructed sexual course of life as registered in cultural history (Boxer & Cohler, 1989; Laumann et al., 1994; Newton, 1993).

But a caution is in order. It is wise to resist the blanket of historical determinism that is implied by the stitching together of cultural stories of sexual history (cf. Foucault, 1980). Porter and Weeks (1991), for instance, relate the remarkable story of a young British man in the 1920s whose family accepted and encouraged his sexual/romantic relation with their younger son.[2] Although such narratives may be very atypical of that cultural epoch, they remind us of the dangers of being excessively reliant upon normative frameworks or categories in interpreting the past.

We have found in our Chicago study that the individual's narrative of sexual development tends over time to submerge what was unique into what was typical of the historical period. Ironically, however, individual misfortunes tend not to be viewed in a normative light, but as "bad luck" or particularistic and coincidental, as if a certain raid on a bar that was raided before should not have resulted in jailing, exposure in the newspapers, or blackmailing as before. Thus coming-of-age boundaries are denoted by virtue of the stories people tell, the events of their sexual histories that they remember, the common events and roadblocks they experienced, such as harassment and discrimination, and their present-day social relations that reflect upon contemporary cultural norms and institutions.

From research in Chicago, we have located a four-category cohort system that defines sexual identity development, comprised of histori-

cal age-groupings: 1900: Cohort One, came of age during or after
World War I (age range 90s); 1940: Cohort Two, came of age during/
after WW II (age range 60s); 1969: Cohort Three, came of age after
Stonewall (age range 40s); 1982: Cohort Four, came of age in the era
of AIDS (age range 20s). In Chicago, before the gay and lesbian movement of the 1960s, homosexuality was confined to the margins of city.
In general, the early cohorts in this century lived dichotomous lives,
their sexuality presumptively defined as heterosexual in public affairs,
while their sexuality and intimate lives were covertly defined as "homosexual," "queer," "faggot," or "fairy." Chauncey's (1994) study of
New York provides a significant glimpse into the limitations of this
dichotomy as expressed in the largest urban center of the country. The
situation was surely different in other parts of the United States, however, both before and after World War II (Berube, 1990; D'Emilio &
Freedman, 1988; Murray, 1996). Growing up before the war left the
mark of blending and resisting to acculturation, according to the person, time, and place. Activism in the late 1950s and 1960s disrupted
this historical stream. Thereafter coming out became the expected and
canonical experience in Cohort Three after this time. But then AIDS
came along in the later 1970s and early 1980s. Whereas in the third
cohort the Stonewall revolution once affected a variety of coming out
relations, today the AIDS epidemic influences the expression of being
gay, of coming out, of having gay sex, through being HIV positive and
negative (well reviewed in Paul et al., 1995; see also Adam, 1987;
Bell & Weinberg, 1978; Bolton, 1992; Brandt, 1988; Crimp, 1990; St.
Lawrence et al., 1990; Turner et al., 1993). "To be designated a 'person
with AIDS'," Peter Nardi (1990: 160) has written, "is to carry a double
stigma: the disease itself and the possibility of being a gay man." In a
medicalized era, these stigmata are viewed both as illness and moral
weakness. Ironically, the AIDS epidemic marks a boundary between
the third and fourth cohorts for reasons having largely to do with active teaching and learning about sexually-transmitted disease.

The most recent gay-identified cohort is unique—the product of gay
and lesbian activism and the offspring of the new culture-building process. Never before in social history have gay and lesbian identified
youth been known; for the first time, persons are expressing their
same-sex desires during the adolescent phase of life.[3] As we shall see,
this poses some significant ironies for the status of gay youth. The com-
mentaries on gay and lesbian youth are generally patriotic in their genuine praise of the courageous youngsters as new citizens of the gay
republic, but ambivalent by virtue of the attitude that the older genera-

tion rarely, if ever, actually meets these strange social creatures. As many adults from our Chicago study commented, "Where are they? I never see them." Such comments reflect the sociological realities of the invisibility of gay youth, but they also represent a different perspective on coming out in the prior generation. As historian Martin Duberman (1990) has suggested, prior to the 1950s, to engage in same-sex desires was to venture from alienation and the solitary existence of the lone wolf into the confines of a secret club: the hidden homosexual networks and murky places of large urban centers (Cain, 1991). The same kind of pattern has been identified in the cultural history of same-gender relations in Chicago (Herdt & Boxer, 1996). Although this torment remains acute for closeted homosexuals today, the presence of gay and lesbian culture offers new opportunities for gay youth to come out.

Research over the past twenty-five years suggests that the mean age of coming out is decreasing in the United States and North America. A variety of studies, mostly clinical at the beginning, demonstrate that the age of expressing same-sex desires (either to the self or to others) has lowered by five years or more (reviewed in Herdt, 1989; see also Bell & Weinberg, 1978; Herdt & Boxer, 1992a, 1993; Murray, 1992). Many conceptual and methodological problems beset such studies, including their retrospective bias, White middle-class bias, and inattention to meanings of being out to self and/or to others.[4] Earlier studies have found that gender influenced processes of coming out as well, with females expressing their identities significantly later than did males. It is increasingly appreciated, however, that such findings are a phenomenon of modern Western society (Cass, 1996), whatever their status for the world system and the globalization of identities (Altman, 1995). In fact, such studies refract the historical experience of the late 1960s and 1970s age cohort, the so-called baby boomers (Kimmel & Sang, 1995).

Our study at the Horizons Social Services Center for gays and lesbians on the north side of Chicago in the late 1980s revealed new developmental milestones leading to coming out at a younger age than before (Herdt & Boxer, 1996). Based upon interviews conducted between 1987 to 1989, our study of young people (mean age of 18.7 years) revealed the first same-sex attraction to occur at 9.5 to 10 years of age, with the first same-sex fantasy at age 11. For males, the first same-sexual activity is at age 13, and for females it is at age 15. Analysis of this and other gender differences showed the powerful effects of role pressures upon young women to conform to reproductive heteronormal roles. With respect to coming out, though, the gender difference evens out by age 16, when disclosure of same-sex desires occurs among boys and girls. It is important to note that youth in general came out to same-aged peers and these friends were themselves inclined to associate with others of like social "status" in the community, suggesting the presence of age-stratification and boundary inclusion in the development of gay identity.

Because the study was based upon a nonrandom sample (though carefully screened), we are sorely aware of its limitations, the special nature of the teens involved, and the highly contextual, particularistic age-historical flavor of the cohort. But that is precisely the point: how culture and historical events, most recently the AIDS epidemic, have influenced the meaning and explanation of sexuality in gay populations. For example, in a recent survey of more than 34,000 Minnesota high school students (mean age of 15 years), 88 percent described themselves as heterosexual, 11 percent were unsure, and 4.5 percent described their fantasies as primarily homosexual (Remafedi et al., 1992). Such a finding suggests that a large pool of persons exist who may experience same-sex desire, but are unsure of how to define or express such feelings. The urban-versus-rural dichotomy is still relevant to sexual identity development in this respect (Laumann et al., 1994. Again, in urban cohorts such as the Horizons group, coming out is no longer typically delayed until college, and certainly not into the later adult years. This, we might posit, is the combined result of the rise of gay culture politics, formation, and migration to the demographically dense gay communities of America, which make same-sex desire more visible and freer to express (Michaels, 1996).

Chicago youth in the process of self-identifying as gay or lesbian have come out to themselves and/or to others by the age of sixteen. The finding derives from our study.[5] The process of identity formation does not match the psychological models of stage development commonly associated with this research area, in part because of the young age, but also because of the omission of cultural context and AIDS concerns in prior studies (see, for example, Troiden, 1988). In Chicago we found that many teens felt themselves to be attracted primarily or even exclusively to the same sex early in development, some as early as age five or six. Nevertheless, cultural barriers made it difficult to express their desires, the more so for females than males. Thus we found that many youth began their self-understanding and narratives by saying that they initially regarded themselves as "bisexual." Later, however, they came to feel that this was a transitional identity, a way station in the process of acculturating into gay/lesbian social roles and institutions. The more they participated in youth group meetings, the more they were incorporated into a circle of gay and lesbian social relations. As a nineteen-year-old White man commented, "As we were coming out, it was easier to say, 'I'm bisexual,' rather than one extreme or the other. It's less threatening." In general, this image of bisexuality is also changing in our society (Herdt & Boxer, 1995). It is likely that a new age-cohort change is enabling larger numbers of teens to self-identify as "bisexual" and to carry forward into adulthood this positive sense of being "less categorized" than before.

These are not only distinctive categorical identity changes and social pathways; they also involve what Goffman (1963) calls divergent "moral careers" in the sexual life course of gay Americans. The social and historical landscape of chronological age and coming out have changed, as we have seen, but to understand the experience of these changes requires an ethnographic account that illuminates how the new cohort is coming out in the era of AIDS, and how this is affecting their moral careers.

Social Rituals of Coming Out

The cultural changes alluded to suggest not only that what was rare (coming out) is now relatively common, but that the folk psychology and ideology of the gay community increasingly expect that to be a "normal and natural" gay is to live an openly gay life. A decade ago, it seemed common to think of the processes of coming out on part with tribal rites of passage as identified in other cultures around the world (Herdt, 1992; Herdt & Boxer, 1996). The idea of course, denotes change in social status, which signals new rights and duties—a new course of moral personhood, dramatically represented in the life-crisis ritual. It is often held that the social ritual reflects and/or protects the existential transformation of the initiate who is coming of age and entering upon the stage of society as an adult actor (Turner, 1967). Both learning and unlearning of social roles and cultural scripts are involved; and the fundamental problem of discontinuity in lesbian and gay lives arises from the presumption of heterosexuality as they grow up (Herdt, 1990). Central to this notion are concepts of dramatic "unlearning" and "relearning" of self and social role through ritual and the "magical thinking" that accompany the passage between normative social states.

Is sexual identity development steady and incremental or is it disrupted, even subject to major developmental barriers and reversals? Benedict (1938) stressed how ritual resocialization might create cultural discontinuities in this sexual developmental cycle of identities and roles. Likewise, I have emphasized what is discontinuous and unlearned in understanding sexual socialization among the Sambia of New Guinea and related societies that utilize same-gender sexual relations in intergenerational systems. They implement marked discontinuity in sexual socialization (Herdt 1981). Historically, some scholars have suggested that the closet bar or covert networks channeled same-sex identities in a similar way, like a ritual passage into clandestine worlds (Read, 1980; Warren, 1977). Today, the political power of the gay/lesbian community suggests that coming out is more of a delayed social puberty rite, a kind of Faustian conversion from heterosexual to gay, which represents social transition into gay and lesbian culture. The emergence of coming out groups in American and other Western cities today embody "coming out" as "lived experience"—the meshing of habitus with cultural ideology in these places.

By "rituals" of coming out, then, I refer to conventionalized social practices that stem from the new gay cultural tradition that celebrates such events as the major site of identity formation and cultural authenticity in entering the gay community (detailed in Herdt & Boxer, 1996). In Chicago, the recurrent ritual practices of gay and lesbian youth include a significant period of secrecy, hiding, and denial, typically resulting in periods of passing as heterosexual; the desire or need to change this life process, which results in a search for new spaces away from home and neighborhood through which to explore forbidden desires; the entry into hidden places or spaces, such as a youth rap group, with the expectations of turmoil and stage fright at being expected to perform a "lesbian or gay" role; and telling stories and confessing one's desires to the group. These practices also include the normalization of this idea of being gay in the process of entering the community and making new friends; the establishment of gay/lesbian friendship and the notion of "family of choice" as being of growing importance in comparison to one's biological family, providing alternative support networks and caretakers or role models; participation in the community activities, including parties and dating; social activism, which becomes increasingly political and makes the self more visible as a player in the community; attending the annual Gay Youth Prom; and marching in the annual Gay Pride Day Parade—a rite of intensification of new social status in gay culture and the community—and an absolute expectation of becoming a full member of the culture.

We observed all these ritual practices in our Chicago study. Situated in the gay neighborhood of the city, the gay and lesbian social services agency (Horizons) depends upon volunteers and the goodwill and interest of neighbors, volunteers, and friends for its existence. One of the key facets of the agency is the youth group that has been prominent in the perceptions of Horizons as a cultural institution that serves the needs of the whole community, drawing together people of different generations and from varied walks of life. For fifteen years the form of these Saturday meetings has been simple: teenagers show up at noon and a group of adult (predominantly gay and lesbian) volunteers from the gay and lesbian community, many of whom have psychological skills or are health care professionals, supervise and facilitate group discussions. Among these discussion topics are the coming out process, AIDS, homophobic problems at school or home, and issues of special interest, such as concerns about and organizing social events.

Gay and lesbian young people undergo ritual passages that are concerned with the "life crisis" of changing from one status position to another in a markedly homophobic society. They grow up with many heterosexual and heterosocial assumptions about their existence and social and moral careers. They must unlearn these notions before learning new ones—the input of gay and lesbian cultural socialization. As young people come out and experience change in social status, they change their inner realities and developmental subjectivities as well. Like every American, they grow up with the immutable sense of being and becoming heterosexual; that is, of being a natural and normal person, classified by the naturalness of feelings, desires, and actions known as heterosocial. Ultimately this sensibility is driven by what we might call a higher-order ideology of reproduction. What they are learning issues from the polarities of male/female, heterosexual/homosexual in American tradition.

To deconstruct these cultural and existential assumptions is among the most difficult tasks of gay and lesbian culture and the project of coming out for the self. The unlearning process includes: (1) unlearning the assumption of heterosexual normalcy; (2) unlearning internal and external homophobia, that is, hatred of one's same-gender desires; (3) unlearning an involuntary "gender reversal," by which the expression of same-sex desire previously meant adopting without exception the meanings, actions, and symbols of the opposite sex; and (4) unlearning heterosocial goals, norms, and social relations, such as the idea of reproductive heterosexual marriage, to construct aspirations as a gay- and lesbian-identified person. The contents of "gay culture" are offered in place of these.

But the practice of deconstructing and unlearning such powerful stereotypes is difficult and leads to many pitfalls, which may be highlighted by understanding the "magical thinking" characteristic of these developmental transitions. By "magical thinking" I mean contagious sympathetic beliefs about homosexuality that stem from the American folk tradition of treating it like a "disease" that one can "catch" in line with the "germ theory" of disease in mass culture. Magical beliefs warn about the dangers of expressing these desires. They are a device of the self to protect the boundaries of a secret inner self, of what young people call their "true self." Such beliefs include a sympathetic/magical idea that by going to a gay community organization, one's gender identity will reverse automatically, ruining the self with women's clothes and makeup (for a man), and other old-fashioned notions of camp. Another common contagious fear is the belief that merely by contacting other gays, their "disease" (i.e., homosexuality) will spread to the self, which will then unwittingly spread to others, such as straight friends and siblings. A common tactic to defend against such fears is to act "heterosexual" and pass as straight, associating with only other straights. This belief is based upon the cultural myth that same-sex desires are "adolescent" desires of a transient nature that will go away, and if the self ignores them, the desire for the opposite sex will grow in their place. Magical fears of contracting AIDS build upon these scripts and remain a powerful deterrent to coming out among youth (see also Marks, 1988; Paul et al., 1995).

Learning to hide one's desires is crucial, especially at home and at school—the two institutions that perpetuate the greatest amount of homophobia in the United States. The role of secrecy, passing, and hiding, are critical here; they have changed dramatically as a function of the historical cohort sequences we have reviewed. Many youth must continue to hide; in our sample, more than half are not out to their parents. Hiding and passing in American high schools (Harbeck, 1991) are the most powerful examples of institutionalized de facto heterosociality and homophobia in the development of youth. Ironically, as Michelle Fine (1992) noted in her study of African American adolescent girls in New York City high schools, it was the gay and lesbian organization in the schools that provided the only situation for a safe, expressive discourse on desire for young American females. Here the young gays and young straight women could begin to become the agents of their own desires. Some youth do come out in school; their experiences are highly variable (boys are targets of more violence, girls have more problems with their families). The Chicago study found that most youth have experienced harassment in school, and when this is combined with harassment and pressure at home, it signals a serious mental health risk, especially for suicide (Remafedi et al., 1992) and sexual risk-taking behavior (Kelly et al., 1990).[6]

On the other hand, cultural discontinuity and personal unlearning are the royal road to learning new roles and prosocial practices in the gay and lesbian community. The prior steps of unlearning—assumptive heterosexuality, homophobia, and so forth—provide the basis for the creation of a new social consciousness and activism. The positive role models provided by the largely White middle-class adult advisers at Horizons are the crucial source of learning here. In general, as we shall see, AIDS sexual education created new contacts with older gay and lesbian advisers in the group. Some of these served as role models for the teens. We found that many younger males became actively involved in AIDS cultural activity after they felt increasingly comfortable being gay-identified in public—surely a powerful indication of a new way to build culture.

AIDS and Gay/Lesbian Culture-Building

The effects of the epidemic upon gay culture-building suggest powerful but subtle processes at work, involving a variety of factors of social differentiation, including ethnicity, gender, social class, and age or inter-generational changes. Since the advent of the AIDS epidemic, gay culture-building has increasingly relied upon symbols whose meanings derive from illness and suffering, as witnessed by the emergence of the Names Project and The Quilt national organization (Paul et al., 1995). To some extent, cultural meanings of loss and grief have long been implicit in the coming out process, though they were typically ignored or ideologically denied in the early radicalism of the Gay Liberation Movement (well reviewed in Crimp, 1990; see also Boxer et al., 1991; Herrell, 1996). The epidemic has infected this process with a different narrative than before; the symbols now ring more of grief. Whether in Quilt tours, candlelight vigils for persons who have died of AIDS, health and support group activities for persons with AIDS or those who are HIV-positive, and so forth, a different tone of sadness and mourning is more present in gay and lesbian cultural practices than before. What was born in a rebellious culture, we might say, has now been fired by grief and transformed into a different social consciousness, more stoic. The national activism of ACT-UP, Queer Nation, and kindred movements, although beyond the purview of this chapter, clearly respond to a different strategy of interventionism than before (de Lauretis, 1991; Murphy & Poirier, 1993). These transformations in cultural processes have created new opportunities for culture-building, including the emergence of intergenerational relationships of learning and unlearning different from those that came before. Although these are unintended consequences of the epidemic, they provide new ideas for thinking about how to live with HIV as an ongoing social problem in the gay and lesbian community (Bolton, 1992; Coxon, 1995; Levine, 1992).

How has HIV/AIDS changed the experience of coming out? Age and intergenerational relations take on a new meaning for gay culture now. We must be careful to separate age, generation, and intergenerational influences for each individual (Boxer & Cohler, 1989). A twenty-year-old coming out in rural Nebraska shares more in common with a twenty-year-old coming out in Chicago than we might think; they are exposed to similar influences, positive and negative, through the media and Hollywood. By comparison, a fifty-five-year-old man who has lived his whole life as a "closet homosexual" is more like his heterosexual peers in public demeanor, social relations, and political attitudes than openly gay peers. He may also be alienated or even hostile toward the openly bisexual or gay people in his city. Another fifty-year-old in the same city, on the cusp of the baby boom generation, has been openly gay for twenty years and, in most respects of his social network and personal life, lives by different standards and attitudes. As they both enter into their older years, however, aging and age-related maturational issues such as retirement planning will begin to affect their lives in similar ways. Or consider a forty-year-old woman who has been married with children but is getting divorced and coming out for the first time; she shares some of the critical problems of adaptation faced by her teenage lesbian counterparts, though with enhanced life experience that they lack. Ironically, though, more than the younger cohort, she may be lacking in a social consciousness and confidence with respect to lesbian and gay culture.

To chart the cultural worlds of such persons affected by the epidemic is to understand how age, generation, and culture interact. Although the number of categories of identity has increased to include queer and bisexual, these young adults still share in the meanings of these identities across space and time, despite their diverse contexts and difficulties in expressing their desires. We need to know who is involved with whom in teaching and education, in the efforts of gay culture to promote safe sex or to protect youth who are coming out. Thus coming out is no longer a single event, but a process of lifelong negotiation, relying upon the practices and ceremonies of the emerging gay culture, which merits microscopic scholarly study.

The association between coming out and AIDS is of special interest. Many stories have appeared in the lesbian and gay press regarding the issue. For example, in a story that anecdotally discusses coming out in the age of AIDS, a writer tells of many negative effects on younger men in San Francisco before and after the epidemic (Marks, 1988). He suggests that it is harder to come out than before and he refers to this as a "generation gap." Thus we are told of a young man who moved from Indiana to Berkeley and radically changed his behavior. "Even as late as the spring of 1986, it didn't change my behavior. But when I moved out here, it did, instantly, and it still is, just because I was no longer in the sanctuary of the Midwest" (Marks, 1988:71). Whatever the merits of this story, it is certain that AIDS has influenced both the process that leads to gay identity, including migration, and the creation of sociosexual networks (Murray, 1992).

Coming out earlier burdens development, now more than ever, because of the epidemic (Boxer & Cohler, 1989). In the prior historical conception of the closet homosexual, the real-life losses and punishments of expressing same-sex desires were generally so great as to thwart coming out. After gay liberation in the 1960s, this created personal reactions, as, for instance, in the clinical cases of Charles Silverstein's (1981) early book. Gay-identified men of this cohort were stridently ideological and angry because of the discrimination and violence to which they had been subjected throughout their lives. Consequently they were in general disinclined to discuss any of the negative aspects of their experience of coming out. The disruption of family or parental bonds, the severing of heterosexual friendships or marriages, the loss of children, and the threat of loss of employment were typically played down during the "golden age" of the early gay movement (Crimp, 1990; Isay, 1988; Levine, 1992). How much more difficult must it have been to deal with the "loss" of physical health through the activities of gay sex that had accompanied their newfound freedom and dignity?

AIDS has changed the loss and grief work—but so has the emergence of gay and lesbian culture. This is because, at the beginning of the liberation movement, there was no explicit "culture" as iconic of haven and home. By creating community centers and institutions, rap groups and newspapers, myriad opportunities for symbolic refuge from a hostile hegemonic culture came into being (Levine, 1992). Ironically, then, with the emergence of a more elaborate symbolic culture came enhanced possibilities for self-reflection and the possibility of accepting certain "losses" as a result of being lesbian or gay. Today there is a relatively powerful gay and lesbian culture in communities throughout the United States, making the acceptance of loss, even personal loss as a result of the epidemic, less lonely, less alienating, sometimes bearable.

In our Chicago study we observed over several years how HIV sexual risk and AIDS in general grew to dominate many of the discourses of the Horizons youth group discussions, both at the level of personal narrative as well as at the rhetorical level of social activism (Herdt & Boxer, 1996). Youth were constantly lectured and preached to regarding what was "safe" and "unsafe" sex. This is understandable in the present climate of opinion and at the present point of the epidemic (Aggleton et al., 1991; Ariss, 1992; Lenderyou, 1994). Volunteers and professionals were sometimes brought into the group, and educational material and special public speakers were provided to promote sex education and self-protection from HIV infection. If one listened closely to these conversations and how to play it "safe" in the sexual socialization of gay and lesbian development, the boundaries of gay culture emerged clearly, as the social goals and moral norms of living a gay life gained respect.

For example, it has not gone unnoticed that some youth who fear the equation of AIDS = gay resort to the provisional or situational use of "bisexual" as a circumlocution around this highly conflictual identity (Herdt & Boxer, 1996). The folklore has it that one must avoid older gay men and bisexuals as being carriers of greater risk of HIV (see also Davies et al., 1993). A moral lesson emerges, albeit filtered through the language of AIDS education: one must know the sexual history of one's partner and be wary of those beyond the norms of gay and lesbian culture. Such a discourse begins to illustrate the ways in which gay youth thus differentiate between heterosexual, bisexual, and gay/lesbian agents based upon life-experience histories and cultural schema.

Another change concerns the responsibility to teach and protect the young, "the symbolic children" of the gay and lesbian movement. Protect them from what? The objective risks of HIV/AIDS infection today, of course, must be seen as primary (Davies et al., 1993). To understand this aspect of changing attitudes, we need to ascertain current barriers to coming out and the assumptions and magical fears that prefigure coming out among youth today.

Gay and lesbian culture, as has been shown elsewhere, is a distinctive symbolic system that is still in the making. As Richard Herrell (1992) has shown in his symbolic analysis of the Gay and Lesbian Pride Day Parade, it appears as much through its construction in these ritual events as through its implicit competition and contrast with the festivals and parades of other ethnic and cultural minorities, such as the Cinco de Maya Day Parade of the Latino community. Along with other social and imaginary communities, and other cultural systems (e.g., Black American culture), these constitute American society as a historic nation/state formation. These cultural minorities operate through key symbols, social roles, and institutions, at the national and local level, but when they create organizational life in bounded locales such as Chicago or New York, they are "sociological" communities in the full sense of face-to-face relations that create meaning, *communitas,* and jural order in everyday life.

Gay men's identities and relationships were born in the rebellious social ferment of the later 1960s, a social and sexual reform movement with roots in the nineteenth century (Weeks, 1985). Many have focused upon the significance of Stonewall as a symbolic watershed in American gay liberation, and rightly so (D'Emilio, 1983). Yet we must not overlook the continuities and contingencies of the prior period that carried over into the 1970s (Chauncey, 1994; Murray, 1996). Of course significant strides were made before by the homophile movement and others who had begun to describe themselves as "gay" rather than "homosexual" (see Bayer, 1989). But this misses the point of how change occurred. "The problem was not an absence of gay politics," D'Emilio (1992: 239) has written. "Rather, pre-Stonewall activists were employing ordinary means to attack an extraordinary situation"—the immense hatred of homosexuals so entrenched in American society that little would shake it loose until the Stonewall riot (see also Herdt & Boxer, 1996). As gay and lesbian culture advanced in the United States of the later twentieth century, it has institutionalized new practices that are becoming traditions, most notably the Gay Pride Day Parade, of course, but also the much vaunted HIV/AIDS support groups for adults and coming out groups for adolescent boys and girls (Paul et al., 1995).

Note that in Chicago, the coming out group for teens and the support groups for HIV-related activities meet in the same space, often in contiguous rooms or the same room on different nights, highlighting the social fact that shared cultural space is constitutive of shared identity and the rise of culture. This is a normalizing process—a symbolic building and political expansion that followed upon activism. It was necessary for the successful creation and transmission of a new culture that spanned age-cohorts and generations. In another way this has occurred concurrently with the creation of the concept of "family of choice." Likewise, Kath Weston's (1990) important study of changing ideas of "family" and coming out to blood kin show how generational changes are being introduced into intimate social relations. This emerging gay culture constructed a new world view, with key collective symbols such as the Gay and Lesbian Pride Parade that were primarily liberationist in their intent. Such was the matter as it existed until the early 1980s, when the historical moment of disease, signified by the erroneous concept of GRID (Gay-Related Immune Defiency) highlighted a new turn in the fates of gay identities and culture.

Learning AIDS and Gay Socialization

Besides learning new social practices and roles, the repertoire of the youths' socialization includes a new kind of sexual socialization into gay and lesbian culture. In its broader sense, we are dealing with what D'Augelli (1996) refers to as the "enhancement" of the development of gay, lesbian, and bisexual youth, their empowerment as intentional agents (Herdt, 1995). Activism not only led to the rise of gay and lesbian culture a generation ago. During the past decade, it was precisely this activity that fueled the emergence of funding for AIDS in support of those suffering from HIV (Crimp, 1990). But how do we link this understanding to a study of AIDS education in the context of gay culture?

Here we can use the ethnography of local gay and lesbian cultural scenes to reveal links between social discourse and ideology about generation and age on the one side, and sexual intimacy and social agency in real-life situations on the other. (Herdt & Stoller, 1990; Herdt & Boxer, 1991; Parker et al., 1991.) This gay sexuality is the link we need to understand how historical cohort, mediated by forms of coming out, is influenced by and is influencing the course of the HIV/AIDS epidemic in the United States. What is critical is how sexual norms, roles, and relationships—what I have called sexual culture—have changed across historical cohorts of younger and older gay men. For instance, all the youth in our study understood the significance of not exchanging body fluids and of using barriers to prevent fluids from entering the body. Their knowledge was much greater than that of their straight peers, according to their own reports (Herdt & Boxer, 1992b).

But gay youth learn a great deal from their peers in coming out and sexual intercourse is indeed an aspect of the experience of many boys and girls who are involved in the Horizons group.

Sexual intercourse was by contrast forbidden with the adults of the Horizons Center. As we reported in our study, a strong taboo had been created within the community about the need to protect youth from sexual victimization, and there was a general concern to ensure that all adult advisers adhered to this rule. A sense of the apocryphal surrounded the age taboo, and stories warned of the dire consequence to all concerned should the taboo be broken. The lesson that we should take from this urgent age-prohibition concerns the cultural imagery that had long disparaged all gays and lesbians as sexually exploitative of children. By implementing the age taboo, the agency was not only protecting itself, but dealing with the hegemony of domination from heteronormal attitudes and norms. We are reminded of this context of Eve Sedgwick's (1991) advice that gays and lesbians not be intimidated by the dominant culture from taking on the responsibility of the socialization of lesbian- and gay-identified teens.

For the vast number of the youths, however, the age restriction was not of concern to them, as they had their own peers and same-aged romantic or sexual partners. In those relations, their concern was with the negotiation of a new country, surrounded as it was by the worries and deadly signs of HIV. Again and again we found that AIDS entered into discourse. Indeed, we found that AIDS had a conscious effect upon the coming out process of virtually all youth, males especially. Jerome, a nineteen-year-old Black, reveals in his narrative the effects of AIDS, both the positive and negative implications for Chicago teens:

> [AIDS] has made it harder . . . to have sex; it's harder to meet people because everyone's so afraid of AIDS. As opposed to what I hear from older people, it was open and you could meet people but now you can't do that. I would be irresponsible. Yeah, I don't look for sex as much as I did 'cause I don't want to die. And when I'm doing things, I don't do the ones that would make me susceptible. It's made me more mature, more monogamous. When I first came out I was all over the place. [But] I visited a guy in the hospital and I saw it was quarantined and that scared the shit out of me. . . . I'm more positive [about myself] because with AIDS, when it first came out, it made me want to say, "God, I wish I wasn't gay." But since it got stronger, I just decided I am what I am, and I'm not going to let it change me—just [change] my practices.

Jerome's narrative is a social commentary not only on his own experience, but on the collective wisdom of the gay and lesbian youth group in Chicago. Let me explain.

Back in the "good old days," as Lonnie, another Black man, put it, his participation in 1979–1980 "meant just to know about sex. I mean that coming out to me was—about sex. To know what it was like to be gay." There was no concept of socializing youth either for dating or attending social events that did not automatically include at least the possibility of sexual encounter during this time. Furthermore, in the prior cohort, virtually all members of the group during Lonnie's time went to gay bars in Chicago, not merely to socialize, but to make sexual contact. By contrast, youth who frequent bars say they are not necessarily expecting to pick up sexual "tricks." Certainly their adolescent folklore tells them that one does not readily find a "partner for life" there. Today, youth are not so much inducted into gay and lesbian culture through bars, as through the cultural institution of Horizons. They use bars less for sex or for picking up sexual partners and more as places to socialize, meet friends, and have fun. As for their gay sexual coming of age, the bars do not define this totally as they did for the age-cohort preceding them, since the bar is no longer their primary cultural space.

It should be noted that there was no teaching about AIDS or "sexual risk" in the prior generation, since there was no concept of "safe sex" as it is currently understood and taught at Horizons. AIDS education did not commence until after 1982–1983. Moreover, there was no explicit discussion of sex, since within the group, sex was perceived to be a matter of private, not public, concern. Here is another marker of cohort differences between the third and fourth groups indicated earlier.

Socialization into gay sexuality must of course deal with the magical contagion of AIDS. In the youth group today, "AIDS = gay" is a homophobic myth of many young people; it is the idea that one can contract the disease merely by being gay or interacting with gays—a common magical idea that youth express upon first entry at Horizons. Many a youth group member has commented soon after entering, "If I am gay, does that mean that I've got AIDS? or "I can't be gay, or else I'll get AIDS." Another version of this myth is that by simply entering the group they will "catch" AIDS, being around so many gays who must "obviously" have the disease. Overcoming the fear that AIDS has spread into their lives is no easy task. Conversely, many a youth has felt at some point that "safe sex" was obtainable—but only with younger people. As one boy expressed it, "If I only sleep with people my own age I am safe." This idea is soon weakened but not eliminated by being educated about "safe" sex in the context of the youth group. Unlearning this attitude is tantamount to unlearning homophobia, and in the context of AIDS sexual socialization, this is a key to positive enculturation into the current gay and lesbian community.

The Horizons institution is dedicated to safe-sex campaigns and AIDS education for youths. The agency prides itself on being a leader in safe-sex education and AIDS awareness, not only within the youth group, but in the wider gay and lesbian community. Horizons runs the AIDS hot line under contract to the state of Illinois. In a study of the sexual practices of Horizons' gay youths, we have found that they have a very high knowledge of what constitutes "safe sex" (Herdt & Boxer, 1992b). Even more important, we have found that they implement this concept of their sexual practice. Even when they practice sexual interaction that has a greater "objective risk" in it, such as anal intercourse, they use condoms and other protective measures at a higher frequency than do their heterosexual peers. Horizons' adolescents talk of "playing it safe" and "knowing who your partner is what s/he has done." Their standard joke was to learn "the catechism of safe sex," which says "Do this and not that"; "on me, not in me."

The youths of today continue to live under the powerful grasp of cultural myths of gay male sexuality. These include such stereotypes as the gay male clone of bathhouse and dirty sex, typified by clone culture folklore and sometimes vilified by moralizing commentators such as the late Randy Shilts (1987). As they enter into the process of sexual socialization at Horizons, there are many kinds of ways of teaching and learning. For instance, how does one date someone of the same sex? How does one kiss someone of the same sex? These sorts of questions are very close to the youths.

Intergenerational relationships between advisers and youths create conflict over the meanings of unsafe sexual practice. Many advisers are in coupled permanent relationships or seeking them. Some do not approve of "casual sex" or "cruising," and they dislike the bars as a place to socialize and seek sexual partners. They have either seen their friends die of AIDS or have known or read about the cases. And yet the adults pride themselves on being democratic, not autocratic, when it comes to teaching. Among the advisers the overriding theme is the operative value of participatory democracy. Consequently, some advisers are hard-pressed to accept diversity of all kinds, including sexuality that involves AIDS risk. Here is a cultural attitude we see reflected in the youths' ambivalent feelings regarding the bars and the change that has occurred in past bar culture.

One of the members of the group, a nineteen-year-old White man from the lower working class, died of AIDS complications in 1987, not long after he returned from the famed March on the Capitol, Washington, D.C. He was said to be somewhat "marginal" in the group. He was involved in S&M; he had a relationship with a gay man in his later forties or early fifties; and he liked to go to leather bars in Chicago. In all of these ways Joey stood out from his peers, and he was outside of the "norm" of the group, in the eyes of the advisers. Could a boy such as Joey be a member of the group and live beyond its sexual norm?

AIDS education is a hallmark for gay culture, but also a bore to the youths at times. After months of continuous AIDS teaching, the youths complain that the adults harp too much on AIDS: they even refer to it sarcastically as the "big 'A.'" When the advisers announce another discussion on AIDS or a film to educate, sighs and moans can be heard in the group. The older members have "heard it all" before. Some young women feel they are less vulnerable to the disease, or that it is of concern only because their male friends in the group may be exposed to the risk. But there is good reason for the adults to be alert: the youths themselves allude to what they call their "vulnerability syndrome"—the threat to their confidence that while nothing can harm them inside the security circle of Horizons, all around them danger lurks on the streets of Chicago. Unlike prior generations of youths, however, this one feels that the cultural notion of "vulnerability" directly challenges the possibility of contracting a fatal sexually transmitted disease. In fact, the "magical" thinking regarding AIDS remains a constant threat, because, of course, unsocialized newcomers are entering the youth group all the time. For example, an eighteen-year-old Black girl who came to the group said, "AIDS has not affected me. I will not involve myself with a bisexual female. I figure that way I'll be safe." She added, "You should leave girls who have sex with guys alone!"

In the prior cohort, a time when coming out was unfettered by AIDS sexual risk, the meaning of coming out was contentious because of homophobia and the dangers of violence and discrimination. We find this repeatedly in interviews with gay men of that cohort in Chicago. For instance, a prominent man in his thirties told me of his struggle to come out around 1974–1975. "I was depressed," he said. "My . . . greatest fear was that I'll lose it all—friends, family, career—lose everything . . . if I come out. [I was] down but happy to be able to use the word 'gay.' [For a time I was] suicidal . . ." Another man, a middle-class Black in his late twenties, gave a long interview in which he told of his coming out. No AIDS content or concerns about HIV were revealed until the very end, when I raised the question. He replied simply that he did not have much sexual activity now.

For contemporary youth, however, fear of HIV/AIDS is a general sign of reluctance to come out; of what, after all, is at stake in living as a gay men in American society. A sixteen-year-old White middle-class boy said this:

> It's [AIDS] demoralized me—there is a big fear now, and if you come out you're really gonna be in for a lot of trouble. Yes, I have to really know the person before I engage in sexual activity. S&M is not included, but I don't prefer that. [I found out about AIDS through the death of] Rock Hudson . . . No, I wasn't aware of it at all until [his death]. [The only way to protect yourself is] no fellatio or any of that shit. It's basically hands-off or a monogamous relationship.

Nonetheless, another nineteen-year-old White working-class man remarked: "AIDS hasn't slowed down my sexual behavior. I'm just more cautious, I guess. It hasn't had an emotional impact on me." Asked if he engages in unsafe sex, he said: "Sometimes. I may come in someone else's mouth. I won't let a guy come in my mouth unless I am certain about him. . . . It depends on the circumstances—how well you know or don't know the other guy. Things like that."

Our AIDS sexual study in Chicago identified three types of concepts of sexual risk among youths that are associated with their identities (Herdt & Boxer, 1992b). One type is "unsafe sex," as defined by most standard criteria. Another type is "safe sex," which by consensual criteria usually requires condom or barrier protection and prohibits exchange of body fluids. A third kind is what we could call "conditional safe sex"—this is sexually riskier than the other types, usually penetrative, but confined to specific circumstances: knowing the other person, using protective devices, and so forth. These distinctions we came to know as the refinements of gay socialization in the time of AIDS.

Again, from standardized self-report measures we know that Horizons' youth engage in what are by today's standards heightened sexual risk-taking. More than two-thirds of the males over eighteen who answered the relevant questions said they had "unsafe sex" at least once in the prior six months. From this same sample, however, we also found that more than 90 percent of these males used a condom to protect themselves when they engaged in these episodes of intercourse.

We may speculate that although the effects of HIV on coming out among these young men are variable, the epidemic has resulted in a central tendency to push them into coming out earlier in their development, with earlier exposure to sexual risk.

As they come of age, today's gay-identified youth are saturated with the awareness of AIDS, which changes their intimate and romantic lives. New studies estimate that 25 percent of individuals infected with HIV between 1987 and 1991 were under twenty-one years of age. Sexual contact accounts for approximately 35 percent of AIDS cases among young people thirteen to nineteen years old, whereas some 70 percent of the instances among men aged twenty to twenty-four are accounted for by sexual infection with HIV (Centers for Disease Control, 1990; Selik et al., 1993). With the heightened risk for HIV infection to heterosexuals, the risk to women—particularly those who are economically underprivileged and often of color—is of greater concern. This enhanced AIDS risk seems to be caused by more sexual risk-taking and ignoring information about safe sex that would protect people from the disease. This is true although society in general and gay and lesbian institutions in particular are more diligent in promoting prevention and as vigilant as ever in teaching safe-sex education. The increased numbers of HIV-positive youths may suggest both that the pattern we observed a few years ago in Chicago no longer protects them, and that a broader range of youths beyond the boundaries of gay and lesbian culture is being exposed to infection.

AIDS and Intergenerational Commitment

Every culture creates a certain climate for social relations, an emotional atmosphere and a worldview—that is, an internal discourse—that influences what people think and say backstage and the mythic images and social conduct they convey to the public. Horizons is but one element of this cultural discourse. The sorts of decisions that are weighed or acted out, and those that are rejected or unconsidered, occur against the rhetorical backdrop of historical and social categories—especially the "homosexual" versus "gay" signifiers—that structure discussions and sentiments that people wring from the discourse. HIV/AIDS has continuously affected the discursive ideology by virtue of how sex education had entered into the prevailing policies and stratagems of collective action.

A long debate has surrounded these issues in the larger gay culture. Critics have pointed out that Shilts (1987) and Larry Kramer (1989) in particular have exaggerated the events of the sexual spread of the disease (Nunokawa, 1991) in a way reminiscent of the pre-AIDS homophobia of the past. Moreover, in a brilliant article, Douglas Crimp (1990) derided Kramer as well as Daryl Yates Rist (1989) for criticizing AIDS activities to the supposed detriment of culture-building. Crimp excoriates Kramer for his impatience with ACT-UP and other groups. AIDS activism was absolutely vital for research and education/caretaking funding and should not be made a scapegoat for the faults of culture-building, Crimp argues. This debate is still suggestive of a lesson for culture-building.

The AIDS epidemic has both facilitated and hindered the task of building a gay and lesbian culture in local communities throughout the United States. Organizing gay and lesbian culture in competition with other groups requires three steps: (1) the creation of institutions such as Horizons through which to socialize and affirm gay and lesbian values and lifeways; (2) the integration of the older generation of gay men and lesbians into the emerging cohort or, at the least, the provision of cultural means to deal with the alienation of the older generation from the young; and (3) the cultural training of the young, new recruits who will transmit social values and cultural rules and beliefs—the utopian ideology—that must endure into the uncertain future. Paradoxically, although AIDS has laid waste to many of the third historical age cohort, and created immense suffering, it has also created the opportunities for a new kind of interaction, including direct teaching and socialization, that was hitherto closed between youth and adults. We have seen this in the description of the youth group.

Nearly three decades of social study have documented the positive effects of identification and participation in gay and lesbian activities. The cultural account might begin with Evelyn Hooker's (1965) article, "Male Homosexuals and Their 'Worlds'," which generally painted a sympathetic portrait of the turmoil of "homosexuals" on the eve of their political transformation in to a minority group seeking justice and social rights. It continues with publications by Hammersmith and Weinberg (1973), whose comparative study of male homosexuals from the United States, Holland, and Denmark found support for the view that "homosexual commitment" to community created positive psychological adjustment. Williams and Weinberg (1974) found from the same study that passing was related to feelings of depression, shame, anxiety, and social awkwardness in interaction, whereas being out was correlated significantly with positive mental health. A study by Greenberg in 1976 showed the positive effect of participation in a gay group for self-esteem in young adult men in Buffalo, New York. Jacobs and Tedford (1980) demonstrated that membership in a gay group in Texas elevated self-esteem. John Alan Lee (1978) showed the positive changes in a small sample of Canadian men who went from being out in a more general or passive way to being publicly out. T. S. Weinberg (1983) showed the relationship between positive sexual experiences and positive social labeling of these experiences. Finally, Troiden and Goode (1980) showed a significant relationship between early high school same-sex experience and a "positive gay identity," even in persons who had not yet experienced same-sex relationships.

A fundamental issue concerns the extent to which the AIDS epidemic has hampered gay/lesbian culture-building over the past decade. Scholars such as Ralph Bolton, Steven Murray, and Martin Levine have suggested a largely negative effect. The grief of caring for the chronically ill person living with HIV and of those who have experienced death due to AIDS complications in friends, lovers, and others in the cultural community are underlined. Surely homophobia, a century old and scarcely less potent for its age, has been crucial to the ways in which the dominant society has understood the issues, as Treichler (1987) has written. On one side, for instance, we have the cynicism of Darrell Yates Rist (1989:13), who wrote, "The ruse that comforts us is that the fight against AIDS and the struggle for gay rights are the same." AIDS has challenged the received ideology of a "community" of gay men and lesbians and their willingness and commitment to forebear in the face of great adversity. We might say that from the anthropological perspective of culture-building, a social consciousness has been created within the gay community. But this social consciousness, as objectified in the Gay and Lesbian Pride Parade, has been co-opted by the seductive embrace of educational campaigns and the "cultural work" of HIV/AIDS (Herrell, 1992). By the earlier 1980s the rhetoric was beginning to change, as exemplified, for instance, by the extraordinary symbol of the Names Project and the Quilt.

The contributions of the community studies in *Gay Culture in America* (Herdt, 1992) stand for a valuable chapter in the newer research literature. We find a trend of listing the positive achievements of gay and lesbian organizations and institutions over the past twenty years. We find a difficulty in the discourse concerning the role of sexuality in this culture, and in the relationships between men and women when it comes to collective social action. But, as Michael Gorman demonstrates for Los Angeles, Richard Herrell shows for Chicago, and Steve Murray argues convincingly for San Francisco, both problems were renegotiated, with new attitudes appended sometime in the late 1980s, at least in those communities. Through the rhetoric directed toward the AIDS epidemic, contested aspects of gay male sexuality and relationships between men and women were largely resolved in favor of a new paradigm, we might call this the "consensual culture contract" of gays.

One example of this contract is the Quilt, a key symbol of AIDS cultural work. The collective activity of creating the symbol and the mourning ritual (Crimp, 1990) of observing it have brought together men and women in a social commemoration of the dead. AIDS work initiated new practices and networks, not always pulling people together, but certainly pulling, with the effect of creating the larger presence of a collective culture. The Quilt was to solidify and sanctify people through the collective grief of a culture too young to have institutionalized grief and loss prior to the epidemic (Gorman, 1992). Thus whatever the contested debate about gay male sexuality and sexual institutions, such as the bathhouses, a new rhetorical focus brought together the sexes and generations in the rebellion against what was perceived as an insensitive government and a formerly disunified polity. A recent ethnographic community study has demonstrated a similar process there (Ariss, 1992). In one of the most comprehensive ethnographic analyses of the effects of HIV on culture formation, Ariss has shown the positive effect of "strategies of resistance" to AIDS on the part of the politically mature gay community in Sydney, Australia (see also Kippax et al., 1990).

Of course, we must recognize the extraordinary diversity of gay culture-building in this respect: today the "multiculturalism" of identities rather than homogeneity of any sort of male "clones" extends beyond the confines of the United States and western Europe and is a matter of significant new cultural revival in many other places. The teaching of gay and lesbian identity, I would argue, is a contingency of politics and a necessity of AIDS. In short, through the epidemic a new basis for the formation of gay social and cultural life emerged; it was created in part by the renunciation of the past and of certain elements of what that heterosexual past represents. But it also signifies the newer forms of coming out, including coming out as HIV positive. The process of coming out symbolically condenses this social history for the earlier historical cohort and the new generation.

Although the gap remains between the diverse age-cohorts spelled out in the Chicago study, new cultural spaces and institutional networks serve to bring younger and older gay men into the same social formation. Differences in belief and attitude mirror diversity in experience and life goals, but HIV/AIDS is a common enemy and symbolic reminder not only of shared same-gender desires, but also of the aspirations of young and old alike to belong to a culture that will comfort and protect, through good times and bad, sickness and health.

Conclusion

AIDS has drawn older and younger men into the development of a common gay culture for the first time in American history. This chapter has reviewed some influences of HIV/AIDS upon the rise of gay and lesbian culture and concomitant changes in coming out across generations of gay men. One might conclude that a sea change has occurred—the transformation from local community to national culture—the theme that I have referred to elsewhere as the shift from *gesellschaften* to *gemenshaften* in culture-building (following F. Toennies). As the culture has become increasingly empowered, the new-found sexuality of gay males across generations has become more a matter of intention and desire to live a "gay life."

> The self-conscious leadership and participation of gay men . . . suggests that individuals actively participate in creating and changing cultural and erotic meanings, particularly when they have a stake in doing so. Safer-sex campaigns reveal active sexual agents with an awareness of their symbolic universe and an ability to manipulate and re-create it, rather than passively receiving sexual enculturation. (Vance, 1991:881)

Ironically, the AIDS epidemic has pushed gay and lesbian culture into efforts (i.e., safe-sex education campaigns) that have definitely affected youths. Precisely how successful the process has been is difficult to assess. Many anecdotal reports suggest a positive effect. Our own study of AIDS-related knowledge and practice among gay adolescents suggests that in the context of Horizons, at least, adults have been very effective in teaching about risk. Recent newspaper reports, however, suggest that such an effect may not be generalizeable and may be reversing in some areas of the country, as evidence points to the emergence of a new and higher rate of HIV infection among young gay men.

In our multidisciplinary project in Chicago, we came to the conclusion that new means of cultural intervention were needed to create a more satisfactory link between social policy and the interventions of gay and lesbian culture. Conflicts between cohorts and generations must be addressed. Unless one addresses the dual problem of teaching and socializing both adults and teenagers as parts of the same functioning whole (also known as culture) one will fail to deal adequately with the risk and the rewards of coming out in the time of AIDS. Both teens and adults are involved in the struggle to deal with homophobia and adaptation in the age of AIDS. The positive images of gay culture supplanted rhetoric that made it unacceptable and even dangerous to be gay or lesbian and to live an open life. This meant that for a whole cohort up to and including the late 1960s, one could not live openly with being gay, except at great price; therefore, one could never work through the problems of loss. After Stonewall another cohort emerged and policitized gay life through activism. In that cohort one could live more openly as a gay person, and the struggles were fewer, but still very great. In the most recent cohort to come of age since 1982, young men live more openly than ever, the product of supporting gay cultural institutions. Indeed, their lives are testimonies to the conviction and hope that gay culture will be there throughout life to comfort and protect them, till death do them part.

Perhaps only the emergence and urgency of HIV prevention could have exercised the necessary power—representational, existential—to overcome the dreaded charge that by educating gay and lesbian youth, adults would be "brain-washing" them or "seducing" them, among other such cultural myths. No doubt this is the chief problem that still confronts gay and lesbian culture in the building of intergenerational relationships. As Eve Sedgwick (1991: 26) has written, "Constructionist arguments have tended to keep hands off the experience of gay and proto-gay kids." Sedgwick warns of the need to counter this fear and to intervene to support the positive social development of youths who would disrupt "the hygienic Western fantasy of a world without any more homosexuals in it." The politics of such interventions are notoriously difficult and filled with potential for upheaval. Nevertheless, as the story of gay and lesbian youth in Chicago has shown, there remains a critical need for the supportive socialization of these youths by the older generation that would guide them as symbolic parents and patrons in a world that is all too often hostile.

Gay and lesbian citizens should take courage from the utopian visions that come down from the nineteenth century and still fan the flames of aspirations for positive change across the generations. Our efforts to support the younger cohort in its nascent struggles of coming out and living with AIDS are generative not only of a commitment to gay and lesbian culture-building, but of the very finest legacy of the American tradition of liberal democracy.

Notes

1. In this chapter I shall emphasize the male intergenerational process, primarily because of the prevalence of HIV among American gay males, but also because the relevant research literature was until recently less developed for lesbians. See, however, the contributions of my colleagues in this volume.

2. "The father suggested that the best thing would be for this younger brother to live with me! Which he did, for many years. Whenever I went to any party or dinner in his parents' house with him I was treated like a sort of son-in-law." (1991: 37) This from the 1920s!

3. Virtually all work on "adolescent" coming out has been done through surveys of adults who remembered their teenage years (reviewed in Boxer & Cohler, 1989). Many of these studies are based on culturally and ethnically limited samples, such as those of Bell and Weinberg (1978), with its limited middle-class minority representation. Besides these sampling issues, there is the methodological problem posed by retrospective distortion introduced from accounts of the past. Such problems are compounded by the changing symbolic meanings of the coming out process across these cohorts.

4. Among these are the sample bias; the tendency to rely upon White middle-class norms; the difficulty of locating predictive variables; the problem that different factors, such as the definition of self-identification, are operationalized in quite different ways across studies; and, of course, the problem of retrospective memory bias—perhaps the great issue in this literature, though usually ignored (reviewed in Boxer & Cohler, 1989).

5. See Herdt and Boxer (1996) for details.

6. In our sample, approximately one-third of all youths attempted to take their own lives at least once before the came to the Horizons group (Herdt & Boxer, 1993).

References

Abramson, Paul, & Herdt, Gilbert. (1990). "The Assessment of Sexual Practices Relevant to the Transmission of AIDS: A Global Perspective." *Journal of Sex Research*, 27 (2), 215–232.

Adam, Barry. (1986). "Age, Structure, and Sexuality: Reflections on the Anthropological Evidence on Homosexual Relations." *Journal of Homosexuality*, 11, 19–33.

Aggleton, Peter, et al. (1991). *AIDS: Working with Young People*. West Sussex, England: AVERT.

Altman, Dennis. (1988). "Legitimation through Disaster: AIDS and the Gay Movement," In E. Fee and D. M. Fox, eds., *AIDS: The Burdens of History*. Berkeley: University of California Press.

———. (1995). "Political Sexualities: Meanings and Identities in the Time of AIDS," In R. Parker and J. Gagnon, (Eds.), *Conceiving Sexuality* (pp. 97–108). New York: Routledge.

Ariss, Robert. (1992). *Against Death*. Doctoral dissertation, University of Sydney, Australia.

Bayer, Ronald. (1989). *Private Acts, Social Consequences: AIDS and the Politics of Public Health*. New York: Free Press.

Bell, Alan P. & Weinberg, M. S. (1978). *Homosexualities: A Study in Diversity Among Men and Women*. New York: Simon & Schuster.

Bellah, Robert, et al. (1985). *Habits of the Heart*. Berkeley: University of California Press.

Benedict, Ruth. (1938). "Continuities and Discontinuities in Cultural Conditioning." *Psychiatry*, 1, 161–167.

Berridge, Virginia. (1996). *AIDS in the UK: The Making of Policy, 1981–1994*. New York: Oxford University Press.

Bérubé, Allan. *Coming Out under Fire*. (1990). New York: Free Press.

Binson, Diane, et al. (1995). "Prevalence and Social Distribution of Men Who Have Sex with Men: United States and Its Urban Centers." *Journal of Sex Research*, 32, 245–254.

Bolton, Ralph. (1992). "Mapping Terra Incognito: Sex Research for AIDS Prevention— An Urgent Agenda for the 1990s." In G. Herdt and S. Lindenbaum (Eds.), *The Time of AIDS* (pp. 124–158). Newbury Park, CA: Sage.

Boxer, Andrew, et al. (1991). "Double Jeopardy: Identity Transitions and Parent-Child Relations among Gay and Lesbian Youth." In Karl Pillemer and K. McCartney (Eds.), *Parent-Child Relations throughout Life* (pp. 59–92). Hillsdale, NJ: Lawrence Earl-baum Associates.

Boxer, Andrew & Cohler, Bertram. (1989). "The Life Course of Gay and Lesbian Youth: An Immodest Proposal for the Study of Lives." In G. Herdt (Ed.), *Gay and Lesbian Youth* (pp. 317–355). New York: Harrington Park Press.

Brandt, A. (1988). "AIDS in Historical Perspective: Four Lessons from the History of Sexually Transmitted Diseases." *American Journal of Public Health*, 78, 367–371.

Brummelhuis, Han ten & Herdt, Gilbert. (Eds.). (1995). *Culture and Sexual Risk*. New York: Gordon and Breach.

Carrier, Joseph & Bolton, R. (1991). "Anthropological Perspectives on Sexuality and HIV Prevention." *Annual Review of Sex Research* 2, 49–76.

Cass, Vivienne. (1996). "Sexual Orientation Identity Formation: A Western Phenome-non." In Robert P. Cabaj & T. S. Stein (Eds.), *Textbook of Homosexuality and Mental Health* (pp. 227–252). Washington, DC: American Psychiatric Press.

Cain, Roy. (1991). "Disclosure and Secrecy among Gay Men in the United States and Canada: A Shift in Views." *Journal of the History of Sexuality*, 2, 25–45.

Carpenter, Edward. (1908 [1984]). "The Intermediate Sex." In *Edward Carpenter: Se-lected Writings, Volume 1: Sex*. London: GMP Publishers Ltd.

Chauncey, George Jr. (1994). *Gay New York*. New York: Basic Books.

Centers for Disease Control. (1993). "Update: Mortality Attributable to HIV Infection/ AIDS among Persons Aged 25–44 Years—United States, 1990 and 1991." *Morbidity and Mortality Weekly Reports*, 42 (25), July 2, 481–486.

Coxon, Anthony P. M. (1995). "The Use of Social Networks as Method and Substance in Researching Gay Men's Response to HIV/AIDS." In R. Parker and J. Gagnon (Eds.), *Conceiving Sexuality: Approaches to Sex Research in a Postmodern World*, pp. 215–234. New York: Routledge.

Crimp, Douglas. (1990). "Mourning and Militancy." In Russell Ferguson, et al. (Eds.), *Out There: Marginalization and Contemporary Culture* (pp. 223–246). Cambridge, MA: MIT Press.

D'Emilio, John. *Sexual Politics, Sexual Communities*. (1983). Chicago: University of Chicago Press.

———. (1992). *Making Trouble: Essays on Gay History, Politics, and the University*. New York: Routledge.

D'Emilio, John & Estelle Freedman. (1988). *Intimate Matters: A History of Sexuality in America*. New York: Harper and Row.

Davies, P. M. et al. (1993). *Sex, Gay Men, and AIDS*. London: Falmer Press.

DeLauretis, Teresa. (1991). "Queer Theory: Lesbian and Gay Sexualities: An Introduc-tion." *Differences*, 3, iii–xviii.

Deisher, Robert. (1989). "Preface." In G. Herdt (Ed.), *Gay and Lesbian Youth* (pp. xiii–xv). New York: Haworth Press.

Duberman, Martin. (1991). *Cures.* New York: Harcourt Brace.

Elder, Glen. (1974). *Children of the Great Depression.* Chicago: University of Chicago Press.

Eyre, Stephen L. (1991). "Emotional Conflict as a Weapon against AIDS." *Anthropology Today,* 7, 2–4.

Farmer, Paul. (1992). *AIDS and Accusation: Haiti and the Geography of Blame.* Berkeley: University of California Press.

Fine, Michele. (1992). *Disruptive Voices: The Possibilities of Feminist Research.* Ann Arbor: University of Michigan Press.

Foucault, Michel. (1980). *The History of Sexuality.* New York: Pantheon.

Fuss, Diana. (Ed.). (1991). *Inside/Out: Lesbian Theories, Gay Theories.* New York: Routledge.

Gagnon, John. (1989). "Disease and Desire." *Daedalus,* 118, 47–77.

Goffman, Erving. (1963). *Stigma.* Toronto: Prentice-Hall.

Gonsiorek, John C. (1993). "Mental Health Issues of Gay and Lesbian Adolescents." In Linda D. Garnets & D. G. Kimmel (Eds.), *Psychological Perspectives on Lesbian and Gay Male Experiences* (pp. 469–485). New York: Columbia University Press.

Gorman, Michael. (1992). "The Pursuit of the Wish: An Anthropological Perspective on Gay Male Subculture in Los Angeles." In G. Herdt (Ed.), *Gay Culture in America* (pp. 87–106). Boston: Beacon.

Greenberg, J. (1976). "A Study of the Self-Esteem and Alienation of Male Homosexuals." *Journal of Psychology* 83, 137–143.

Harbeck, Karen M. (Ed.). (1991). *Coming Out of the Classroom Closet.* New York: Haworth Press.

Harry, Joseph. (1974). "Urbanization and the Gay Life." *Journal of Sex Research,* 10, 238–247.

Herdt, Gilbert. (1981). *Guardians of the Flutes.* New York: McGraw-Hill.

———. (1987). *Sambia: Ritual and Gender in New Guinea.* New York: Holt, Rinehart and Winston.

———. (1990). "Developmental Continuity as a Dimension of Sexual Orientation across Cultures." In David McWhirter, J. Reinisch, & S. Sanders (Eds.), *Homosexuality and Heterosexuality: The Kinsey Scale and Current Research* (pp. 208–238). New York: Oxford University Press.

———. (1992). "Introduction." In G. Herdt & S. Lindenbaum (Eds.), *The Time of AIDS* (pp. 3–26). Newbury Park, CA: Sage.

———. (1993). "Introduction." In G. Herdt (Ed.), *Ritualized Homosexuality in Melanesia* (pp. vii–xliv). (Paperback edition.) Berkeley: University of California Press.

———. (1995). "The Protection of Gay and Lesbian Youth." *Harvard Educational Review,* 65, 315–321.

Herdt, Gilbert. (Ed.). (1989). *Gay and Lesbian Youth.* New York: Haworth.

———. (Ed.). (1994). *Third Sex, Third Gender.* New York: Zone Books.

———. (Ed.) (in press). *Sexual Cultures and Migration in the Era of AIDS.* New York: Oxford University Press.

Herdt, Gilbert & Boxer, A. (1991). "The Ethnographic Study of AIDS." *Journal of Sex Research,* 28, 171–189.

———. (1992a). "Introduction: Culture, History, and Life Course of Gay Men," in G. Herdt (Ed.), *Gay Culture in America* (pp. 1–28). Boston: Beacon Press.

———. (1992b). "Sexual Identity Development and AIDS Sexual Risk." In T. Dyson (Ed.), *Sexual Behavior and Networking: Anthropological and Socio-Cultural Studies on the Transmission of HIV.* Liege, Belgium: Ordina Editions.

———. (1995). "Bisexuality: Toward a Comparative Theory of Identities and Culture." In R. Parker & J. Gagnon (Eds.), *Conceiving Sexuality* (pp. 69–84). New York: Routledge.

————. (1996). *Children of Horizons: How Gay and Lesbian Youth Are Forging a New Way Out of the Closet*. Second edition. Boston: Beacon Press.

Herdt, Gilbert & Lindenbaum, S. (Eds.). (1992). *The Time of AIDS: Theory, Method, and Practice*. Newbury Park, CA: Sage.

Herdt, G. & Stoller, R. J. (1990). *Intimate Communications: Erotics and the Study of Culture*. New York: Columbia University Press.

Herek, Gregory M. (1996). "Heterosexism and Homophobia." In R. Cabaj & T. Stein (Eds.), *Textbook of Homosexuality and Mental Health* (pp. 101–114). Washington, DC: American Psychiatric Press.

————. (1990). "Illness, Stigma, and AIDS." In Paul T. Costa, Jr. & Gary R. Vanden Bos (Eds.), *Psychological Aspects of Serious Illness: Chronic Conditions, Fatal Diseases, and Clinical Care*. Washington, DC: American Psychological Association.

Herrell, Richard K. (1992). "The Symbolic Strategies of Chicago's Gay and Lesbian Pride Day Parade." In G. Herdt (Ed.), *Gay Culture in America* (pp. 225–252). Boston: Beacon.

————. (1996). "Sin, Sickness, Crime: Queer Desire and the American States." *Identities*, 2 (3), 272–300.

Hooker, Evelyn. (1965). "Male Homosexuals and Their 'Worlds.'" In J. Marmor (Ed.), *Sexual Inversion: A Modern Appraisal*. New York: Basic Books.

Isay, Richard. (1988). *Homosexual Development*. New York: Farrar, Straus, & Giroux.

Jacobs, John & Tedford, W. (1980). "Factors Affecting the Self-Esteem of the Homosexual Individual." *Journal of Homosexuality*, 5, 373–382.

Kelley, Jeffrey A. et al. (1990). "Psychological Factors That Predict High-Risk Versus AIDS Precautionary Behavior." *Journal of Consulting and Clinical Psychology*, 58, 117–120.

Kennedy, Elizabeth L. & Davis, M. D. (1993). *Boots of Leather, Slippers of Gold: The History of a Lesbian Community*. New York: Penguin.

Kimmel, Douglas C. & Sang, B. E. (1995). "Lesbians and Gay Men in Midlife." In A. R. D'Augelli & C. J. Patterson (Eds.). (1995). *Lesbian, Gay, and Bisexual Identities over the Lifespan* (pp. 190–214). New York: Oxford University Press.

Kinsey, Alfred et al. (1948). *Sexual Behavior in the Human Male*. Philadelphia: W. B. Saunders.

Kippax, S. et al. (1990). "The Importance of the Gay Community in the Prevention of HIV Transmission: Social Aspects of the Prevention of AIDS Project." *Report No. 7*. Sydney: Macquarie AIDS Research Unit.

Knauft, Bruce M. (1993). *South Coast New Guinea Cultures: History, Comparison, Dialectic*. New York: Cambridge University Press.

Kramer, Larry. (1989). *Reports from the Holocaust: The Making of an AIDS Activist*. New York: St. Martin's Press.

Laumann, Edward O. et al. (1994). *The Social Organization of Sexuality: Sexual Practices in the United States*. Chicago: University of Chicago Press.

Lee, John Alan. (1978). "Going Public: A Study in the Sociology of Homosexual Liberation." *Journal of Homosexuality*, 3, 49–78.

Levine, Martin. (1992). "Birth and Death of the Gay Clone." In G. Herdt (Ed.), *Gay Culture in America* (pp. 68–86). Boston: Beacon Press.

Lenderyou, Gill. (1994). "Sex Education: A School-Based Perspective." *Sexual and Marital Therapy*, 9, 127–144.

Marks, Robert. (1988). "Coming Out in the Age of AIDS: The Next Generation." *Outlook*, (Spring), pp. 66–74.

Michaels, Stuart. (1996). "The Prevalence of Homosexuality in the United States." In R. Cabaj and T. Stein (Eds.), *Textbook of Homosexuality and Mental Health* (pp. 43–64). Washington, DC: American Psychiatric Press.

Mohr, Richard. (1992). *Gay Ideas*. Boston: Beacon Press.

Murphy, Timothy F. (1991). "No Time for an AIDS Backlash." *Hastings Center Report,* 21, 7–11.

Murphy, Timothy F. & Poirier, Suzanne. (Eds.). (1993). *Writing AIDS: Gay Literature, Language, and Analysis.* New York: Columbia University Press.

Murray, Stephen O. (1992). "Components of Gay Community in San Francisco." In G. Herdt (Ed.), *Gay Culture in America* (pp. 107–146). Boston: Beacon Press.

———. (1996). *American Gay.* Chicago: University of Chicago Press.

Nardi, Peter M. (1990). "AIDS and Obituaries: The Perpetuation of Stigma in the Press." In D. Feldman (Ed.), *Culture and AIDS* (pp. 159–168). New York: Praeger.

Newton, Esther. (1993). *Cherry Grove, Fire Island: Sixty Years in America's First Gay and Lesbian Town.* Boston: Beacon Press.

Nunokawa, Jeff. (1991). "All the Sad Young Men: AIDS and the Work of Mourning." In D. Fuss (Ed.), *Inside/Out: Lesbians Theories, Gay Theories* (pp. 311–323). New York: Routledge.

Parker, Richard. (1987). "Acquired Immunodeficiency Syndrome in Urban Brazil." *Medical Anthropology Quarterly,* 1, 155–175.

Parker, Richard, Herdt, Gilbert, & Caballo, Manuel. (1991). "Sexual Culture, HIV Transmission, and AIDS Research." *Journal of Sex Research,* 28 (1), 75–76.

Patton, Cindy. (1990). *Inventing AIDS.* New York: Routledge.

Paul, Jay et al. (1995). "The Impact of the HIV Epidemic on U.S. Gay Male Communities," In A. R. D'Augelli & C. Patterson (Eds.), *Lesbian, Gay, and Bisexual Identities over the Lifespan: Psychological Perspectives* (pp. 347–396). New York: Oxford University Press.

Piontek, Thomas. (1992). "Unsafe Representations: Cultural Criticism in the Age of AIDS." *Discourse,* 15(1), 128–153.

Plummer, Kenneth. (1991). "Speaking Its Name: Inventing a Gay and Lesbian Studies." In K. Plummer (Ed.), *Modern Homosexualities.* New York: Routledge.

Porter, Kevin & Weeks, Jeffrey. (1991). *Between the Acts: Lives of Homosexual Men 1885–1967.* New York: Routledge.

Read, Kenneth E. (1980). *Other Voices.* Novato, CA: Chandler and Sharpe.

Remafedi, Gary et al. (1992). "Demography of Sexual Orientation in Adolescents." *Pediatrics,* 89 (4), 714–721.

Rhode, Deborah L. (Ed.) *Theoretical Perspectives on Sexual Difference.* New Haven, CT: Yale University Press.

Rist, Darrell Yates. (1989). "AIDS as Apocalpyse." *Christopher Street,* 11, 11–14.

Rubin, Gayle S. (1997). "Elegy for the Valley of Kings. AIDS and the Leather Community in San Francisco, 1981–1996." In Levine, Martin P., Nardi, Peter M., & Gagnon, John H. (Eds.), *In Changing Times: Gay Men and Lesbians Encounter HIV/AIDS.* Chicago: University of Chicago Press.

Sedgwick, Eve Kosofsky. (1991). "How to Bring Your Kids Up Gay." *Social Context,* 18–27.

Selik, R. M. et al. (1993). "HIV Infection as Leading Cause of Death among Young Adults in US Cities and States." *Journal of the American Medical Association,* 269, 299–194.

Shilts, Randy. (1987). *And the Band Played On.* New York: St. Martin's Press.

Silverstein, Charles. (1980). *Man to Man: Gay Couples in America.* New York: William Morrow.

Stein, Edward. (1990). "Conclusion: The Essentials of Constructions and the Construction of Essentialism." In E. Stein, *Forms of Desire: Sexual Orientation and the Social Constructionist Controversy.* New York: Garland Publishing.

Tremble, Bob et al. (1989). "Growing Up Gay or Lesbian in a Multicultural Context," in G. Herdt (Ed.), *Gay and Lesbian Youth* (pp. 253–268). New York: Haworth.

Troiden, Richard. (1988). *Gay and Lesbian Identity.* New York: Prentice-Hall.

Troiden, Richard & Goode, E. (1980). "Variables Related to Acquisition of Gay Identity." *Journal of Homosexuality*, 5, 383–392.

Turner, Charles et al. (1989). *AIDS: Sexual Behavior and Intravenous Drug Use*. Washington, DC: National Academy Press.

Turner, Victor. (1967) "Les Rites des Passage." In *The Forest of Symbols*, pp. 93–111. Ithaca, NY: Cornell University Press.

Vance, Carole S. (1991). "Anthropology Rediscovers Sexuality: A Theoretical Comment." *Social Science and Medicine*, 33, 875–884.

Weeks, Jeffrey. (1985). *Sexuality and Its Discontents*. London: Routledge and Kegan Paul.

Warren, Carol A. B. (1977). "Fieldwork in the Gay World: Issues in Phenomenological Study." *Journal of Social Issues*, 33, 93–107.

Weinberg, George. (1972). *Society and the Healthy Homosexual*. New York: St. Martin's Press.

Weinberg, Thomas S. (1983). *Gay Men, Gay Selves*. New York: Irvington.

Weinberg, Martin S. & Williams, Colin J. (1974). *Male Homosexuals: Their Problems and Adaptations*. New York: Oxford University Press.

Weston, Kath. (1990). *Families We Choose*. New York: Columbia University Press.

ELEVEN   **AIDS-Related Risks and Same-Sex Behaviors among African American Men**

JOHN L. PETERSON

M ale same-sex behavior represents a significant risk factor for HIV transmission among African Americans. Over 10 percent of all AIDS cases in the United States contracted through male-male sexual contact have occurred among African American men (Centers for Disease Control and Prevention [CDC], 1995). Among African Americans, the proportion of AIDS cases attributed to male homosexual/bisexual activity (36 percent) is almost equal to that attributed to injection drug use (38 percent) and higher than that attributed to heterosexual contact (12 percent; CDC, 1993). Within their respective racial categories, more African Americans (41 percent) than Hispanics (31 percent) and Whites (21 percent) reported bisexual activity when they engaged in male-male sexual contact (Chu, Peterman, Doll, Buehler, & Curran, 1992). In comparison to Whites, African American females have a higher rate of AIDS cases attributed to sex v h a bisexual man (Chu et al., 1992; Doll et al., 1992), which sup-)rts the suspicion that male bisexual activity may be a major secondary source of HIV transmission risk for African American women.

However, after a decade of the AIDS epidemic, it is striking that there has been minimal AIDS prevention research among homosexually active African American men. One explanation for this neglect is that emphasis for prevention research has been on HIV prevention among heterosexual African Americans. HIV transmission in African American communities is primarily viewed as a problem among injection drug users (IDUs). This misperception may have developed from the focus in the mass media on racial differences in AIDS cases associated with injection drug use. The disproportionate number of cases of AIDS among African Americans was attributed primarily to HIV

Reprinted by permission of Sage Publications, from Gregory M. Herek and Beverly Greene (Eds.). 1995. *AIDS, Identity, and Community: The HIV Epidemic and Lesbians and Gay Men.* Thousand Oaks, CA: Sage.

transmission among heterosexual drug users and their sexual partners (Bakeman, McCray, Lumb, Jackson, & Whitley, 1987). This transmission route was further responsible for most AIDS cases among infants and children. Also, the limited visibility of homosexuals in the African American community may have led to the impression that gay people are not a significant segment of the general African American population (Herek & Glunt, 1991; Mays & Cochran, 1987) and the tendency to ignore the fact that transmission through homosexual behavior accounts for the second highest proportion of AIDS cases among African Americans. Consequently, when social and political resources were finally marshaled to demand a response to the epidemic in the African American population, the emphasis was on prevention research among heterosexual drug users.

However, a second explanation is that the influence of homophobia—both on homosexually active African American men and the general African American community—contributed to homosexually active men being ignored in AIDS prevention research among African Americans (Dalton, 1989; Icard, 1985–1986). The AIDS-related stigma associated with homosexuality may have diminished support among heterosexual African Americans for HIV prevention research that recognized the prevalence of homosexual activity. Moreover, among homosexually active African American men, including those who self-identify as gay, fear of homophobia and strong attachment to the minority community may have been strong disincentives to respond to the AIDS epidemic as primarily a gay issue. The absence of national gay leaders and large gay constituencies in the African American population offered few opportunities to mobilize support for HIV/AIDS prevention research among men at risk through homosexual behavior. As a result, few demands were made on researchers by homosexually active African American men regarding AIDS prevention.

A third reason for this neglect could be that advocacy for AIDS prevention by White gay men rarely included mention of minority gay men. The relatively high degree of community organization among White gay men in urban areas enabled them, understandably, to respond to the threat of HIV/AIDS. However, little of the effort to change high-risk behavior among gay men focused on African American men in the gay community or homosexually active men in the African American community. As a result, little attention was drawn by White gay men to the prevention needs of African American men.

Hence this chapter is prompted by the lack of prevention research among African American men who engage in male-male sexual contact. The chapter begins with a presentation of the scant existing data on the prevalence of high-risk sexual behaviors among homosexually active African American men. Then the factors that may be associated with HIV risk reduction in these men are discussed. The chapter concludes with a discussion of methodological issues and the need for future studies in this population.

HIV High-Risk Same-Sex Behavior among African American Men

Several reviews have noted the paucity of data on HIV risk reduction among homosexually active minority men (Coates, 1990; Fisher & Fisher, 1992; Hays & Peterson, 1994; Kelly & Murphy, 1992). What we know about AIDS-related risk behavior in homosexually active African American men is derived from only a few recent studies. Admittedly, the majority of AIDS case in the United States still occur among White gay and bisexual men; the epidemic has escalated and continues to exact a profound toll from this population (CDC, 1995). Whereas White gay and bisexual men have demonstrated significant reduction in HIV risk behaviors, however, the limited available data do not permit researchers to determine whether African American men have experienced similar behavior changes. Also, because most study samples have consisted predominantly of Whites, they have lacked sufficient African American participants to examine HIV risks and determinants separately by racial group. However, the few studies with large samples of homosexually active African American men indicate that high-risk sexual behavior is quite prevalent among these men.

With my colleagues at the UCSF Center for AIDS Prevention Studies, I examined high-risk sexual behavior and condom use among African American gay and bisexual men (Peterson et al., 1992). Data were obtained from the first wave of the African American Men's Health Project, an ongoing longitudinal survey in the California cities of San Francisco, Oakland, and Berkeley. The present data are based on interviews with the first two hundred fifty respondents recruited in 1990 from bars, bath houses, and erotic bookstores and through African American newspapers, health clinics, and personal referrals from study participants.

Respondents were asked to report the frequency of anal intercourse and condom use in the previous six months with both their primary and secondary male sexual partners. *Primary partner* was defined as the respondents' main male sexual partner, with whom they lived or to whom they had a special commitment; *secondary partner* was defined as all other sexual partners. All sexual activities were stated in language that used culturally familiar terms (e.g., "butthole" for rectum). Of the men who engaged in anal intercourse within the past six months (73 percent), over half reported having had unprotected anal intercourse: 22 percent with their primary sexual partner and 35 percent with their secondary sexual partners. A nontrivial minority of the total sample had engaged in unprotected vaginal intercourse with primary (7 percent) or secondary (12 percent) female partners. These data demonstrate a substantially higher prevalence of unprotected anal intercourse (52 percent) among African American men than the rate previously reported among White gay and bisexual men in the San Francisco Bay Area (15 percent to 20 percent) (Ekstrand & Coates, 1990; McKusick, Coates, Morin, Pollack, & Hoff, 1990).

Mays (1993) conducted a national mail survey of HIV risk behaviors among 889 African American gay and bisexual men in the United States. Participants were obtained largely through questionnaires mailed to various organizations that included or served African American gay and bisexual men. The organizations then distributed the questionnaires to potential participants. Among the sexually active men, 31 percent of the participants reported that they had engaged in combined unprotected receptive and insertive anal intercourse to climax within the prior month.

Doll et al. (1992) reported data on HIV risk behaviors among 209 HIV seropositive male blood donors, most of whom were African American (59 percent) and self-identified as bisexual (44 percent). Among the sample, 73 percent of homosexually identified, 62 percent of bisexually identified, and 29 percent of heterosexually identified men reported that they had engaged in unprotected anal intercourse with men during the year before their last blood donation.

Data reported by McKirnan, Stokes, Doll, and Burzette (1994) reveal similarly elevated levels of high-risk sexual behavior among bisexually active men in Chicago. Participants in their sample (N=536) of African American (52 percent) and White (48 percent) bisexually active men were recruited from bars, print advertisements, community outreach, and personal referrals by respondents. Although there were no ethnic differences in unprotected anal intercourse during the prior six months, 31 percent of participants reported at least one instance of unprotected anal intercourse with a male and 42 percent reported at least one instance of unprotected vaginal or anal intercourse with a female. Also, African American respondents were much more likely to report both male and female partners, whereas Whites were more likely to report exclusively male partners. Similarly, though to a lesser extent, African American respondents were somewhat more likely than Whites to report at least one instance of unprotected penetrative sex with both a male and a female or with a female only. White respondents were more likely to report no risk behavior or risk behavior with men only.

Taken together, these studies establish that high levels of HIV risk behavior occur among African American men who engage in male-male sexual contact. However, it is also necessary to understand the correlates of these high-risk behaviors. Such information is important not only because it enables us to understand risk-taking, but also because it can provide suggestions about how to design behavioral interventions. In the following section, I discuss the limited existing research on the factors that may possibly influence whether or not homosexually active African American men engage in high-risk behavior.

Factors Associated with High-Risk Same-Sex Behavior among African American Men

African American men who engage in male-male sexual contact may manifest distinctive individual, interpersonal, and contextual characteristics that affect their levels of HIV risk and the types of interventions needed to change their high-risk behavior. Most of these factors are described in major theoretical models employed to explain HIV risk behavior, such as the health belief model (Rosenstock, Strecher, & Becker, 1994), social cognitive theory (Bandura, 1989, 1994), reasoned action theory (Fishbein & Middlestadt, 1989; Fishbein, Middlestadt, & Hitchcock, 1994), the AIDS Risk-Reduction Model, or ARRM (Catania, Kegeles, & Coates, 1990), and diffusion theory (Dearing, Meyer, & Rogers, 1994). Recently, some researchers (Mays & Cochran, 1993) have argued that some of these theories are inadequate for understanding high-risk behavior among African Americans. However, others (Jemmott & Jones, 1993) have suggested that these theories may be useful for AIDS prevention research in African American populations but that various determinants of risk behavior may differ in such populations from those in White populations. Obviously, it is an empirical question whether these theories are capable of explaining HIV risk behaviors across race and ethnicity. Consequently, conclusions are not possible until adequate data are available.

Individual Factors

Sexual Orientation. Personal definitions of sexual identity may be particularly relevant to describing the same-sex behavior of African American men. These men confront strong negative attitudes toward homosexual behavior in the African American community (Klassen, Williams, & Levitt, 1989) because of the acceptance of Judeo-Christian views in African American religion and traditional gender roles in the African American family (Peterson, 1992). Because of the stigma attached to homosexuality in African American culture and because of the absence of a formal Black gay subculture to buffer gay intolerance, bisexuality has been suggested as commonly preferred over homosexuality as an expression of sexual identity (Doll, Peterson, Magana, & Carrier, 1991). Studies consistent with this suggestion have found that African American men who had engaged in male-male sexual contact were more likely than others to report their self-identity as bisexual rather than homosexual (McKirnan, Stokes, & Burzette, 1992; McKirnan et al., 1994; Stokes, McKirnan, & Burzette, 1992, 1993). It is possible that many African American men who engage in same-sex behaviors do not consider themselves to be homosexual, depending on the meaning of or reasons for their sexual behavior (Blumstein & Schwartz, 1977; Humphreys, 1970; Reiss, 1961). Some of these men may engage in recreational homosexual behavior to satisfy physical pleasure or in situational homosexual behavior for economic reasons, such as in male prostitution or during imprisonment (DeLamater, 1981; Wooden & Parker, 1982). Other men may protect themselves from the inference of homosexual identity by engaging exclusively in anonymous sex (Humphreys, 1970) or in homosexual activities that they consider to be associated with a masculine role, such as the insertive role in oral and anal sex (Carrier, 1985; Parker, 1985).

Moreover, fear of the possible disclosure of their homosexual behavior may increase the likelihood that some homosexually active African American men engage in high-risk sexual behavior (Mays & Cochran, 1987; Mays, Cochran, & Bellinger, 1992; Peterson, Fullilove, Catania, & Coates, 1989; Peterson et al., 1992). African American gay and bisexual men with greater discomfort about publicly disclosing their homosexual behavior were more likely to engage in unprotected anal intercourse than were men who did not experience such discomfort (Peterson et al., 1992). Also, bisexual African American men who did not disclose their homosexual behavior to female partners—compared to those who did disclose—were more self-homophobic, perceived less acceptance of their homosexuality by friends, family, and neighbors, had more female partners, and used condoms less often with their female partners (McKirnan et al., 1994).

Social Background. Variations in social background, especially education and income, may have important consequences for African

American men's involvement in same-sex behavior. High-risk sexual behavior was strongly associated with marginal status (e.g., low income, being paid for sex, or injection drug use) in our study of African American gay and bisexual men (Peterson et al., 1992). Similarly, Mays (1993) found that African American gay and bisexual men with lower income, less education, and more unskilled occupations were more likely than others to engage in unprotected anal intercourse. However, McKirnan et al. (1994) found, even after controlling for sociodemographic variables, that African American bisexual men were more likely than White bisexual men to have received money or drugs from a male for sex or to have given money or drugs to either a male or female for sex. Other data by McKirnan and Peterson (1989a, 1989b) have revealed a complex relationship between substance use and HIV/AIDS risk behavior. These researchers found that men who used drugs or alcohol to reduce anxiety related to their sexuality were more likely to engage in high-risk sex, independent of the amount of substances consumed. Among bisexual men who were more self-homophobic, substance use was significantly associated with both high-risk sexual behavior and sexual behavior in general. No such relationship was found for those low in self-homophobia. Consequently, the social diversity among African American men who engage in homosexual behavior may account for substantial differences in HIV risk behaviors across social strata.

Interpersonal Factors

Perceived Risk. Typically, it has been assumed that the perception of risk for HIV infection is associated with reduction of HIV risk behaviors. It is unclear to what extent African American men who engage in homosexual behavior may deny their risks of HIV infection, especially if they reside outside AIDS epicenters or outside White gay neighborhoods. Those who deny their susceptibility are unlikely to modify their behavior if, as argued by some theorists (Rosenstock et al., 1994), personal susceptibility is judged less on the basis of individual behavior than on the basis of the social group(s) with whom people identify. This argument suggests that the concentration of AIDS cases among gay males and IDUs may prompt individuals who are not members of these specific groups to deny their HIV risk despite their involvement in high-risk behaviors. Consistent with this reasoning, Stokes et al. (1993) found that bisexual men with low identification with the gay community expressed less perceived vulnerability to AIDS than did those with high identification. However, our data (Peterson et al., 1992) showed that even African American gay and bisexual men who correctly perceived themselves at risk for HIV infection still engaged in high-risk sexual behavior, suggesting that efforts to increase risk perceptions are necessary but not sufficient to produce changes in behavior.

Normative Beliefs. It has been suggested that social norms regarding HIV risk behaviors influence whether individuals are likely to engage in those behaviors (Dearing et al., 1994; Fishbein & Middlestadt, 1989; Fishbein et al., 1994). Our study examined the relationship between AIDS ethnocentric beliefs and high-risk sexual behavior among African American gay and bisexual men (Peterson et al., 1992). AIDS ethnocentrism refers to race-relevant beliefs that African Americans may espouse about the AIDS epidemic. Examples include the beliefs that African American men are at risk for HIV/AIDS only if they have sex with White men and that AIDS is a plot of the federal government to cause genocide among African Americans. We failed to find an association between ethnocentric beliefs and participation in unprotected anal intercourse. However, our results provided support for the association between perceived norms and HIV high-risk behavior. The men who were more likely to use condoms had stronger beliefs that condom use was normative among their peers in the community. The data from this study suggest that high-risk sexual behavior among African American gay and bisexual men is influenced more by general normative beliefs about condoms than by race-specific beliefs about AIDS.

Behavioral Beliefs. An important behavioral belief regarding HIV high-risk behavior concerns the consequences of HIV risk reduction for sexual enjoyment (Catania et al., 1989; Catania, Kegeles, & Coates, 1990). Our data suggest that expectations about the positive or negative consequences of safe-sex practices are associated with unprotected anal intercourse among African American gay and bisexual men (Peterson et al., 1992). The men who were more likely to use condoms had more positive expectations about using condoms.

Control Beliefs. Perceived efficacy or the belief about one's ability to practice safe sex during a sexual encounter is one type of control belief that has been hypothesized to be important in reducing high-risk same-sex behavior (Bandura, 1989, 1994). Our data provided support that perceived self-efficacy is related to HIV risk behavior among African American gay and bisexual men (Peterson et al., 1992). The men's perceived self-efficacy to use condoms was strongly associated with their reports of condom use. Men who had stronger beliefs that they could practice safe sex were more likely than others to use condoms.

Contextual Factors

Sexual Venues and Social Networks of African American Men. Because HIV risk behaviors occur within a social context, it is appropriate to consider the locales in which homosexually active African American men find their potential sexual partners. Men who self-identify as gay are likely to use gay social networks (e.g., gay bars, friendships, social cliques, and private house parties), whereas men who engage in male-male contact but do not identify as gay may rely more on meeting potential partners in venues that are less embedded in gay-identified networks (e.g., parks, public restrooms, the sex industry). Also, the rates of HIV risk behavior may vary among the locales in which homosexually active African American men meet to form sexual liaisons because the norms regarding sexual behavior differ across social contexts and consequently affect the tendency toward sexual risk taking. Data have revealed that the setting in which men met their sexual partners is a strong predictor of high-risk sexual behavior (McKirnan et al., 1992). For example, men who met their partners in bars were more likely to have engaged in high-risk sexual behavior than were men who met their partners through friends; this finding was unrelated to differences in alcohol consumption between venues.

Resources for Help-Seeking and Social Support. It is important that African American men who engage in high-risk behavior obtain the social support they need to change their behavior. The resources that should be developed and offered to these men may be suggested from our data on help-seeking patterns among men who engage in high-risk sexual behavior (Peterson et al., 1995). We examined the extent and effectiveness of help seeking and its association with HIV status. Data were collected from 318 African American gay and bisexual men in the San Francisco Bay Area. One third of the sample reported seeking help regarding their HIV risk behavior. Peers (e.g., lovers and friends) and professionals (e.g., physicians and counselors) were the most widely sought sources of help as well as the sources perceived to be the most helpful. HIV-seropositive men were more likely to seek help than were men who were HIV seronegative or who did not know their HIV status. The seropositive men were least likely to seek help from family members and least likely to perceive family members as helpful with their concerns about their high-risk sexual behavior. The latter finding may result from the family's difficulty in accepting the men's sexual lifestyle, the men's limited involvement with their family in order to avoid disclosure or discussion of their homosexual behavior, or to the family's lack of familiarity with AIDS and gay issues.

The high rate of HIV risk behaviors among African American men who engage in male-male sexual contact warrants the development of controlled intervention trials that can help them modify their risk behaviors. Similar to the sparse data on risk factors, there have been few studies of evaluated trials of HIV risk reduction among homosexually active African American men. Given the level of risk behaviors, the most urgent need is for studies that design and evaluate the influence of behavioral interventions to reduce high-risk behavior in this population. In the following section, I discuss the limited data that exist on intervention studies among homosexually active African American men.

Intervention Studies among African American Men Who Engage in Same-Sex Behavior

With my colleagues I examined the impact of what, to our knowledge, is the only HIV risk-reduction study designed to change high-risk sexual behaviors among African American gay and bisexual men (Peterson et al., 1994). Based on extensive pilot research, we developed a rationale for altering the spread of HIV infection in this population. We hypothesized that a successful intervention would have to accomplish multiple goals:

- Reduce the men's discomfort about their homosexuality and increase their sense of pride associated with their sexual status within the African American community.
- Improve their cultural misperceptions of risk-reduction information and ineffective condom use skills.
- Strengthen their beliefs that condom use should become normative in the African American gay subculture.
- Increase their ability to obtain social support regarding their risk behaviors.
- Enhance beliefs in their ability and expectations to use condoms through improved self-regulatory behavior.
- Provide opportunities for them to acquire strategies for risk reduction that would consequently bolster their beliefs in the efficacy of risk-reduction techniques.

Participants were 318 African American men recruited in the San Francisco Bay Area in 1990 and 1991 during the first wave of the African American Men's Health Project described earlier in this chapter. Following their baseline interview, participants were randomly assigned to either a single- or triple-session experimental intervention group or to a waiting-list control group. They were then reinterviewed 12 and 18 months later. Participants in the waiting-list control group received the intervention of their choice after completing their final follow-up interview. Men in the triple-session intervention condition attended a series of three weekly 180-minute group sessions. Men in the single-session intervention condition attended one 180-minute group session. Both intervention conditions had identical components except that the single-session intervention occurred in a more abbreviated group format. All training materials, videotapes, games, and role-plays were extensively pilot tested for their accuracy and their cultural relevance for African American gay and bisexual men. For example, all videos depicted only African American men and included content on issues and experiences related to the men's same-sex attitudes and behaviors expressed in culturally appropriate language.

The intervention model examined in this study was derived from social learning and cognitive-behavioral principles applied to HIV risk reduction. In small groups of ten to twelve members, study participants initially engaged in group discussion. The discussion, which was designed to improve self-identity and social support for HIV risk reduction, was designed to promote participants' pride as racial and sexual minorities and their understanding about the possible consequences of poor self-identity for risk-taking behaviors. This component was followed with HIV risk education in which participants received AIDS information and engaged in skills training procedures, such as modeling and feedback, regarding condom use. The final intervention component provided participants with training to develop assertiveness to follow risk-reduction guidelines and strengthen their commitment to sustaining HIV risk-reduction activities. This session included role-play rehearsal exercises on sexual assertiveness and communication. Participants also shared strategies that they had used to change their high-risk behaviors in the past, and they made verbal commitments to maintain changes that occurred during the intervention. Over half (53 percent) of the participants in the triple-session condition and 46 percent of participants in the single-session condition attended the intervention. There were no significant differences between study conditions in loss to follow-up or in loss to follow-up by baseline risk behavior.

An "intention to treat" procedure was employed whereby data from all subjects obtained at follow-up were included in the data analysis. Results revealed that participants in the triple-session intervention greatly reduced (50 percent) their frequency of unprotected anal intercourse; this change was maintained through the 18-month follow-up. However, levels of risk behavior decreased only slightly at both follow-ups for the single-session intervention group and remained constant across both follow-up evaluations for the control group. These results suggest that multiple-session intervention approaches are more warranted than single-session approaches for risk reduction with African American gay and bisexual men. Our study design does not permit us to identify which components were most responsible for changes in risk behavior. Because interventions had the same components, however, the differences between the effects of these interventions are probably attributable to greater exposure to the intervention in the multiple-session condition.

These findings demonstrate that homosexually active African American men—at least those who self-identify as gay or bisexual—can make substantial changes in HIV high-risk sexual behaviors when they are exposed to skills-building, cognitive-behavioral group interventions. The findings also suggest that only interventions that occur over more than one occasion will be sufficient for high-risk men to acquire and successfully adopt the skills they need to change their risk behaviors.

Methodological Issues and Future Research Needed

Although existing studies are few in number, they have important implications for future research with homosexually active African American men. They suggest some important issues that should be considered in the design and implementation of risk-reduction interventions for these men. The most prominent issues for consideration are sampling approaches for recruitment, the ethnic validity of instruments, and the cultural relevance of interventions.

Sampling Approaches for Recruitment

Differences in sexual identity among African American men who engage in same-sex behavior suggest that many men at risk of HIV infection may be ignored if interventions target only those who self-identify as gay. Also, fear of condemnation of homosexual behavior in the African American community may lead many men to engage in homosexual behavior covertly and to be reluctant to participate in interventions that require them to disclose their homosexual activities. Hence multiple recruitment procedures and incentives may be required to reach this diverse population of African American men. In addition to bars and clubs, private house parties may be especially useful venues in which to reach these men. Recruitment through street outreach in parks, adult public restrooms, and erotic bookstores may yield samples of men who engage in male-male sexual contact who would not be reached otherwise. Additionally, media recruitment may be extremely useful through newspaper ads. It is a mistake, however, to rely exclusively on ads in gay publications, which tend to bias sampling toward African American men who primarily self-identify as gay. In addition to these, advertisements are effective in general population newspapers, including major African American newspapers and free weekly neighborhood newspapers.

Many African American men who engage in same-sex activity may have a low income level or may engage in prostitution and injection drug use. Consequently, successful recruitment may require that eligible participants be offered financial incentives such as money or redemption vouchers to exchange for housing, food, and social services. Those men less involved in the White gay community will have less access to formal gay institutions, such as gay newspapers and social organizations (Peterson & Marin, 1988). Last, "snowball" sampling, in which participants refer other potentially eligible men, may be helpful to recruit men who are members of study participants' social networks.

Ethnic Validity of Instruments

In addition to the serious methodological problems in much AIDS behavioral research (Catania, Gibson, Chitwood, & Coates, 1990), the issue of ethnic validity is especially important to studies that include minority participants. The assessment of correlates and determinants of outcome variables can involve substantial measurement error if the instruments used to assess these variables lack ethnic validity. Typically, measures originally developed with White participants are administered to African American respondents with little or no revision. Before doing so, however, major effort should be made to pilot test and appropriately adapt these measures for ethnically diverse populations. At a minimum, the items in culturally appropriate measures should include the specific wording and language used in African American populations. More important, it would be helpful to conduct validity studies to determine the stability of the factor structure of scales. Hence researchers should carefully examine the ethnic validity of the instruments used in studies with African American men.

Design of Interventions

The number of controlled outcome studies is too small, and it is inappropriate to rely on the one available study to determine the effectiveness of these interventions. A substantial increase in intervention research is needed to guide the development of prevention programs to limit further HIV transmission among homosexually active African American men. In the design of these interventions, it is very important that they include components intended to enhance self-identity and social support for overcoming the AIDS-related stigma attached to homosexual behavior. Male-male sexual contact violates traditional norms about gender role behaviors and is perceived as a threat to the institution of the family because of the shortage of marriageable men in African American society. Cultural beliefs about conventional sex roles equate masculinity with exclusive sexual interest in women and violations of these role expectations are perceived to limit propagation of the African American population. Insofar as these negative views are internalized (self-homophobia), African American men may be motivated to avoid recognition of their HIV risks and efforts to change high-risk behaviors. Hence behavior change interventions need to reduce the psychological discomfort that African American men may experience about their homosexual behavior. For men who self-identify as gay or bisexual, the interventions should include activities to promote feelings of self-pride in their sexual orientation. Whether men self-identify as heterosexual, bisexual, or gay, interventions need to reduce the possible negative consequences of poor sexual identity for risk-taking behavior.

Also, interventions should be implemented with procedures uniquely suited for African American men. They should include materials culturally relevant to these men and expressed in culturally appropriate language. For example, visual materials such as videos and pictures should only depict African American men, and all written documents should convey information in the language most commonly used by, and at the education level of, the specific target population.

Also, group facilitators should be matched in race and gender to those of the participants unless future research confirms the absence of significant race and gender effects of facilitators. Thus, the format and delivery of interventions should be tailored appropriately for African American men.

Last, there is a pressing need for studies to examine the effectiveness of community-level interventions to reach larger numbers of people more quickly than is possible through individual-level approaches. Typically, diffusion interventions are designed to promote behavior changes through the adoption of new reference group norms by the members of social networks (Dearing et al., 1994; Kelly & Murphy, 1992). Among African American men, individuals who self-identify as gay may be reached through the social influence of opinion leaders in their informal gay networks, such as African American gay bars or private house parties. Homosexually active men who identify as bisexual or heterosexual may be reached more effectively by messages diffused through their network of sexual contacts, such as members of the sex industry or gay sexual partners.

Summary

The prevention of HIV infection among African American men who engage in homosexual behavior is of sufficient importance to warrant serious research attention. However, since the epidemic's onset, there has been a neglect of empirical research in this population. In this chapter, various explanations were offered for this neglect, including emphasis on prevention research among high-risk African American heterosexuals, suppression of demands for research among homosexually active African American men because of the AIDS-related stigma of homosexuality, and the neglect of the needs of African American men in advocacy for prevention research by White gay men.

The chapter also discussed the few available studies concerning homosexually active African American men. Data for these studies were obtained from samples in the San Francisco Bay Area, in Chicago, at blood donation sites across the United States, and in various organizations for homosexually active African American men throughout the country. Across studies, results uniformly revealed that high-risk sexual behavior is quite high among these men. Discussion also focused on possible factors that have been found to influence whether or not these men engage in safer sex. Findings indicated various correlates of high-risk behavior, including individual factors such as sexual identity, education, and income; interpersonal factors such as perceived risk, normative beliefs, behavioral beliefs, and control beliefs; and contextual factors such as sexual venues, social networks, and resources for help seeking and social support.

Discussion next focused on research that involved controlled intervention trials designed to modify high-risk behaviors among homosexually active African American men. In the one intervention study available, findings demonstrated that cognitive-behavioral interventions that emphasize skills training can produce substantial changes in HIV high-risk sexual behaviors among homosexually active African American men.

The chapter concluded with discussion of methodological issues in research and future studies needed with homosexually active African American men. Discussion focused on sampling approaches for recruitment, ethnic validity of instruments, and cultural relevance in the design of behavior change interventions. Much more research is needed to adequately determine the factors associated with HIV risk behaviors, the appropriate approaches for risk-reduction interventions, and the effectiveness of different types of interventions for behavior change. However, unless there is a substantial increase in AIDS prevention research among these men, the unrelenting spread of HIV will not be abated in this population even at the end of the second decade of the AIDS epidemic.

References

Bakeman, R., McCray, E., Lumb, J. R., Jackson, R. E., & Whitley, P. N. (1987). "The incidence of AIDS among Blacks and Hispanics." *Journal of the National Medical Association, 79,* 921–928.

Bandura, A. (1989). "Perceived self-efficacy." In V. Mays, G. Albee, & S. Schneider (Eds.), *Primary Prevention of AIDS: Psychological Approaches* (pp. 93–110). Newbury Park, CA: Sage.

Bandura, A. (1994). "Social cognitive theory and the exercise of control over HIV infection." In R. DiClemente & J. Peterson (Eds.), *Preventing AIDS: Theories and Methods of Behavioral Interventions* (pp. 25–59). New York: Plenum.

Blumstein, P., & Schwartz, P. (1977). "Bisexuality: Some social psychological issues." *Journal of Social Issues, 33,* 30–45.

Carrier, J. M. (1985). "Cultural factors affecting urban Mexican male homosexual behavior." *Archives of Sexual Behavior, 5,* 103–24.

Catania, J. A., Coates, T. J., Kegeles, S., Ekstrand, M., Guydish, J., & Bye, L. (1989). "Implications of the AIDS risk reduction model for the homosexual community: The importance of perceived sexual enjoyment and help-seeking behaviors." In V. Mays, G. Albee, J. Jones, & J. Schneider (Eds.), *Psychological Approaches to the Prevention of AIDS* (pp. 242–261). Newbury Park, CA: Sage.

Catania, J. A., Gibson, D. R., Chitwood, D. D., & Coates, T. J. (1990). "Methodological problems in AIDS behavioral research: Influences on measurement error and participation bias in studies of sexual behavior." *Psychological Bulletin, 108,* 339–362.

Catania, J., Kegeles, S., & Coates, T. (1990). "Towards an understanding of risk behavior: An AIDS risk reduction model (ARRM)." *Health Education Quarterly, 17,* 381–399.

Centers for Disease Control and Prevention. (1995, February). *HIV/AIDS Surveillance.* Atlanta, GA: Author.

Chu, S. Y., Peterman, T. A., Doll, L. S., Buehler, J. W., & Curran, J. W. (1992). "AIDS in bisexual men in the United States: Epidemiology and transmission to women." *American Journal of Public Health, 82,* 220–224.

Coates, T. J. (1990). "Strategies for modifying sexual behavior for primary and secondary prevention of HIV disease." *Journal of Consulting and Clinical Psychology, 58,* 57–69.

Dalton, H. (1989). "AIDS in blackface." *Daedalus, 118,* 205–227.

Dearing, J. W., Meyer, G., & Rogers, E. M. (1994). "Diffusion theory and HIV risk behavior change." In R. DiClemente & J. Peterson (Eds.), *Preventing AIDS: Theories and Methods of Behavioral Interventions* (pp. 79–93). New York: Plenum.

DeLamater, J. (1981). "The social control of sexuality." *Annual Review of Sociology, 7,* 263–290.

Doll, L. S., Peterson, J., Magana, J. R., & Carrier, J. M. (1991). "Male bisexuality and AIDS in the United States." In R. Tielman, M. Carballo, & A. Hendriks (Eds.), *Bisexuality and HIV/AIDS* (pp. 27–39). Buffalo, NY: Prometheus.

Doll, L. S., Peterson, L. R., White, C. R., Johnson, E. S., Ward, J. W., and the Blood Donor Study Group. (1992). "Homosexually and nonhomosexually identified men who have sex with men: A behavioral comparison." *Journal of Sex Research, 29,* 1–14.

Ekstrand, M. L., & Coates T. J. (1990). "Maintenance of safer sexual behaviors and predictors of risky sexual behaviors and predictors of risky sex: The San Francisco Men's Health Study." *American Journal of Public Health, 80,* 973–977.

Fishbein, M., & Middlestadt, S. (1989). "Using the theory of reasoned action as a framework for understanding and changing AIDS-related behaviors." In V. Mays, G. Albee, & S. Schneider (Eds.), *Primary Prevention of AIDS: Psychological Approaches* (pp. 93–110). Newbury Park, CA: Sage.

Fishbein, M., Middlestadt, S., & Hitchcock, B. J. (1994). "Using information to change sexually transmitted disease-related behaviors: An analysis based on the theory of reasoned action." In R. DiClemente & J. Peterson (Eds.), *Preventing AIDS: Theories and Methods of Behavioral Interventions* (pp. 61–78). New York: Plenum.

Fisher, J., & Fisher, W. A. (1992). "Changing AIDS risk behavior." *Psychological Bulletin, 111,* 455–474.

Hays, R., & Peterson, J. (1994). "HIV prevention for gay and bisexual men in metropolitan cities." In R. DiClemente & J. Peterson (Eds.), *Preventing AIDS: Theories and Methods of Behavioral Interventions* (pp. 267–295). New York: Plenum.

Herek, G., & Glunt, E. K. (1991). "AIDS-related attitudes in the United States: A preliminary conceptualization." *Journal of Sex Research, 28,* 99–123.

Humphreys, L. (1970). *Tearoom Trade: Impersonal Sex in Public Restrooms.* Chicago: Aldine.

Icard, L. (1985–86). "Black gay men and conflicting social identities: Sexual orientation versus racial identity." *Journal of Social Work and Human Sexuality, 4,* 83–93.

Jemmott, J. B., & Jones, J. M. (1993). "Social psychology and AIDS among ethnic minority individuals: Risk behaviors and strategies for changing them." In J. B. Pryor & G. D. Reeder (Eds.), *The Social Psychology of HIV Infection* (pp. 183–224). Hillsdale, NJ: Lawrence Erlbaum.

Kelly, J. A., & Murphy, D. A. (1992). "Psychological interventions with AIDS and HIV: Prevention and treatment." *Journal of Consulting and Clinical Psychology, 60,* 576–585.

Klassen, A. D., Williams, C. J., & Levitt, E. E. (1989). *Sex and Morality in the U.S.* Middletown, CT: Wesleyan University Press.

Mays, V. M. (1993, June). *High risk HIV-related sexual behaviors in a national sample of U.S. Black gay and bisexual men.* Paper presented at the Ninth International Conference on AIDS, Berlin.

Mays, V. M., & Cochran, S. D. (1987). "Acquired immunodeficiency syndrome and Black Americans: Special psychosocial issues." *Public Health Reports, 102,* 224–231.

Mays, V. M., & Cochran, S. D. (1993). "Applying social psychological models to predicting HIV-related sexual risk behaviors among African Americans." *Journal of Black Psychology, 19,* 142–151.

Mays, V. M., Cochran, S. D., & Bellinger, G. (1992, June). *Factors Influencing AIDS Risk perception of Black Gay Men.* Paper presented at the Eighth International Conference on AIDS, Amsterdam.

McKirnan, D. J., & Peterson, P. L. (1989a). "AIDS-risk behavior among homosexual males: The role of attitudes and substance abuse." *Psychology and Health, 3,* 161–171.

———. (1989b, June). *Tension Reduction Expectancies Underlie the Effect of Alcohol on AIDS Risk Behavior Among Homosexual Males.* Paper presented at the Fifth International Conference on AIDS, Montreal.

McKirnan, D. J., Stokes, J. P., Doll, L., & Burzette, R. G. (1994). *Bisexually active men: Social characteristics and sexual behavior.* Manuscript submitted for publication.

McKirnan, D. J., Stokes, J. P., & Burzette, R. G. (1992, June). *Self-Identification Among Bisexual Men: Effects of Psychological Well-Being and HIV Risk.* Paper presented at the Eighth International Conference on AIDS, Amsterdam, The Netherlands.

McKusick, L., Coates, T. J., Morin, S., Pollack, L., & Hoff, C. (1990). "Longitudinal predictors of reductions in unprotected anal intercourse among gay men in San Francisco: The AIDS Behavioral Research Project." *American Journal of Public Health, 80,* 1–8.

Parker, R. (1985). "Masculinity, femininity, and homosexuality." *Journal of Homosexuality, 11,* 155–164.

Peterson, J. L. (1992). Black men and their same-sex desires and behaviors. In G. Herdt (Ed.), *Gay Culture in America: Essays From the Field* (pp. 147–164). Boston: Beacon.

Peterson, J. L., Coates, T. J., Catania, J. A., Middleton, L., Hilliard, B., & Hearst, N. (1992). High-risk sexual behavior and condom use among gay and bisexual African American men." *American Journal of Public Health, 82,* 1490–1494.

Peterson, J. L., Coates, T. J., Catania, J. A., Hilliard, B., Middleton, L., & Hearst, N. (1995). "Help-seeking for AIDS high risk sexual behavior among gay and bisexual African American men." *AIDS Education and Prevention, 7,* 1–9.

Peterson, J. L., Coates, T. J., Hauck, W. W., Catania, J. A., Daigle, D., Middleton, L., Hilliard, B., & Hearst, N. (1994). *An HIV Prevention Strategy for African American Gay and Bisexual Men.* Manuscript submitted for publication.

Peterson, J. L., Fullilove, R., Catania, J., & Coates, T. (1989, June). "*Close Encounters of an Unsafe Kind: Risky Sexual Behaviors and Predictors Among Black Gay and Bisexual Men.*" Paper presented at the Fifth International Conference on AIDS, Montreal.

Peterson, J. L., & Marin, G. (1988). "Issues in the prevention of AIDS among Black and Hispanic men." *American Psychologist, 43,* 871–877.

Reiss, A. J. (1961). "The social integration of queers and peers." *Social Problems, 9,* 102–119.

Rosenstock, I. M., Strecher, V. J., & Becker, M. H. (1994). "The health belief model and HIV risk behavior change." In R. DiClemente & J. Peterson (Eds.), *Preventing AIDS: Theories and Methods of Behavioral Interventions* (pp. 5–24). New York: Plenum.

Stokes, J. P., McKirnan, D. J., & Burzette, R. G. (1992). *Behavioral Versus Self-Labelling Definitions of Bisexuality: Implications for AIDS Risk.* Paper presented at the Seventh International Conference on AIDS, Amsterdam, The Netherlands.

———. (1993). "Sexual behavior, condom use, disclosure of sexuality, and stability of sexual orientation in bisexual men." *Journal of Sex Research, 30,* 203–213.

———. (1994). *Female Partners of Bisexual Men: What They Don't Know Might Hurt Them.* Manuscript submitted for publication.

Wooden, W. S., & Parker, J. (1982). *Men Behind Bars: Sexual Exploitation in Prison.* New York: Plenum.

NOTES ON CONTRIBUTORS

BARRY D. ADAM is professor of sociology at the University of Windsor (Ontario, Canada) and the author of *The Survival of Domination* (Elsevier, 1978) and *The Rise of a Gay and Lesbian Movement* (Twayne, 1995). He has also published articles on new social movement theory, on television news coverage of Nicaragua, on the Sandinista Defense Committees, and on the social organization of homosexuality in such journals as *Medical Anthropology, Canadian Review of Sociology and Anthropology, Critical Sociology, Dialectical Anthropology,* and *Comparative Studies in Society and History.*

LOURDES ARGUELLES is professor of education at the Claremont Graduate School and a psychotherapist in private practice.

RAFAEL MIGUEL DIAZ is adjunct associate professor at the Center for AIDS Prevention Studies at the University of California, San Francisco. He is studying HIV prevention in Latino gay/bisexual men, attempting to identify sociocultural barriers to safer sex practices in that population and developing culturally relevant risk-reduction interventions. When he was at Stanford University, he conducted research on childhood bilingualism and on the early development of self-regulation in children with impulsivity and attentional dysfunctions.

JOHN H. GAGNON is professor of sociology at the State University of New York at Stony Brook. Previously he was Senior Research Sociologist and member of the Board of Trustees of the Institute for Sex Research. He has been a visiting professor at Harvard University, Princeton University, and the University of Essex and an Overseas

Fellow at Churchill College, Cambridge. He is a Fellow of the American Association for the Advancement of Science and is the author or coauthor of *Sex Offenders* (Harper and Row, 1965), *Sexual Conduct* (Aldine, 1973), *Human Sexualities* (Scott, Foresman, 1977), *Life Designs* (Scott, Foresman, 1978), *The Social Organization of Sexuality* (University of Chicago Press, 1994), and *Sex in America* (Little, Brown, 1994). He has also coedited several books, including *Conceiving Sexuality* (Routledge, 1995) with Richard Parker and has written many scientific articles.

GILBERT HERDT is an anthropologist, professor of human development, and director of the Center on Culture and Mental Health at the University of Chicago, where he has taught since 1985. He has written or edited fifteen books and numerous articles, including *Guardians of the Flutes* (third edition, University of Chicago Press, 1994), *Rituals of Manhood* (University of California Press, 1982), *Ritualized Homosexuality in Melanesia* (University of California Press, 1984), *The Sambia: Ritual and Gender in New Guinea* (Holt, Rinehart, and Winston, 1987), *Ritual Secrecy and Cultural Reality* (Cambridge University Press, in press), *Third Sex, Third Gender: Beyond Sexual Dimorphism in Culture and History* (Zone Books, 1994), *Children of Horizons* (Beacon Press, 1993), and most recently, *Same Sex, Different Cultures* (Westview Press, 1997). His recent work on HIV/AIDS, prevention, and sexuality began with a large funded project on gay and lesbian youth development, community, and history in Chicago from 1987 to 1990.

GREGORY M. HEREK is a research psychologist at the University of California, Davis. Among the recent books he has edited or coedited are *Hate Crimes: Confronting Violence Against Lesbians and Gay Men* (Sage, 1992), *AIDS, Identity, and Community: Psychological Perspectives on the HIV Epidemic and Lesbians and Gay Men* (Sage, 1995), and *Out in Force: Sexual Orientation and the Military* (University of Chicago, 1996). In addition to an ongoing study of public reactions to AIDS, his current empirical research includes studies of the impact of the AIDS epidemic on gay and bisexual men and of the mental health consequences of violence against lesbians and gay men.

NAN D. HUNTER is associate professor of law at Brooklyn Law School. She was the founder and first director of the American Civil Liberties Union (ACLU) AIDS Project and the ACLU Lesbian and Gay Rights

Project. From 1993 to 1996, she served as deputy general counsel to the U.S. Department of Health and Human Services. She has written extensively on civil rights law and health law.

MARTIN P. LEVINE was on leave from Florida Atlantic University when he died from complications of AIDS on April 3, 1993. From 1978 to 1990 he taught at Bloomfield College and was a researcher at Memorial-Sloan Kettering Cancer Center in New York on a study of sexual activity among gay men during the AIDS epidemic. He wrote many articles on gay topics, including several on "gay clones," based on his dissertation research. He was the editor of *Gay Men: The Sociology of Male Homosexuality* (Harper & Row, 1979) and a cofounder of the Sociologists' Lesbian and Gay Caucus of the American Sociological Association and the Society for the Study of Social Problems.

PETER M. NARDI is professor of sociology at Pitzer College/The Claremont Colleges. He coedited *Growing Up Before Stonewall: Life Stories of Some Gay Men* (Routledge, 1994) and edited *Men's Friendships* (Sage, 1992) as well as a special issue of *California Sociologist* on AIDS (11, 1–2, 1988). He is politically active in the gay community, having served as chair of the Sociologists' Lesbian and Gay Caucus of the American Sociological Association and the Society for the Study of Social Problems, cochair of the Los Angeles Gay Academic Union, and copresident and board member of the Los Angeles Chapter of the Gay and Lesbian Alliance Against Defamation. He serves as book review coeditor of *GLQ: A Journal of Lesbian and Gay Studies* and special features coeditor (with Beth E. Schneider) of *Sexualities*.

JOHN L. PETERSON is associate professor of psychology in the Community Psychology Graduate Program at Georgia State University. His areas of interest are prevention research, stress, and coping research related to HIV/AIDS among African Americans and the effects of experimental interventions to change high-risk behaviors. His publications include articles in the *American Journal of Public Health, AIDS, American Journal of Community Psychology*, and a chapter in *Gay Culture in America*, edited by Gilbert Herdt. He coedited *Preventing AIDS: Theories and Methods of Behavioral Interventions* (Plenum, 1994).

ANNE RIVERO is a licensed clinical social worker at Kaiser Permanente Mental Health Clinic in Montclair, California.

GAYLE S. RUBIN teaches women's studies at the University of California, Santa Cruz.

BETH E. SCHNEIDER is professor of sociology and women's studies at the University of California, Santa Barbara. She is the editor of *Gender & Society* and special features coeditor (with Peter Nardi) of *Sexualities*. She has coedited (with Joan Huber) *The Social Context of AIDS* (Sage, 1992) and (with Nancy Stoller) *Women Resisting AIDS: Feminist Strategies of Empowerment* (Temple University Press, 1995). She has also written extensively on the sexualization of the workplace, lesbians' experience at work, and the contemporary women's movement. She served for four years as president of the Board of Directors of the Gay and Lesbian Resource Center, the parent organization of the AIDS Counseling and Assistance Program of Santa Barbara County.

NANCY E. STOLLER is professor of community studies and sociology at the University of California, Santa Cruz. From 1984 to 1987, she worked at the San Francisco AIDS Foundation, for which she founded and directed the Women's Program. She is coeditor (with Beth E. Schneider) of *Women Resisting AIDS: Feminist Strategies of Empowerment* (Temple University Press, 1995) and author of the forthcoming *Lessons from the Damned: Queers, Whores, and Junkies Respond to AIDS* (Routledge, 1997).

INDEX